Frontiers in General Surgery

Frontiers in General Surgery

Edited by

D. W. Jirsch

Consultant General Surgeon, St Michael's Hospital, Toronto
Associate Professor of Surgery, University of Toronto, Ontario, Canada

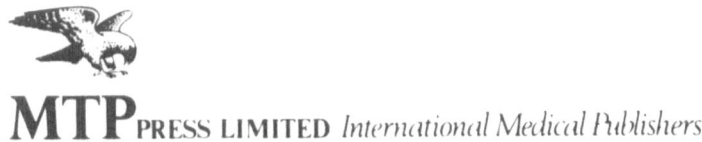

MTPPRESS LIMITED *International Medical Publishers*

Published by
MTP Press Limited
Falcon House
Lancaster, England

British Library Cataloguing in Publication Data

Frontiers in general surgery.
  1. Surgery
  I. Jirsch, D. W.
  617   RD31

    ISBN-13: 978-94-011-6644-7   e-ISBN-13: 978-94-011-6642-3
    DOI: 10.1007/978-94-011-6642-3

Butler & Tanner Ltd,
Frome and London

Contents

List of contributors   vii

Foreword   ix

1 The surgeon and endoscopy for gastrointestinal disease:
W. I. Wolff   1

2 Diagnosis of intra-abdominal disease by computerized axial
tomography: *J. R. Haaga, R. J. Alfidi and J. M. Shuck*   41

3 Angiography in diagnosis and control of bleeding:
T. E. Gallant, A. J. Greenfield and C. A. Athanasoulis   85

4 Oncofetal antigens in gastrointestinal cancer: *E. D. Holyoke*   123

5 Adjuvant therapy of gastrointestinal carcinoma:
F. J. Ansfield and G. Ramirez   143

6 Combined modality (adjuvant) therapy in breast cancer:
K. Cowan and M. Lippman   163

7 Principles of intravenous hyperalimentation:
M. Deitel and I. Sanderson   181

8 Drug treatment of peptic ulcer disease:
D. C. Carter and D. H. Osborne   219

9 Recent realizations in the surgical treatment of ascites:
H. H. Leveen   257

10 The continent ileostomy:
I. M. Gelernt, J. J. Bauer, B. A. Salky and I. Kreel   313

11 Surgical management of supra-ampullary biliary obstruction
in adults: *S. S. Hanna, S. Wilson and D. W. Jirsch*   331

Index   381

List of Contributors

R. J. ALFIDI
Department of Radiology
University Circle
Cleveland, OH 44106, USA

F. J. ANSFIELD
Department of Human Oncology
Oncology Associates, S.C.
2315 North Lake Drive
Milwaukee, WI 53211, USA

C. A. ATHANASOULIS
Department of Radiology
Massachusetts General Hospital and
Harvard Medical School
Boston, MA 02114, USA

J. J. BAUER
Department of Surgery
Mount Sinai School of Medicine
1 Gustave Levy Plaza
New York, NY 10029, USA

D. C. CARTER
University Department of Surgery
Royal Infirmary
Glasgow, G4 0SF, Scotland

K. COWAN
Medicine Branch
National Cancer Institute
National Institutes of Health
Bethesda, MD 20205, USA

M. DEITEL
Surgeon, St. Joseph's Health Centre
30 The Queensway
Toronto, Ontario M6R 1B5, Canada

T. E. GALLANT
Department of Radiology
Massachusetts General Hospital and
Harvard Medical School
Boston, MA 02114, USA

I. M. GELERNT
Department of Surgery
Mount Sinai School of Medicine
1 Gustave Levy Plaza
New York, NY 10029, USA

A. J. GREENFIELD
Department of Radiology
Massachusetts General Hospital and
Harvard Medical School
Boston, Massachusetts 02114

J. R. HAAGA
Department of Radiology
University Circle
Cleveland, OH 44106, USA

S. S. HANNA
Department of General Surgery and the
University of Toronto
Sunnybrook Medical Centre
2075 Bayview Avenue
Toronto, Ontario M4N 3M5, Canada

E. D. HOLYOKE
Department of Surgical Oncology
Roswell Park Memorial Institute
666 Elm Street
Buffalo, NY 14263, USA

D. W. JIRSCH
Department of General Surgery
St. Michael's Hospital and the University of Toronto
30 Bond Street
Toronto, Ontario M5B 1WB, Canada

I. KREL
Department of Surgery
Mount Sinai School of Medicine
1 Gustave Levy Plaza
New York, NY 10029, USA

H. H. LEVEEN
Department of Surgery
Medical University of South Carolina
171 Ashley Avenue
Charleston, SC 29403, USA

M. LIPPMAN
Medicine Branch
National Cancer Institute
National Institutes of Health
Bethesda, MD 20205, USA

D. H. OSBORNE
University Department of Surgery
Royal Infirmary
Glasgow, G4 0SF, Scotland

G. RAMIREZ
Department of Human Oncology
University of Wisconsin
Clinical Science Center K4-634
600 Highland Avenue
Madison, WI 53792, USA

B. A. SALKY
Department of Surgery
Mount Sinai School of Medicine
1 Gustave Levy Plaza
New York, NY 10029, USA

I. SANDERSON
Hyperalimentation Services
Northwestern General Hospital
Toronto, Canada

J. M. SHUCK
Department of Radiology
University Circle
Cleveland, OH 44106, USA

S. WILSON
Department of Radiology
and the University of Toronto
Sunnybrook Medical Centre
2075 Bayview Avenue
Toronto, Ontario M4N 3M5, Canada

W. I. WOLFF
Department of Surgery
Beth Israel Medical Center
Mount Sinai School of Medicine
10 ND Perlmon Place
New York, NY 10003, USA

Foreword

Recent developments have favourably and extensively altered general surgical practice. As editor I have happily been able to select certain topics of new and major interest for detailed discussion and have thus had the opportunity to collect these authoritative submissions within the covers of one text.

The range of topics is broad. Endoscopy has changed the nature of both investigation and treatment of much gastrointestinal disease and the therapeutic uses of endoscopy continue to grow. That sophisticated new tool of the radiologist, computerized axial tomography, has revolutionized the diagnosis of intra-abdominal disease, very often permitting precise localization of hitherto occult disease, and, as might be expected, it has become helpful in determining both the nature and extent of surgical and other therapy. Although an invasive procedure, intra-abdominal angiography has similarly come of age as a means of localizing gastrointestinal haemorrhage and controlling such bleeding. Unfortunately, intra-abdominal malignancy continues to be a major source of concern to the general surgeon and the discovery that such tumours are associated with unusual markers, termed oncofetal antigens, suggests that early diagnosis and early detection of recurrence may yet be feasible. Adjuvant or post-surgical therapy is an exciting development in terms of prolonging the disease-free interval in women with breast cancer limited to regional lymph nodes. Equally efficacious therapy is not yet available for patients with gastrointestinal cancer, highlighting the need for more specific drugs and drug combinations. Intravenous hyperalimentation can reverse progressive malnutrition and permit survival in patients with a variety of diseases that would have been once untreatable. Pharmacologists have been busy and productive and several drugs have changed our approach to peptic ulcer disease; gastric surgery is much less often necessary unless drug therapy has proven inadequate or if fear of malignancy is present. Patients with ascites that did not respond to dietary restriction and diuretics were once untreatable; the development of a catheter system

which reintroduces ascitic fluid into large veins has changed this.
Ulcerative colitis, a frequent disease of youth, may require proctocolectomy and before the advent of the continent ileostomy, such patients
wore a permanent external bag. For these and other ileostomy patients,
a continent intra-abdominal reservoir has been of inestimable benefit.
Bile duct obstruction above the ampulla, whether due to stone, stricture
or neoplasm, may prove difficult in diagnosis and treatment but ultrasonography, computerized axial tomography and other contrast studies
have revolutionized such diagnosis. It is possible to treat retained biliary
tract stones and strictures although prevention remains paramount and
tumour blockage of the biliary tree has similarly become amenable to
specific, technically advanced therapy.

   Although these topics may be considered as examples of current clinical achievement, they enlarge our horizons for further discovery. As
editor, my approach to the selection of both topics and authors has been
an eclectic one. To some extent I would hope that the material is both
provocative and informative. The chapters succeed, I believe, in describing areas of progress and concern germane to current surgical practice.

Toronto, Canada   D. W. JIRSCH
December 1980

1
The surgeon and endoscopy for gastrointestinal disease

W. I. WOLFF

INTRODUCTION

Advances in instrumentation have brought a new dimension to the diagnosis and clinical management of diseases of the alimentary tract. The flexible fibre-optic endoscopes which have become available during the past two decades are responsible for a veritable explosion in the field of endoscopy, obviously satisfying a long-felt need for direct examination of the interior of the digestive hollow viscera – a need never adequately fulfilled by rigid instruments. In expert hands these flexible endoscopes offer the opportunity for examination on an ambulatory basis with only topical anaesthesia, little discomfort to the patient, and, what is most important, a remarkably high degree of safety.

It is reasonable to state that, at the present time, endoscopic evaluation has achieved equal status with roentgenographic examination in terms of relative importance in diagnosing diseases of the digestive tract. This high level of reliability has been reached primarily as the result of two factors:

(1) advances in the quality and variety of instruments available to the clinician, and, more importantly;
(2) an enormous increase in the number of trained and experienced endoscopists who are capable of performing skilful and safe studies.

These two methods of disease diagnosis, i.e. radiography and endo-

1

scopy, are not competitive but rather complementary[1]. Usage of both modalities can provide a higher degree of accurate diagnosis than was formerly possible and has resulted in markedly improved patient care. In addition, the modern endoscopist and radiologist are prepared to offer not only diagnostic services but also important therapeutic opportunities, such as colonoscopic removal of large bowel polyps; gastroscopic laser or electrocauterization of points of gastrointestinal haemorrhage; reduction of intussusception or volvulus; radiologically controlled transcatheter vascular blockades of demonstrated sites of active bleeding, and others.

Indeed, the state of the art is such that those involved in direct patient care, be they primary care physicians, internists, surgeons, pediatricians or radiologists, should have a good working knowledge of what endoscopy has to offer so that they will know which patients can benefit and when to call upon the endoscopist. Surgeons who do not do endoscopy or who have not had the opportunity to have reliable endoscopic support available often fail to realize the very considerable advantages endoscopically derived data contribute in terms of deciding upon the nature, timing and extent of the surgical procedure to be undertaken. For example, the 'blind gastrectomy' for upper gastrointestinal haemorrhage is (or should be) an obsolete operation; emergency portosystemic shunting operations for massive bleeding are now performed much less frequently since it has been recognized that patients with documented oesophageal varices may well be bleeding from other sources; complex operations on the jaundiced patient are better planned and executed when the site, extent and nature of the obstructing lesion have been defined by endoscopic retrograde cholangiopancreaticography, possibly abetted by transhepatic 'skinny' needle hepatic ductography; the patient with sigmoid colon obstruction in the presence of known diverticulitis may have an associated carcinoma which the colonoscopist can see and biopsy, and so forth.

What endoscopic skills the surgeon himself should acquire is a consideration still in evolution. Unfortunately, surgeons for the most part have been slow in accepting an active role in learning such techniques. When we introduced endoscopic examination of the entire colon using the fibre-optic colonoscope in 1969[2], most surgeons regarded the procedure as a *tour de force*. Even when we began to remove colonic polyps endoscopically that same year and in ever-increasing numbers thereafter[3-11], there were only a handful of surgical centres whose leaders had the perspicacity to recognize the potential of the technique and to organize programmes in surgical endoscopy[12,13]. As a result, endoscopy of the alimentary tract is now largely in the hands of gastroenterologists, with surgeons climbing on the bandwagon in notable numbers only during the past few years. Since such examinations do not fall rightfully into the province of any specialty group exclusively, it behooves the surgeon to develop his own skills in the method or, at the very least, to possess a first-hand familiarity with its potentialities and its limitations[14-16].

Endoscopic study has particularly important implications with respect to alimentary tract cancer[8-11,17,18]. The information gained often enables the clinician to act promptly and decisively. Early cancers of the oesophagus or stomach can be detected and proven by direct biopsy or cytological brushings well before they are demonstrable by the usual radiological techniques[19]. We have repeatedly mentioned in our publications examples of colonic cancer diagnosed by colonoscopy when the barium enema was read as negative. When the radiological study is interpreted as indeterminate, endoscopy frequently can settle the issue. Positive radiological findings are confirmable by biopsy and identification of false-positives can prevent an unnecessary operation.

OESOPHAGOSCOPY

Modern gastrointestinal endoscopy can be said to have originated with Kussmaul who, in 1868, assisted by a professional sword-swallower, passed a 24-30 cm hollow tube into the gullet and peered through it by the light of an oil-lamp and a reflector[20]. Stoerk, an Austrian laryngologist, in 1881 examined the oesophagus with rigid tubes[21], but Mikulicz, a well-remembered Polish surgeon, is credited with developing the principle of rigid tube gastroscopy[22]. By 1917, there were enough specialists in the USA interested in the subject to form the 'Association of American Peroral Endoscopists'. Four years later this became the 'American Bronchoscopic Society', and, later on, 'The American Broncho-Esophagological Association', in recognition of the importance of advances in knowledge of diseases of the upper food passages[23]. Prominent among practitioners of the art was Chevalier Jackson, a Philadelphia surgeon who, in 1907, published the first textbook on the subject entitled *Tracheo-Bronchoscopy, Esophagoscopy and Gastroscopy*[24].

Henning, in 1932, formalized the application of endoscopy to gastroenterological problems[25], but the real impetus towards upper gastrointestinal endoscopic study came from the work of Schindler and his disciples beginning in the early 1920s[26]. Rigid scopes were required for oesophageal examinations and even Schindler and Wolf's semiflexible gastroscope[27] never found popular acceptance. Rigid tube oesophagoscopy requires considerable technical skill and proficiency and is currently performed chiefly by thoracic surgeons and otolaryngologists whose training dates back a few decades. The procedure is uncomfortable for the patient – therefore, frequently calling for general anaesthesia – and patient acceptance is often poor, so that it lends itself poorly to repeat or serial examinations. This picture has been radically and rapidly altered by the appearance of flexible fibre-optic endoscopes. Introduced by Hirschowitz and co-workers in 1958[28], these instruments brought about what is described by Colcher as an 'explosion' in the field of endoscopy[29] and marked the emergence of a new specialty in medicine – *gastrointestinal endoscopy*.

Oesophagoscopy, as currently practised, is a simple, safe and minimally distressing procedure carried out under light topical anaesthesia and usually as part of a more complete study known as *oesophagogastro-duodenoscopy* (EGD)[8]. Examination is abetted by short-acting intravenously administered light sedation and is readily accomplished on an ambulatory basis, often as not as an office procedure. As a rule it takes under 30 min to carry out a complete study of the structures mentioned[8,30]. In Japan, where the incidence of malignant disease of the stomach and oesophagus is high, a request for endoscopic examination may be initiated by the patient when he first experiences indigestion; examination may be carried out in mobile endoscopic units transported in specially equipped vans, similar to those used in the USA for chest roentgenography. Patients readily seek evaluation at one of these at the first signs of digestive indisposition.

Oesophagoscopy is best performed with a 'forward-looking' endoscope. The patient lies comfortably on his left side and is asked to swallow as the instrument is introduced. By gentle insufflation with air the visualization of the oesophageal lumen through the dilated gullet is far superior to that afforded via the rigid scope advanced through the collapsed organ. Peristaltic action can be observed and motility disorders are often recognizable. In the absence of an incompetent cardiac sphincter mechanism or obstruction, only swallowed saliva occupies the lumen and this is easily aspirated. Gastro-oesophageal reflux is readily observed and an incompetent cardiac sphincter appears patulous for long periods. Elevation of the 'Z-line', representing the zone of mucosal change from stratified squamous to gastric epithelium, denotes the presence of a hiatal hernia and associated oesophagitis can be recognized grossly and confirmed by biopsy.

Washings may be taken for cytological study and brushings and biopsy under direct observation are easily and safely performed. Endoscopy can detect small, presumably early, cancers which may be missed in the contrast oesophagram[16] and it should, therefore, be recommended early whenever there is persistent or recurrent dysphagia[31]. Maimon *et al.* report a group of cases in which positive cytological specimens were obtained without a detectable neoplasm by either endoscopic or radiological study[32]. Overt cancers were not found in some of these patients until several months later.

For suspicious lesions both direct biopsy and brushings are recommended. The value of the latter depends largely on the availability of a skilled cytologist to interpret the material obtained. The value of the former may be limited by the superficial nature of the small specimens obtainable. A negative biopsy, therefore, should not lull the responsible physician into a false sense of security, and it is the endoscopist's duty to advise the clinician of the limitations of the technique. It is not uncommon to encounter areas of oesophageal narrowing that are treated for long periods as benign strictures before cancer is diagnosed. Cancers, particularly those originating near the cardia, may extend proximally in a submucosal plane and produce only narrowing and dysphagia[33,34] and will be missed if the biopsy is not taken deep enough[35]. If this fact is kept in mind and the patient re-examined with the old, rigid-type scope – which permits larger and deeper biopsy – such errors are less apt to occur[8].

Oesophagoscopy is of value to the surgeon in following the effectiveness of radiation therapy to an oesophageal carcinoma, where it may assist in determining whether or not resolution is complete. Occasionally, this may be a factor in terms of whether or not resectional surgery is warranted. Post-oesophagectomy patients not infrequently develop problems at the anastomosis; oesophagoscopy may be critical in determining whether a narrowing is inflammatory in nature or the result of a recurrent cancer. Under any circumstance, it permits oesophageal dilatation either under direct intraluminal observation or under fluoroscopic control. Oesophagoscopic biopsy plus cytological specimens obtained by the brush technique can provide histologically confirmed diagnoses in over 90% of instances[36–38].

Dilatation of oesophageal strictures, particularly very narrow ones, should be attempted only by experienced endoscopists. The concurrent use of fluoroscopy can be quite helpful. Oesophagoscopy is useful in evaluating upper gastrointestinal bleeding (*see below*); in achalasia[39,40]; for diagnosing reflex oesophagitis[41]; for improving recognition of benign oesophageal strictures[42] and webs or rings[43], and the treatment thereof[44].

GASTROSCOPY AND DUODENOSCOPY

As previously noted, Schindler introduced the semiflexible gastroscope in 1932 and over the next three decades he and his disciples promoted its use[26,27]. Wide acceptance of gastric endoscopy did not occur, however, until the modern era was heralded by the development of a truly flexible fibre-optic instrument in 1958 by Hirschowitz and co-workers[28,45,46]. The Japanese deserve the credit for the rapidity with which the art advanced and they are responsible for the introduction of numerous innovations, both in technique and in instrumentation. Undoubtedly they were stimulated by pressing clinical needs based on the very high incidence of gastric and oesophageal cancer in their land[29,47,48] A number of excellent monographs and texts on the subject of gastroscopy are available[18,49-56].

While the indications for *oesophagoscopy* in the era of rigid instrumentation were, as previously pointed out, primarily a strong suspicion of organic disease, the reasons for undertaking *gastroscopy* became, as described by Palmer and Boyce[57], 'simply the known or suspected presence of organic stomach disease and the presence of some systemic diseases which may be accompanied by important gastric complications'. Today the excellence, ease, safety and fruitfulness of the method in experienced hands is such that it constitutes a diagnostic measure of prime order, on equal footing with the standard radiological upper gastrointestinal series. By-products of the technique are: (1) ready and safe examination of the oesophagus on the way down; and (2) extension of the examination by passing the instrument through the pyloric sphincter into the duodenum.

Gastroscopy is usually performed as an ambulatory procedure, under topical pharyngeal anaesthesia and light intravenous analgesia and sedation.

Instruments have progressed from the simple device first used by Hirschowitz and the gastro-camera (a small camera enclosed within the tip of the endoscope which took colour photographs of the gastric interior)[8] to a wide variety of forward-looking and side-viewing highly flexible endoscopes, some under 1 cm in diameter. There are no longer any 'blind' areas and retrograde viewing of the cardia from within the stomach lumen is accomplished easily. A biopsy channel permits brush and forceps biopsies and insertion of a wire snare for cautery excision of polypoid lesions. Grasping devices are obtainable for the removal of foreign bodies, even in small children[58], and for guiding the tip of a long intestinal tube such as the Miller–Abbott, Cantor or Dennis types, into the duodenum. Electrocautery probes or laser beam waveguides can be introduced for electro- or photo-coagulation of appropriate lesions such as bleeding sites or vascular anomalies (*see below*)[59-66].

Complications with modern instruments in experienced hands are most uncommon.

Despite remarkable technical advances, the diagnostic accuracy of upper gastrointestinal endoscopy is still largely dependent upon the skill, knowledge and experience of the specialist doing the examination. This is also true, of course, in radiology. As in radiology, permanent records may be made of endoscopic findings by the use of one of the various cameras on the market which fit to the eyepiece of the scope and permit continuous viewing and instantaneous picture-snapping during the examination. Ciné studies are also readily obtained and small, light television cameras are available to make videotape recordings or to project the endoscopic scene, while performed, to large audiences via video-monitors.

Basic admonitions

When the recommendation for upper gastrointestinal endoscopy of a particular patient originates from a physician other than the endoscopist, under no circumstances should the latter regard himself, or be regarded, as a mere technician performing a requested procedure. There must always be a consultative aspect to the referral in which the clinical problem is reviewed, the indications analysed, the aims recorded and the risks considered. The results of the patient's complete physical examination, and his previous laboratory reports, must be transmitted. The presence and seriousness of systemic disease states, particularly cardiopulmonary disease or diabetes, must be known and the endoscopist should be advised of any history of allergies or drug sensitivities. As examples, we know of diabetics who became acidotic or who had insulin reactions associated with fasting in preparation for a procedure scheduled late in the day; and of narcotic users who developed alarming systemic reactions when naloxone hydrochloride (Narcan) was injected intravenously and thoughtlessly as a routine measure on completion of a study.

The possibility of transmission of disease through the instruments or by exposure of the examiner should always be contemplated, particularly infectious hepatitis or resistant pulmonary tuberculosis.

The presence of early pregnancy should be known or considered. Endoscopy is often preferable to X-ray study in the diagnosis of urgent or recurrent gastrointestinal illness in pregnant females, to avoid unnecessary radiation exposure to the fetus.

Indications

In addition to the general statement of Palmer and Boyce referred to previously, specific indications for upper gastrointestinal endoscopy other than those already suggested will be briefly considered. A number of oesophageal problems have already been alluded to. *Diverticula*, pulsion or traction, demonstrated by radiological means do not, *per se*, require endoscopy but their presence may be a matter of interest and even concern should gastroscopy be contemplated for another condition. Patients with *hiatal hernias* may be endoscoped prior to corrective surgery to establish the presence and extent of *oesophageal reflux* whose existence can usually be noted radiologically when sought after, but whose effects on the oesophageal mucosa are not as readily apparent as by endoscopy. Known episodes of *bleeding*, persistent unexplained *anaemia* and the radiological demonstration of *ulceration* warrant endoscopic study. *Persistent heartburn* or *upper abdominal pain* not responding to medical measures and with negative X-ray studies may call for endoscopy.

Duodenal ulcers, diagnosed radiologically, usually do *not* require endoscopy, but one of the contributions of the method has been to demonstrate the presence of *duodenitis* when no ulcer crater could be seen radiologically[67]. *Duodenal deformity* without radiological demonstration of an ulcer crater is a valid indication, as would be duodenal disease which does not respond appropriately to medical treatment. For the surgeon, it is helpful to have endoscopy done prior to *contemplated surgical intervention*, both to document the fact that an active duodenal ulcer is responsible for the patient's symptoms and to disclose the existence of other lesions which may modify or change the surgical approach.

Gastric ulcers, of course, present a different problem. Although *gastric carcinoma* is on the decline, it must still be considered, and one need not enter into the controversy over whether chronic benign gastric ulcers become malignant or are that way from the start[33,68]. It is generally accepted that gastric ulcers should be followed both radiologically and endoscopically[68]. Indeed, it has been claimed that when gastric ulcer is diagnosed radiologically, there is a 'clarion call' for the endoscopist.

Any *tumour* or *mass* seen radiologically in or abutting on the stomach or duodenum calls for endoscopy. This will help to establish its nature and can prove useful to the surgeon in other ways. For *extra-gastric masses* it will help to define the degree of gastric wall involvement, if any, and its extent when present. For a highly situated benign tumour, such as a *leiomyoma*, it can provide information as to whether or not the cardia is clear and, hence, the best surgical approach. *Pseudo-masses* may turn out to be large folds when flattened out by air insufflation during endoscopy.

Endoscopy is useful in evaluating problems relating to the *post-surgical stomach*. *Marginal ulcers*[8] and *suture granulomas*[69] may be revealed only by direct examination; *alkaline gastritis* (or oesophagitis) may be suggested; and *cancer* developing in a gastric stump may be identified[70,71].

Endoscopy is extremely useful when applied to *bleeding problems*, whether they are acute and massive or recurrent, covert or suggested only by chronic anaemia. Certain lesions, such as *erosive gastritis* or *Mallory–Weiss tears*[72] will not be seen on conventional X-ray examinations. This subject will be discussed later, in greater detail.

Therapeutic indications include the presence of *foreign bodies* requiring removal, *gastric polyps* which may be excised by the snare electrocautery technique, bleeding lesions, and the need to advance a long intestinal tube.

Gastric neoplasms

Adenocarcinoma, polyp, leiomyoma and leiomyosarcoma are among the more important neoplasms of the stomach indentifiable by endoscopy.

Formerly diagnosed usually at an advanced stage[73], most clinicians claim that *gastric cancer* can now be diagnosed much earlier, thanks to gastroscopy[74]. The limitations of radiology in detecting early gastric cancer are generally accepted[19,75]. Endoscopic disclosure of 'early' lesions has, however, introduced new elements of conflict. The gross appearance of an 'early' lesion is by no means characteristic[76] and multiple brushings, washings and biopsies may be required for diagnosis[16,70]. (Even advanced cancers may present problems[77].) Apparently, there is no clear understanding of just what is meant by 'early gastric cancer' and Hirschowitz suggests that a serious difference in interpretation of histology may exist between American and Japanese pathologists[78]. In essence then, and contrary to popular belief, the documented evidence that gastroscopy really provides earlier diagnosis of gastric cancer still leaves much to be desired. For an erudite discussion of this interesting subject and an analysis of its controversial aspects, the recent monograph by Johansen is recommended[79].

Gastroscopy has contributed to identification of inflammatory conditions such as Crohn's disease[80], but here again the biopsy process is quite superficial and is usually not decisive in establishing the nature of the changes seen.

Gastric polyps may produce bleeding and require removal on that basis[81,82], but once detected, concern usually centres about whether or not a given polypoid lesion is malignant or premalignant. Here again, biopsy, because of its superficial and random nature, seldom provides a satisfactory answer[81,83]. Success with snare-cautery resection of colonic polyps via the colonoscope (*see below*), however, has led to electrosurgical removal of polypoid lesions from the stomach, as reported by Classen and Demling in 1971[84], and this has now been established as a safe and effective procedure when properly applied[85–89], and preferable to biopsy. Further surgical efforts will depend upon the pathological findings.

Duodenal neoplasms

As noted, gastro-duodenoscopy can usually shed light on the presence and nature of duodenal inflammatory conditions, with the caveats already noted in the case of gastric lesions. While duodenal neoplasms are rare, and 35 tumour types have been identified[90], fibre-optic endoscopy has contributed considerably to their detection, to indication of their probable pathological nature and to the appropriate surgical approach[91].

Discussion of ampullary and periampullary lesions will be covered under ERCP.

Other applications

Ingestions of *corrosive chemicals* are well recognized as diagnostic and therapeutic challenges to the surgeon. Fibre-optic endoscopy has proven to be of considerable value in estimating the location and extent of the chemical burn injury, in following its progress and in arriving at a decision in terms of treatment.

Ingestion of *alkalis* results primarily in oropharyngeal and oesophageal mucosal destruction, while *concentrated acids* tend to spare the oesophagus (or affect it only superficially) and produce a coagulative necrosis of the stomach epithelium. Pyloric stenosis, requiring surgical intervention, may be a late result. With lye injuries, the extent and depth of the corrosive injury to the oesophagus depends on the nature, amount and concentration of the ingested agent.

Most agree that oesophagoscopy should be performed *early* after the corrosive injury and, today, use of the slim, pediatric type of endoscope is preferable. Early endoscopy probably has its greatest usefulness in identification of patients who have sustained little or no injury, thereby obviating the need for further treatment. Usually the burn has occurred to its maximal degree by the time the patient reaches the hospital and no additional areas will become involved.

With rigid instrumentation, endoscopy should stop at the upper level of burn, to avoid any chances of perforation. With the flexible, slim instrument, there is more leeway, especially when the oesophageal component is minimal. Excessive air insufflation should be avoided. Acid ingestion may cause rapid gastric wall necrosis[92] so that, unless endoscopy is done *very early*, it is probably best deferred until the patient is out of immediate danger, and then to help plan appropriate therapy[93].

Haller and associates, based on experimental studies and experience with 285 corrosive burn injuries, perform endoscopy within 12 h and again following ciné fluoroscopy 3 weeks later, if indicated[94]. Further endoscopic examinations are carried out at 2–4-week intervals as warranted. Since most centres see only occasional cases, it will take some time before the proper role of fibre-optic endoscopy in corrosive injuries can be determined.

ENDOSCOPY IN GASTROINTESTINAL BLEEDING

Optimal management of gastrointestinal bleeding has long been a problem for all clinicians and a matter of special interest to surgeons. When the cause of the bleeding episode has been established, the surgeon may be called in either to bring about control of continuing loss of circulating volume or for definitive management of the underlying disease process. The surgical measures indicated in a given situation are determined by:

(1) the rapidity of blood loss,
(2) the effectiveness of replacement therapy,
(3) the nature of the pathological process contemplated, and
(4) the age and general condition of the patient.

When the cause of bleeding is undetermined or obscure, the challenge to the surgeon becomes far more difficult and is greatest when the haemorrhagic episode is acute and massive. In most if not all of these bleeding episodes, endoscopy has proved to be a measure of very considerable value, both diagnostically and therapeutically.

Superior care of the haemorrhaging patient requires the services of an interdisciplinary team of experts whose efforts must be integrated and brought to bear with appropriate timing and logical sequence. Surgeons are able to play their most effective role when they are brought in early in the consultative phase and thus able to see and follow the patient from the time he enters the hospital. They are, by training and experience, prepared to manage rapid losses of blood volume and to make decisions promptly. As part of the investigative and decision-making process, they should either themselves perform endoscopy or make every effort to be present if this procedure is performed by another. Under either circumstance, they need to be conversant with the technique and its potential contributions when employed early and aggressively in addressing the haemorrhagic incident.

Upper gastrointestinal bleeding

The occurrence of haematemesis or the presence of bloody material in a nasogastric tube aspirate almost invariably signifies a bleeding source located proximal to the ligament of Treitz. Once a rapid history has been obtained from the patient or his associates and measures to control shock have been instituted, upper gastrointestinal endoscopy appears to offer the greatest chance for successful and accurate early diagnosis.

An approach first suggested by Carter and Zamcheck[95] and long espoused by Palmer[96,97] and others, early aggressive endoscopic analysis of a bleeding episode has for some years been justified on the basis of its established safety and proven high percentage of correct diagnoses. The validity of this tactic became even more impressive with the advent of flexible fibre-optic instruments[8,98].

The advantage of early identification of the bleeding site and source reasonably closely, anatomically speaking, has long been stressed by surgeons, going back to the reports by Allen[99] and Welch[100]. Excessive delays before corrective surgical intervention are thought to be associated with increased morbidity and mortality. Moreover, the frustration to the surgeon of operating upon a bleeding patient and finding that the bleeding has ceased with the source still indeterminate[101] is almost entirely eliminated.

Endoscopic examination can be carried out at the bedside or in the emergency department. What unfavourable reports do exist in the literature, reflect clinical experience prior to the past decade[102]; recent reviews are almost uniformly favourable[97,102–105]. A fact to be emphasized is that to be of value the endoscopic examination must be done *during* the acute bleeding phase. Delays of even 1 or 2 days may lead to an incorrect diagnosis[98,106] Unremitting, vigorous bleeding as an obstacle to successful examination should be a problem for an experienced endoscopist in under 1% of cases. If the precise bleeding point cannot be identified, the study should at least indicate whether the bleeding is coming from the lower oesophagus, from the proximal or the distal stomach, from a level beyond the pylorus, or from multiple sites and sources. Armed with reasonably accurate knowledge of the cause and location of the vascular leak, the surgeon can decide on the immediacy of action and the type of the surgical procedure best suited for the case in question.

Largely as a result of the early and judicious use of endoscopy, certain facts have become better appreciated:

(1) bleeding episodes often result from pathologicial changes which are quite superficial and not demonstrable by customary radiological means, such as with erosive or haemorrhagic gastritis, arterio-venous malformations, and other vascular anomalies;
(2) bleeding sites are often multiple rather than single[105];
(3) there may be a combination of factors involved, such as reflux oesophagitis in a patient with oesophageal varices; and
(4) a patient does not always bleed from a known possible aetiology in that individual, such as a previously proven duodenal ulcer[8,105].

Not only is upper gastrointestinal endoscopy for haemorrhage diagnostically valuable, but it also has important therapeutic implications.

The use of electrocautery recommended by Papp[60,87] and Colpicelli *et al.*[64] or laser coagulation, as suggested by Waitman and associates[66] and Silverstein *et al.*[62], offer the clinician an opportunity to control the bleeding when the source is superficial and the rate of bleeding is not excessive. At present, Waitman and associates, at our institution, apply laser photocoagulation to a variety of bleeding sources. While it is too early to evaluate adequately its effectiveness, there have to date been no complications[65]. In the non-acute bleeder, it appears to be an excellent method for dealing with either single or multiple vascular malformations.

Endoscopy can and should be judiciously combined with angiographic techniques. Having an endoscopic diagnosis prior to angiography aids the angiographer by permitting immediate *selective* catheterization and, possibly, control of bleeding by vasopressin infusion of the artery supplying the bleeding site.

Endoscopy plays an equally important role in the management of patients whose bleeding has stopped, or of those who have sustained recurrent intermittent haemorrhages or occult bleeding of undetermined origin. This statement applies to any part of the gastrointestinal tract. Even the small bowel can be examined using a special instrument designed by Shinya which resembles a long intestinal tube[8]. This is passed like a Cantor or Miller-Abbott tube and allowed to advance and traverse the entire small bowel until it enters the caecum, which usually requires about 48 h. Then it is slowly withdrawn with the examiner carefully studying the interior of the small intestine gently distended by careful air insufflation.

It is important to note, however, that while an early aggressive endoscopic programme for the management of *massive* upper gastrointestinal haemorrhage yields the highest rate of accurate diagnosis of any method, reduces the number of blood transfusions required, and results in earlier and more precise surgical intervention, there is, as yet, no proof that it affects ultimate patient mortality.[107] With the widespread availability of trained endoscopists that now exists, the compelling need for a prospective randomized study to clarify this issue is quite apparent.

Lower intestinal bleeding

In bleeding of lower alimentary tract origin endoscopy is not as useful a tool during the acute bleeding phase as it is in upper gastrointestinal bleeding. Unless the colon can be adequately cleansed, visibility may be impaired and proper advancement of the scope may be difficult. During active haemorrhage, routine radiographic or angiographic methods would appear to be safest and most likely to prove diagnostic. Transcatheter infusion of vasopressin can usually provide temporary cessation of bleeding[108]. Recent experience moreover suggests that transcatheter embolization may provide more permanent control of haemorrhage[109].

Once bleeding has been stopped by either method, gentle saline or tap-water irrigations can often clear the colon adequately for endoscopic investigation. Todd and Forde found colonoscopy of value in 9 out of 21 patients with active lower gastrointestinal bleeding and in a number of those with chronic bleeding and negative radiological studies[110]. We have reported on cases of recurrent bleeding resulting from angiodysplastic lesions detectable only by the endoscopic route[111] and many reports of unusual vascular lesions are currently appearing[112,113].

Since angiographic vasopressin infusion or transcatheter embolization has the potential hazard of producing bowel ischaemia[109], colonoscopy offers an attractive means of examining the bowel wall if it is done carefully and without excessive air insufflation. Intraoperative per anal colonoscopy is sometimes of value in identifying or localizing vascular lesions at the time of laparotomy for surgical removal, in our own experience and as reported by others[114,115].

ENDOSCOPIC RETROGRADE CHOLANGIOPANCREATOGRAPHY (ERCP)

Shortly after the introduction of fibre-optic gastroscopy, Hirschowitz and associates reported a 50% success rate in entering the duodenum and before long this became a routine component of upper gastrointestinal endoscopy. A flow of reports from Japan[116,117] discussed efforts to visualize and cannulate the ampulla of Vater, an effort which had begun with the report of Watson in 1965[118]. Apparently, the first *endoscopic* effort to cannulate and visualize, by injection of contrast substances, the biliary and pancreatic ducts was that of McCune and coworkers in 1968[119]. For this purpose the side-viewing endoscope is required. Although an arduous and time-consuming procedure when introduced, this procedure soon gained clinical acceptance as a result of the persistent work of Japanese endoscopic groups led by Oi[117], Takagi[120], and others. Its very considerable practical value, as demonstrated by Cotton and co-workers in England[121,122], Blumgart in Scotland[123], Vennes and Silvis in the USA[124], and Classen and associates in West Germany[125], led to widespread adoption by gastroenterologists, surgeons and radiologists. Today, endoscopic retrograde cholangiopancreatography (ERCP) can be performed by most experienced endoscopists[126] and has been associated with striking new developments to be discussed below.

ERCP can be offered to patients on an ambulatory basis, but brief hospitalization is preferred because of occasional untoward sequelae.

General anaesthesia is not required, but a small intravenous dose (2–5 mg) of diazepam is administered at the onset, meperidine (25–50 mg) intravenously as required for discomfort during the procedure and glucagon (0.5–1.0 mg) to provide duodenal relaxation. Image intensifier fluoroscopy and facilities for high-quality radiography are requisite.

When pathological changes in the periampullary area are seen on direct observation, biopsy or washings for cytologic study may be all that is called for and cannulation under such circumstances may be unnecessary. Indeed, local tumours may preclude such accomplishment. However, tissue confirmation is regarded as mandatory since local inflammatory change can simulate cancer[127], when no tumour as such is visible. A method of needle biopsy of the pancreatic head via the endoscope has been reported with a high rate of success[128]. However, it is likely that this approach will fail to realize its promise because of the advent of percutaneous needle biopsy guided by computerized axial tomographic (CAT) scanning[129, 130], a simpler and equally safe method.

ERCP is an important modality in the differential diagnosis of *obstructive jaundice* as stressed by Blumgart[131] and is a method which can be utilized to opacify even a non-dilated biliary ductal system where percutaneous transhepatic cholangiography (PTC) may fail. Even when the latter is feasible, combining the information obtainable through both types of study offers a means of delineating both the proximal and distal extent of biliary ductal obstruction as we have pointed out[132]. For the surgeon planning an attack on ductal lesions, this can be most helpful[133].

The very considerable delays which may be involved in determining whether jaundice is 'medical' or 'surgical' such as may occur with intrahepatic cholestasis, hepatocellular disease caused by drugs, alcohol, virus, metastatic disease, and primary biliary neoplasm or inflammatory disease[134] are sources of great frustration to surgeons. These can often be eliminated by judicious early use of ERCP.

Extrahepatic biliary obstruction is best assessed first by sonographic and scanning techniques. The demonstration of masses or calculi and the presence of a proximal dilated ductal system can then be followed by endoscopy and cannulation to pinpoint the level of obstruction and its likely cause.

ERCP has other diagnostic contributions of value to the surgeon, as indicated by Braasch and Gregg[135]. In the presence of the *postcholecystectomy syndrome*, ERCP may support or challenge the diagnosis by delineating the residual anatomy. This can range from a normal ductal system to the presence of gallbladder remnants, cystic duct stumps, retained or recurrent stones or stenotic areas.

Pancreatography

Diseases of the pancreas have long constituted a challenge to the clinician because of the relative inaccessibility of the organ. Use of non-invasive techniques such as sonography and computerized tomography, and of invasive methods such as angiography and guided needle biopsy has proved of enormous value in recent years. However, ability to cannulate, irrigate and opacify the pancreatic ductal system via the endoscope has also been a major advance.

Cytological analysis of ductal secretions can establish the presence of pancreatic cancer[136]. Ductograms can assist in differentiating between neoplastic and inflammatory change. The surgeon may be helped greatly for, as stated by Rodney Smith: 'The indication for surgery should be clear and the correct operation ... selected for each individual patient[137].' A 'road map' is provided and, according to Warren, 'with this information now available before operation in most instances, the pancreatic surgeon is better equipped to anticipate and to plan the approach in treatment of both neoplastic and inflammatory disorders[138].

Interpretation of pancreatograms is improving[139], and has shed light on the progressive nature of both pancreatitis and neoplastic disease. These facts have led to better classification and more precise clinical management[140, 141]. The difficulty the surgeon has in differentiating between pancreatic cancer and chronic pancreatitis at laparotomy, the hazards of biopsy and the anguish of deciding whether radical resection is or is not warranted are notorious and make prior knowledge most welcome.

Therapeutic applications

The remarkable diagnostic usefulness of duodenal fibre-endoscopic examination has been eclipsed by the dramatic therapeutic applications which have emerged during the past 5 years. By a variety of techniques skilful endoscopists can not only demonstrate the presence, number and location of retained or recurrent stones in the major biliary ducts, but can also bring about their removal, thus avoiding the need for major abdominal, reoperative surgery[142].

By a technique introduced in Japan[139], efforts were first directed at inserting a Dormier-type basket via the biopsy channel of the endoscope through the sphincter to crush or remove calculi. As difficulties were encountered, either from a stenosed or tight sphincter or in reducing the stones to manageable size, a technique of endoscopic sphincterotomy using a wire and electrocautery current was perfected.

This produces a cut of approximately 15 mm through the papilla into the ampulla, permitting the withdrawal of stones using the Dormier basket or allowing their spontaneous passage over the next few days[143]. Large numbers of cases have now been reported from a number of clinics using this technique, as applied early on by Classen and Demling[144]. A recent report by Reiter et al.[145] from West Germany covers 1403 patients who underwent endoscopic papillotomy with a complication rate of 7.3% and a mortality of 1.5%. Stones were retrieved in 32% of cases and expelled spontaneously in 54%. Safrany describes an experience with the method in 562 patients with successful results in all but 29. Complications occurred in 6.9% and the mortality rate was 1.0%[146].

These remarkable developments in biliary endoscopic surgery, now being conducted at a number of centres, are not only favoured as measures for *post*-cholecystectomy patients with retained or recurrent calculi, but have recently been extended to include the poor-risk patient with gallbladder *in situ* and obstructive cholestasis or cholangitis. Relief of the obstruction by endoscopic sphincterotomy can significantly alleviate the acute emergency situation and may, on occasion, prove definitive. The incidence of biliary stricture following endoscopic sphincterotomy should be under 0.5%[147]. Refinements in technique now suggest that endoscopic 'papillotomy' may preserve sphincter function as compared with endoscopic 'sphincterotomy' and may have, therefore, certain advantages[148], but many authors use the terms interchangeably.

CHOLEDOCHOSCOPY

Gallstones are a common and important medical problem. According to Orloff, over 1 million operations are performed in the world each year for gallstones; more than 100,000 of these have calculi in the ductal system, and at least 15,000 patients each year have retained or recurrent bile duct stones after surgery[149]. The 10–13% of patients who are found to have retained stones early after choledocholithotomy can have their numbers reduced by proper surgical technique and intraoperative cholangiography[150]. Operative biliary endoscopy, introduced as far back as 1923 by Bakes[151], can further reduce the incidence of retained stones and is being practised with increasing frequency[152-157].

Two types of endoscopes are available – a flexible one and a rigid, angled choledochoscope. The latter appears preferable, providing better illumination and visualization and a variety of accessory instruments for stone manipulation and removal under endoscopic control. The technique, well described by Berci and co-workers, is readily mastered and appears to merit wider usage[158], as suggested by the discussions of Schein[159] and Warshaw[160].

COLONOSCOPY

Endoscopic examination of the large bowel is traceable to ancient history[161, 162] and Hippocrates is reported as having used a rectal speculum[162]. Riding astride horses or donkeys was probably a common cause of ano-rectal problems.

Desormeaux is regarded as the initiator of the modern era, describing an instrument for rectocolic examination in 1853[161] which was subsequently improved upon by Dr Howard Kelly of Baltimore[8]. The latter device was the forerunner of the conventional rigid sigmoidoscope.

For information relating to the status of the large bowel beyond the 25 cm range of the rigid sigmoidoscope – a level of insertion inconsistently achieved – the clinician was dependent upon the contrast enema until 10 years ago. When flexible fibre-optic instruments came upon the scene, efforts were made to study the large bowel but initial attempts were uniformly discouraging[163-168]. However, in 1969 Overholt[169] showed that it was possible to reach the sigmoid colon with such a scope and, starting in June of 1969, Wolff and Shinya[2] demonstrated that fibre-optic endoscopic examination of the entire colon was both feasible and safe. By the end of that year we had successfully carried out over 100 deep colonoscopies and introduced the practice of endoscopic polypectomy[3]. Accumulated experience and the availability of longer colonoscopes proved the enormous value of complete examination of the entire colon from caecum to rectum by the endoscopic route. 241 successful examinations were performed in the first 18 months without morbidity or mortality. By 1976, 7000 procedures had been performed with no deaths and but one perforation requiring operative intervention[170].

Instruments

At the present time excellent fibre-optic colonoscopes are obtainable through four major manufacturers, the Olympus Company of America, The American Cystoscope Manufacturers Inc. (ACMI), the Machida Co. and Fujinon. The instruments come in a variety of lengths and with a wide assortment of accessory devices about which the manufacturers' brochures should be sought for detailed information. In general, two scopes are favoured, a long scope of about 186 cm in length capable of reaching the caecum, and a medium scope of 105–110 cm in length which can be introduced to the transverse colon and a little beyond. Recently, the manufacturers and others have promoted a fibre-optic sigmoidoscope 60–70 cm in length as a suggested replacement for the traditional rigid sigmoidoscope[171-174].

These various instruments plus the fibre-optic light source, suction apparatus and accessories constitute a sizable financial investment. Expert care in their maintenance and cleansing is called for if expensive repairs and costly loss of availability (while out for repair) are to be avoided. With the rising costs of medical care individual physicians have a responsibility, in an institutional setting, to see that breakage is kept to a minimum and that newer instrument models with minor refinements are not frivolously requisitioned. Knowledgeable assistants, particularly specially trained nurses, are an essential ingredient to run a proper endoscopic unit or practice[175].

Technique

Diagnostic colonoscopy is readily accomplished on an out-patient basis as an ambulatory procedure. A thoroughly cleansed bowel is imperative and to persist in efforts at examining an ill-prepared colon is to court disaster. Either additional enemas should be administered to the patient or the preparation regimen should be continued for another 24 h, regardless of the inconvenience involved. A clean colon is not difficult to achieve on the regimen described in previous publications[176].

General anaesthesia is not required and, in our opinion, is contraindicated. Mild, intravenously administered analgesia and sedation, usually meperidine (Demerol) and diazepam (Valium) in doses adjusted to the patient's need, suffice. Intravenous injections of glucagon are frequently used to relax spastic areas and thereby facilitate passage of the instrument.

In expert hands, and with a bowel properly prepared, complete study should not exceed 1 h. At the conclusion of the examination most patients are given one ampoule (0.4 mg) of naloxone hydrochloride (Narcan) intravenously and are able to leave the unit for their home after adequate surveillance for another hour.

Fluoroscopy

In our early efforts, undertaken when introduction of the scope beyond the level of the sigmoid colon had not been successfully accomplished by any others, we utilized image-intensifier fluoroscopy as an aid in advancing the colonoscope and to determine its location[3, 4, 176, 177].

With increasing experience it was shown to be required less and less frequently. Today many successful colonoscopists utilize it rarely, if at all[173, 178, 179]. However, we believe that image-intensifier fluoroscopy can be of considerable assistance to someone learning the art of colonoscopy and that it can expedite examination in difficult cases for even an experienced endoscopist[180]. Fluoroscopy is required if one employs the stiffening or splinting device[8, 176], which greatly shortens the time required to examine the right colon and caecum. In addition it allows the examiner to verify the level of insertion and the exact location of the tip of the instrument. When one is studying a patient whose contrast enema indicates the presence of a dubious or puzzling finding, such verification enables the examiner to concentrate on the proper zone and satisfy the clinical issues involved.

Diagnostic indications

At present colonoscopy stands on even footing with the contrast enema as a diagnostic modality. We regard the two methods, as we always have, as complementary and not competitive procedures. Since there are more radiologists than experienced colonoscopists available, radiological study usually comes first, chronologically, but there is no reason why this must be so and colonoscopy is a valid primary study. If the barium study is reported as negative or inconclusive the clinician must base a decision for or against a subsequent endoscopic procedure on the merits of the individual case, recognizing that several groups have supported our early study[1] showing that important incremental data are often provided through colonoscopy[180–182]. The following settings would favour subsequent colonoscopy:

(1) the X-ray study is equivocal;
(2) the X-ray is negative in the presence of continued symptoms;
(3) the X-ray study is negative when there is a history of bleeding, occult blood in the stool or persistent unexplained anaemia;
(4) the X-ray study is positive, to confirm the findings (false positives);
(5) the X-ray study is positive for cancer, to identify undemonstrated synchronous cancer or polyps, prior to surgery;
(6) the X-ray study is positive, to obtain specimens for tissue diagnosis (inoperable cases, suspected metastatic involvement, etc.);
(7) the X-ray study is positive for polyp, to identify malignant changes or disclose the presence of additional polyps or cancer; and
(8) the X-ray study is positive for inflammatory disease, to confirm the diagnosis, to clarify the extent of the disease process and to obtain biopsies.

Examples of each of these are to be found in our previous publications[6–9, 17, 197b].

Other diagnostic indications include:

(1) routine screening examinations in patients at high risk for colorectal cancer;
(2) routine follow-up in patients with previous surgery for cancer or

polypectomy, in patients with rising carcinoembryonic antigen (CEA) levels, in patients with multiple or recurrent polyps and in patients with inflammatory bowel disease;

(3) as part of a complete evaluation of certain disease states, such as Osler–Weber–Rendu syndrome.

Biopsy

Biopsy at any level of insertion is possible with special flexible biopsy forceps supplied by the instrument manufacturers. These forceps are rather small, measuring 2–3 mm in diameter when closed and 6–8 mm when fully opened. (Placing a closed biopsy forceps tip alongside a given lesion permits the endoscopist to estimate its size.) The biopsy taken is rather superficial, which sometimes limits its effectiveness but at the same time protects against perforation. In inflammatory bowel disease the site of biopsy must be selected carefully and, because it is superficial, it is often not pathognomonic. For polyps a biopsy is only of benefit when evaluated against the background of other findings, since the sample taken represents only a tiny fraction of the whole. Even if positive for cancer one cannot tell from the biopsy alone if the cancer is *in situ* or *invasive*, a critical distinction (see below).

The biopsy procedure is eminently safe: we have performed several thousand without incident.

Colonoscopy and colorectal cancer

Colonoscopy has two important roles with respect to colorectal cancer:

(1) earlier detection of established cancers – thereby permitting curative surgery to be undertaken at a more favourable stage of the disease; and

(2) the detection and removal of precancerous lesions, notably the common neoplastic or adenomatous polyp.

In terms of established cancer the potential contributions of colonoscopy become apparent when certain facts are considered. First, cancer of the colon and rectum constitutes one of the two commonest visceral cancers in both sexes. Second, it is constantly on the increase, particularly with respect to the colon. This means that relatively fewer tumours can be picked up by digital or routine sigmoidoscopic examination. Third, the stage of disease at the time of detection has not changed appreciably in almost three decades, an important consideration in a condition which can be cured only by surgery, and one in which localized disease (Dukes A category) is associated with prolonged survival in over 80% of instances[183–185]. Fourth, cancers of the colon missed on contrast enema can be detected endoscopically[1, 8, 11, 17]. Fifth, the nature of suspicious changes discovered by contrast enema can be definitively diagnosed immediately, rather than by a policy of waiting and repeating the radiological studies after an interval. Sixth, cancers not infrequently exist in association with other disease processes, such as diverticulitis, polyps, etc. which may dominate radiological interpretation.

Endoscopic polypectomy

We introduced the procedure of endoscopic removal of colonic polyps using a snare-cautery device inserted via the biopsy channel of the colonoscope, doing the first procedure in September 1969[2, 3]. Since then our reported series has grown progressively[5–7, 10, 11, 17]. Our latest report, entitled, 'Morphology, anatomic distribution and cancer potential of colonic polyps: an analysis of 7000 polyps endoscopically removed'[186], discusses significant clinical aspects of the problem.

The importance of endoscopic polypectomy rests upon the relationship between polyps and colorectal cancer. Once a highly controversial subject, with many experienced pathologists questioning the relationship[187–189], the weight of evidence as presented by Morson[190, 191], Enterline and associates[192], Lane and associates[193, 194b], and others now strongly suggests that most, if not all, colorectal cancers originate in polyps.

Two matters require clarification in any discussion of the subject. Just what kind of 'polyps' are we talking about?; and what constitutes 'malignancy' in a polyp?

Table 1 Current and old terminology of colorectal polyps

Current terminology	Old terminology
Non-neoplastic	
Juvenile polyp	retention polyp
Hyperplastic polyp	metaplastic polyp
Neoplastic	
Tubular adenoma	adenomatous polyp
Villous adenoma	papillary polyp
Villotubular adenoma	villoglandular polyp
Polypoid carcinoma	malignant polyp

Much of the past confusion had its origin in lack of uniformity in terminology and nomenclature. Only true *neoplastic* polyps – those formerly referred to as adenomatous polyps or adenomas – have any malignant potential. If, as Fenoglio and Lane state[193] , 90% of polyps are of the *hyperplastic* variety and these do not become malignant, then the issues become more straightforward. And if one discards the widely held belief that adenomatous polyps and villous tumours are entirely distinctive, and accepts the careful studies by Morson and co-workers indicating that these are merely variants of a common category of epithelial neoplasms, with many intermediate forms, then understanding of the subject takes another forward step. We have found that classifying polyps into the major categories listed in Table 1 provides a common ground for discussion. Our histological analysis of polyps endoscopically removed, which included only polyps 0.5 cm in diameter or larger, proved 5786 of 7000 to be neoplastic polyps or adenomas. The major grouping is shown in Table 2. The histological categories are seen in Table 3. Since most polyps, when examined carefully and in multiple sections, have both tubular and villous components this categorization becomes somewhat arbitrary. A polyp that is 75% or more tubular, histologically, is listed as tubular adenoma; one which is 75% or more villous is called a villous adenoma; those remaining are identified as villotubular adenomas. (Other pathologists may use different percentages.)

Table 2 Histological analysis of 7000 polyps endoscopically removed

Non-neoplastic polyps	1173	
Neoplastic polyps	5827	
Adenomas		5786
Polypoid carcinomas		41
TOTAL	7000	

Table 3 Histological types of 5786 neoplastic polyps (adenomas) removed endoscopically

	No.	%
Tubular adenomas	3725	64.3
Villotubular adenomas	1542	26.7
Villous adenomas	519	9.0
TOTAL	5786	100

Our findings have consistently borne out the fact that villous adenomas have the highest incidence of malignant change, and rightly require the most vigorous therapeutic attack. Villotubular polyps are next in frequency of carcinomatous change and tubular adenomas the lowest (Table 4). So much for the individual polyp. In terms of the total

cancer problem, tubular and villotubular adenomas are equally important because of their relatively greater frequency of occurrence.

Table 4 The frequency of malignant change in 5786 adenomas removed endoscopically

	No.	Percentage with cancer in situ	Percentage with invasive cancer
Tubular adenomas	3725	12	3
Villotubular adenomas	1542	11	8
Villous adenomas	519	15	10
TOTAL	5786	12	5

Malignant polyps

Colonoscopy and electrocautery removal of polyps is now practised extensively[85,178-180,194-197]. Since biopsy alone is patently indecisive, only
total excision of the polyp provides unequivocal information relative to
the clinical situation. A compelling need for uniform guidelines in terms
of what is meant by the term 'malignancy' has become apparent.
Answers have been available for some time, however, through the
excellent reports of Morson and co-workers at St Mark's Hospital in
London, Lane and associates at Columbia-Presbyterian in New York,
and Enterline and associates at the University of Pennsylvania. Any
cancer which has not penetrated the muscularis mucosae of the polyp is
regarded as *cancer in situ*. Such cancers have never been known to
metastasize, and complete polyp removal is all the treatment that is
required. Only when the malignant cells have penetrated the muscularis mucosae can the tumour be regarded as 'invasive' and only under
this circumstance should the polyp be called 'malignant'. This distinction is essential.

Conflicting reports in the literature are largely the result of differences
in what authors decide to employ as criteria for use of the term 'malignant' or 'cancer' in a polyp and whether their background data cover all
polyps or only the neoplastic variety. One cannot emphasize too
strongly the importance of direct consultation between the surgeon and
the pathologist before arriving at a decision with respect to patient management when a polyp is termed malignant or when a given lesion has
been incompletely excised.

There is no question that the frequency of both cancer *in situ* and
invasive cancer is directly related to polyp size and to the quantitative
presence of a villous configuration. Morson[33,190] reports for all adenomas taken together, an incidence of invasive cancer of 1.3% for
lesions under 1–2 cm in diameter, of 9.5% for lesions 1–2 cm in diameter,

and of 46% for those over 2 cm. Our own figures for 7000 polyps (which apply only to polyps endoscopically removed) are 0.5%, 4.7% and 10.8%. There are understandable differences to be expected in material obtained in recent years from endoscopic units and that collected over a longer period, with the majority of specimens obtained by colotomy, colectomy or post-mortem examination.

With respect to histological patterns, villous lesions, particularly large ones, carry the highest risk of invasive cancer with villotubular adenomas lower, and tubular adenomas lowest cancer risk. Our own studies show these incidences to be 12.4%, 8.5% and 3.2% respectively, but, again, apply only to tumours lending themselves to endoscopic resection.

The problem of 'malignant' polyps

Our views on this subject have been described in previous publications[10,197]. In situ cancers require no other treatment than complete polyp removal. They have never been known to metastasize. If invasive cancer is reported, consultation with the pathologist should be sought. He can analyse the situation most informatively when the polyp has been carefully fixed and cut in appropriate coronal sections. For pedunculated polyps with well-differentiated cancer confined to the head and adequate clearance between the point of maximal invasion and the level of snare cautery resection, we feel that no additional surgical measures are required. When the cancer is poorly differentiated, comes close to the line of resection, or shows vascular or lymphatic permeation, further measures must be considered and depend on individual patient factors. Broad-based or sessile polyps, particularly those subjected to piecemeal removal, and polypoid carcinomas require a more aggressive attitude, but may be followed and treated endoscopically in the very-poor-risk patient. As elsewhere in surgery, proper management requires judgment, weighing all factors in any given case.

Special applications of colonoscopy

Availability of instruments and the acquisition of requisite skills by individuals at most medical centres has resulted in a number of interesting applications of the method. Ghazi, Shinya and Wolff used the method to correct a recurring sigmoid volvulus[198] and this has since been reported by others[199]. Shinya was able to remove a gold dental crown from the terminal ileum[176] and other foreign bodies have been similarly removed[200]. Colonoscopy has proved useful in decompressing massive caecal dilatation associated with non-organic obstruction in our hands and as reported by Kukora and Dent[201], and Bachulis and Smith[202].

Hunt and associates examined localized strictures of the colon in 154 patients and, by providing an accurate diagnosis, estimated that unnecessary laparotomy was avoided in over half[203]. Wilson *et al.* have used *intraoperative* colonoscopy to remove a polyp via the endoscope at laparotomy, after freeing-up blocking adhesions[204]. We have not yet found this necessary. Others have utilized intraoperative colonoscopy at laparotomy to solve special problems. Folkman first reported the efficacy of this manoeuvre to delineate, by transillumination, several vascular malformations in the bowel wall, having threaded the colonoscope all the way up to the duodenojejunal junction[114].

Colonoscopy as a screening technique for colorectal cancer

There are, as yet, no really satisfactory studies attempting to judge the potential value of colonoscopy as a screening method for earlier detection of colorectal cancer. There is reason to believe that most colorectal cancers are rather slow-growing: it has been estimated that there is probably about a 4-year interval from the beginning of a cancer to the appearance of clinical symptoms.

Theoretically then, if cancers can be detected during this asymptomatic period, more should be discoverable and treatable at a surgically favourable stage of the disease. The evidence to support this concept is indirect. Bolt[205], reviewing 18 335 traditional-type sigmoidoscopies in asymptomatic individuals, reports detection of cancer in 1 out of 435. Moreover, he claims that a 5-year salvage rate of nearly 88% was achieved in this group of patients, as opposed to only 50% for those with symptoms. Gilbertsen and co-workers have long maintained that routine proctosigmoidoscopy is an effective preventive measure for cancers of the distal large bowel[184, 206]. Additionally, they have shown that an assiduously followed programme of early detection and removal of adenomas and other polyps could sharply reduce the anticipated incidence of distal colorectal cancers by about 85%. Those tumours which were encountered are reported as having been small and sharply localized.

Most agree that proctosigmoidoscopy can be carried out satisfactorily and safely by practising physicians without a need for extensive special training. This, of course, is not true of colonoscopy. The number of adequately trained colonoscopists is limited and the risks involved are apparently considerably higher. We do not yet know what the yield might be if routine screening examinations were performed in patients at high risk, much less in a completely asymptomatic group. Lastly, we do not know if the costs required would justify the expense involved.

INFLAMMATORY BOWEL DISEASE

A large variety of inflammatory or pseudo-inflammatory conditions involve the alimentary tract. Some are specific for particular organs, such as the 'Barrett' oesophagus[207,208], Ménétrier's disease of the stomach, or moniliasis affecting both; some are specific and involve all sections, albeit with differing frequency such as Crohn's disease; and some are gut manifestations of a systemic condition, such as Whipple's disease or scleroderma.

All of these conditions have benefited from the use of fibre-optic endoscopy. In inflammatory bowel disease the extent of colonic involvement is determined more accurately than by X-ray study[1,180] and the course of the condition under treatment followed more closely. Biopsy for confirmation of diagnosis is possible and sometimes critical, such as in chronic ulcerative colitis where it can affect the need for and timing of surgery[209]. Since biopsy is superficial and small, it may not allow one to differentiate between the superficial changes of chronic ulcerative colitis and the transmural involvement of Crohn's disease, but the gross appearance of the latter may be characteristic in some cases[54,210]. The value of endoscopic biopsy in Crohn's disease in various parts of the alimentary tract is discussed by Geboes and co-workers[211].

FIBRE-OPTIC SIGMOIDOSCOPY

Instrument manufacturers and a number of clinicians have recently been promoting a fibre-optic 'sigmoidoscope', an instrument similar to the colonoscope but only 40–60 cm in length[171,174,212–215]. There exists currently a state of confusion on this subject so that the pros and cons should briefly be reviewed.

It is not clear whether proponents of flexible sigmoidoscopy intend it to supplement or replace traditional rigid proctosigmoidoscopy. The disadvantages of the latter procedure are that it is uncomfortable, and that full insertion to a depth of 25 cm is not commonly achieved. (Madigan and Halls claim that the average sigmoidoscopist inspects principally the distal 15–18 cm of large bowel[216].) Also, as a result of changes in the distribution of colorectal cancer to higher levels[217,218] fewer cancers can be detected by the traditional approach.

On the positive side are the following facts: the instruments are widely available and relatively inexpensive; most physicians have been trained to use them; the cost of examinations on a large scale can be kept reasonably inexpensive (Gilbertsen, at the time of his report estimated the cost of a proctosigmoidoscopic examination to be only $11.73)[208]; the procedure has proved to be practical and of benefit used as a screening method in large-scale protocols[206, 219-221].

Among the objections to routine proctosigmoidoscopy as a screening procedure are:

(1) it is not feasible for large segments of the population in terms of time and manpower; and
(2) patients are highly resistant for reasons of discomfort as well as aesthetic considerations[220].

Studies in multiphysician trials by Bohlman et al.[171] and Marks et al.[213] indicate that flexible instrument examination is more complete, more comfortable and more productive. On these bases alone it would appear to be advantageous. However, the instruments and accessories are far more highly priced, running into several thousands of dollars; breakage is more frequent; and when the instruments need repair, the price is again high and they are lost from service for weeks to months. The added expenses will inevitably be passed on to the public, adding further to the high cost of medical care. If used in an institutional setting, where individual accountability for the instruments will assuredly be of lower order and where responsibility for their care and maintenance can easily be the lot of untrained personnel part of the time, the added expenses may more than outweigh the theoretical benefit.

Another question, as posed by Christie[222], is who should do flexible sigmoidoscopy? If made available to all surgeons, internists and primary-care physicians, will not all the above caveats be greatly magnified? The complication rate can also be expected, of course, to rise considerably. On the other hand if, as suggested, flexible sigmoidoscopy is restricted to those experienced in colonoscopy and fibre-optic endoscopy in general, be they gastroenterologists, surgeons or others, would not the patient's interests be better served if he had more complete colonoscopy?

Until the above issues are resolved it would appear prudent not to switch over to flexible sigmoidoscopes as rapidly as the purveyors of these instruments would have us do.

LAPAROSCOPY (PERITONEOSCOPY)

Laparoscopy, first described in 1902, is a relatively simple, safe and highly informative endoscopic modality that has largely been overlooked by general surgeons. Since the method is now widely utilized by gynaecologists, the required equipment is available in most hospitals. Fibre-optic lighting equipment provides excellent illumination. Our experience using the method has been reported[223-225] and we have found that performance of the examination under local anaesthesia is associated with no significant complications and is well-accepted by patients.

Laparoscopy can be quite helpful in determining whether or not a formal laparotomy is required, and often, its employment can obviate the need for bigger and riskier operations[226-228]. Diagnostically, we have employed it:

(1) for evaluation of hepatic disease;
(2) for determination of the presence or absence of primary or metastatic intraperitoneal neoplasm,
(3) for ascertainment of the cause of ascites,
(4) for establishment of the nature of abdominal masses,
(5) for staging lymphomatous diseases,
(6) seeking a cause for abdominal pain, and
(7) in looking for a diagnosis in fever of unknown origin.

In short, laparoscopy may prove valuable in many cases in which exploratory laparotomy is the next step. In 35% of 140 patients analysed by us, laparoscopy resulted in a notable alteration in the thrust of strictly medical management and, in an additional 18%, contemplated major resectional surgery was revealed as unwarranted.

Laparoscopy allows one to obtain adequate biopsy specimens in many instances. Contraindications are few and include extreme obesity, intestinal obstruction, acute peritonitis and large hiatal hernias.

It is fair to point out, however, that with wider availability of computerized axial tomography (CAT), the indications for laparoscopy will probably diminish. The information provided by this remarkable radiological diagnostic technique will obviate the need for peritoneoscopy and other invasive forms of study in many instances. Moreover, guided by the computerized image, needle-aspiration biopsy in almost any part of the abdomen now appears feasible[129, 130].

OVERVIEW

The last two decades have produced a veritable explosion in the field of endoscopy with the introduction and development of fibre-optic instruments. The literature is already voluminous and increasing almost geometrically, with a host of new specialty journals appearing on the scene in response to the pressures of reports from multiple centres.

At present, most procedures are carried out by gastroenterologists, with surgeons constituting only a small percentage of endoscopists. A previous lack of availability of suitable training programmes on a national basis is slowly being alleviated. It is advisable that more surgeons become familiar with the art if they are to take advantage of its potential contributions to a fuller degree. Certainly, they have a responsibility to familiarize themselves with the indications for its use, its reliability and its limitations. Exposure to fibre-optic endoscopy should be an integral part of every surgical training programme, with opportunities to perform the less hazardous and intricate procedures. Surgeons should develop expertise in performing those endoscopic procedures most pertinent to their particular area of interest. Chairmen of services should consider an endoscopic unit as part of their departmental organization.

Hospitals have a stake in providing adequate facilities for the performance of endoscopic procedures and trained, reliable personnel to assist and to care for patients and the expensive equipment required. Use of the procedures should be encouraged but not overutilized for financial gain. Patient areas have to be made available which allow as many examinations as possible to be done on an out-patient basis, with adequate safeguards for preoperative and postoperative supervision and care, to avoid medical and medicolegal complications.

The profession has an obligation to press for serious scientific studies and reports based on carefully designed protocols embracing adequate controls. Surveys by questionnaire, without documentation, have little merit. As stated previously by us, 'It is hoped that this very promising new modality will not have its reputation tarnished by misapplications and abuse . . . what is needed are honest facts and figures[8].'

References

1   Wolff, W. I., Shinya, H., Geffen, A. *et al.* (1975). Comparison of colonoscopy and the contrast enema in 500 patients with colorectal disease. *Am. J. Surg.*, **129,** 181
2   Wolff, W. I. and Shinya, H. (1971). Colonofiberoscopy. *J. Am. Med. Assoc.*, **217,** 1509
3   Wolff, W. I. and Shinya, H. (1971). Colonofiberoscopy: diagnostic modality and therapeutic application. *Bull. Soc. Int. Chir.*, **5,** 525
4   Wolff, W. I. and Shinya, H. (1973). A new approach to the management of colonic polyps. In Hardy, J. D. and Zollinger, R. M. (eds.). *Advances in Surgery*. Vol. 7. (Chicago: Year Book Medical Publishers)
5   Wolff, W. I. and Shinya, H. (1973). Polypectomy via the fiberoptic colonoscope. *N. Engl. J. Med.*, **288,** 329
6   Wolff, W. I. and Shinya, H. (1973). A new approach to colonic polyps. *Ann. Surg.*, **178,** 367
7   Wolff, W. I. and Shinya, H. (1973). Colonofiberscopic management of colonic polyps. *Dis. Colon Rectum*, **16,** 87
8   Wolff, W. I. and Shinya, H. (1978). Modern endoscopy of the alimentary tract. In *Current Problems in Surgery*. (Chicago: Year Book Medical Publishers, Inc.)
9   Wolff, W. I. and Shinya, H. (1974). Earlier diagnostic of cancer of the colon through colonic endoscopy (colonoscopy). *Cancer*, **34,** 912
10   Wolff, W. I. and Shinya, H. (1975). Definitive treatment of 'malignant' polyps of the colon. *Ann. Surg.*, **182,** 516
11   Wolff, W. and Shinya, H. (1975). Endoscopic polypectomy: therapeutic and clinico-pathologic aspects. *Cancer*, Suppl. **36,** 683

12 Dunphy, J. E. (1973). In discussion of paper by Wolff and Shinya, *Ann. Surg.*, **178**, 377

13 Moore, F. D. (1973). In discussion of paper by Wolff and Shinya. *Ann. Surg.*, **178**, 376

14 Dent, T. L. (1973). The surgeon and fiberoptic endoscopy. *Surg. Gynecol. Obstet.*, **137**, 278

15 Gaisford, W. D. (1975). The surgical gastroenterologist. *Surg. Gynecol. Obstet.*, **140**, 86

16 Smith, L. E. (1976). Fiberoptic colonoscopy: complications of colonoscopy and poly-pectomy. A symposium. *Dis. Colon. Rectum*, **19**, 407

17 Kobayashi, S., Prolla, J. C. Winns, C. S. *et al.* (1970). Improved endoscopic diagnosis of gastro-esophageal malignancy. *J. Am. Med. Assoc.*, **212**, 2086

18 Wolff, W. I. and Shinya, H. (1978). The impact of colonoscopy on the problem of colo-rectal cancer. In Ariel, I. M. (ed.). *Progress in Clinical Cancer*, Vol. VII, pp. 51–69. (New York: Grune & Stratton, Inc.)

19 Nelson, R. S. (1970). *Endoscopy in Gastric Cancer.* (New York: Springer-Verlag)

20 Kussmaul, A. (1868). Über Magen spiegelung. *Ber. Dtsch. Naturforsch. Gen. Freiberg*, **5**, 112

21 Stoerk, C. (1881). An examination of esophagus with laryngoscope. *Wien. Med. Wochenschr.*, **25**, 706

22 Mikulicz-Radecki, J. von (1881). Zur Technik der Gastroskopie und Oesophagos-kopie. *Wien. Med. Press*, **22**, 1438

23 Jackson, C. (1938). Broncho-esophagology postulated. Semasiologic observations. *Ann. Otol. Rhinol. Laryngol.*, **47**, 1049

24 Jackson, C. (1907). *Tracheobronchoscopy, Esophagoscopy and Gastroscopy.* (St Louis: The Laryngoscope Co.).

25 Henning, N. (1932). About one new esophagoscope for use in the internal medicine clinic. *Klin. Wochenschr.*, **11**, 1673

26 Schindler, R. (1950). *Gastroscopy, The Endoscopic Study of Gastric Pathology*, 2nd Edn. (Chicago; University of Chicago Press)

27 Schindler, R. (1932). Ein vullig ungerfährliches, flexibles Gastroskip. *Münch. Med. Wochenschr.*, **79**, 126

28 Hirschowitz, B. I., Curtiss, L. E., Peters, C. W. and Pollard, H. M. (1958). Demon-stration of a new gastroscope – the fiberscope. *Gastroenterology*, **35**, 50

29 Colcher, H. (1971). Editorial: Progress in gastrointestinal endoscopic instrumentation in the past decade. *Gastrointest. Endosc.*, **17**, 169

30 Lopresti, P. A., Ciforelli, P. S., Dixit, N. *et. al.* (1971). Successful examination of the esophagus and stomach with a new fiberoptic instrument. *Gastrointest. Endosc.*, **17**, 103

31 Hirschowitz, B. (1970). Progress in esophagoscopy. *Endoscopy*, **2**, 75

32 Maimon, H. N., Dreskin, R. B. and Cocco, A. E. (1974). Positive esophageal cytology without detectable neoplasm. *Gastrointest. Endosc.*, **20**, 156

33 Morson, B. C. and Dawson, I. M. P. (1972). *Gastrointestinal Pathology* (Oxford: Black-well Scientific Publications).

34 Scanlon, E. F., Morton, D. R. and Walker, J. M. (1955). The case against segmental resection for esophageal carcinoma. *Surg. Gynecol. Obstet.*, **101**, 290

35 Flick, A. L. (1971). Editorial: fiberoptic controlled biopsy–cytology: emergence into maturity. *Endoscopy*, **18**, 35

36 Bruni, H. C. and Nelson, R. S. (1975). Carcinoma of the esophagus and cardia. *J. Thorac. Cardiovasc. Surg.*, **70**, 367

37 Kobayashi, S., Yoshii, Y. and Kasugai, T. (1972). Selective use of brushing cytology in gastrointestinal strictures. *Gastrointest. Endosc.*, **19**, 77

38 Yoshii, V., Kuno, N., Yagi, M. *et al.* (1971). Endoscopic biopsy and cytology in esop-hageal and gastric carcinoma with the fiberesophagoscope. *Gastrointest. Endosc.*, **17**, 150

39 Ortega, J. A. (1977). Endoscopic diagnosis and treatment of achalasia. *Gastrointest. Endosc.*, **24**, 19
40 Rinaldo, J. A. Jr., Biederman, M. A. and Gelzayd, E. (1976). The relative application of endoscopy and other diagnostic measures in achalasia. *Gastrointest. Endosc.*, **22**, 145
41 Johnson, L. F., De Meester, T. R. and Haggitt, R. C. (1976). Endoscopic signs for gastroesophageal reflux objectively evaluated. *Gastrointest. Endosc.*, **22**, 151
42 Hiatt, G. A. (1977). The roles of esophagoscopy vs. radiography in diagnosing benign peptic esophageal strictures. *Gastrointest. Endosc.*, **23**, 194
43 Arvanitakis, C. (1977). Lower esophageal ring: endoscopic and therapeutic aspects. *Gastrointest. Endosc.* **24**, 17
44 Folkman, M. J. (1973). In discussion of paper by Wolff and Shinya, *Ann. Surg.*, **178**, 377
45 Hirschowitz, B. I. (1961). Endoscopic examination of the stomach and duodenal cap with the fiberoscope. *Lancet*, **1**, 1074
46 Hirschowitz, B. I., Balint, J. A. and Fulton, W. F. (1962). Gastrointestinal endoscopy with the fiberscope. *Surg. Clin. N. Am.*, **42**, 1081
47 Doll, R., Muir, C. and Waterhouse, J. (1970). *Cancer Incidence in Five Continents.* Vol. II (Berlin: Springer-Verlag)
48 Gregor, D. (1972). Epidemiology of gastric cancer. *Recent Advances in Gastroenterology*, 2nd Edn. (Baltimore: Williams & Wilkins Co.).
49 Berci, G. (1976). *Endoscopy.* (New York: Appleton-Century Crofts)
50 Berry, Leonides H. (1974). *Gastrointestinal Pan-Endoscopy.* (Springfield, Ill: Charles C. Thomas)
51 Brühl, W. and Krentz, K. (1970). *Clinical Gastrology: A Manual and Atlas* (Stuttgart: Georg Thieme Verlag)
52 Colcher, H. (1974). Endoscopy of the stomach and duodenum. In Bockus, H. (ed.). *Gastroenterology.* 3rd Edn., pp. 454–474. (Philadelphia: W. B. Saunders Co.)
53 Demling, L., Ottenjann, M. and Elsted, K. (1972). *Endoscopy and Biopsy of the Esophagus and Stomach* (Philadelphia: W. B. Saunders Co.)
54 Ottenjann, R. and Classen, M. (Eds.) (1979). *Gastroenterologische Endoskopie.* (Stuttgart: Ferdinand Enke)
55 Salmon, P. R. (1974). *Fibre-optic Endoscopy* (London: Pitman Medical Publishing Co.)
56 Silverstein, F. E. and Rubin, C. E. (1976). The new look into the gastrointestinal tract. *Disease-a-Month.* (Chicago: Year Book Medical Publishers, Inc.)
57 Palmer, E. D. and Boyce, H. W. Jr (1964). *Manual of Gastrointestinal Endoscopy.* (Baltimore: Williams & Wilkins Co.)
58 Ghazi, A., Tan, S. S. and Wolff, W. I. (1979). Pediatric fiberoptic instruments: application in removal of foreign body in children's stomachs. *N.Y. State J. Med.*, **79**, 384
59 Frühmorgen, P., Bodem, F., Reidenbach, H. D. *et al.* (1976). Endoscopic laser coagulation of bleeding gastrointestinal lesions with report of the first therapeutic application in man. *Gastrointest. Endosc.*, **23**, 73
60 Papp, J. P. (1975). Electrocoagulation in upper gastrointestinal hemorrhage: a two-year experience. *Gastroenterology*, **68**, A-183
61 Papp, J. (1976). Endoscopic electrocoagulation of upper gastro-intestinal hemorrhage. *J. Am. Med. Assoc.*, **236**, 2076
62 Silverstein, F., Rubin, C. E. and Auth, D. C. (1975). Fiberendoscopic control of experimental gastric bleeding by laser photocoagulation. *Gastroenterology*, **68**, A-189
63 Silverstein, F. E., Auth, D. C., Rubin, C. E. *et al.* (1976). High power organ laser treatment via standard endoscopes. *Gastroenterology*, **71**, 558
64 Volpicelli, N. A., McCarthy, J. D., Bartlett, J. D. *et al.* (1978). Endoscopic electrocoagulation: alternative to operative therapy in bleeding peptic ulcer disease. *Arch. Surg.*, **113**, 483

65 Waitman, A. M. (1980). Personal communication
66 Waitman, A. M., Spira, I., Chryssanthon, C. P. *et al.* (1975). Fiberoptic coupled organ laser in the control of experimentally produced gastric bleeding. *Gastrointest. Endosc.*, **22**, 78
67 Whitehead, R., Roca, M., Meikel, D. D. *et al.* (1975). Histologic classification of duodenitis in fiberoptic biopsy specimens. *Digestion*, **13**, 129
68 Siegel, H. I. (1978). Gastroscopy and gastric cancer. In Ariel, I. M. *Progress in Clinical Cancer*. Vol. VII, pp. 45–49. (New York: Grune & Stratton, Inc.)
69 Hoare, A. M. and Alexander-Williams, J. (1977). Thread sutures seen on gastroscopy: do they cause ulcers or indigestion? *Br. Med. J.*, **2**, 996
70 Domellof, L., Eriksson, S. and Janunger, K. G. (1975). Late occurrence of precancerous changes and carcinomas of the gastric stump after Billroth II resection. *Acta Chir. Scand.*, **141**, 292
71 Schrumpf, F., Serck-Hansen, A., Stadaas, J. *et al.* (1977). Mucosal changes in the gastric stump 20 to 25 years after partial gastrectomy. *Lancet*, **2**, 467
72 Pagel, J., Lindkaer-Jensen, S. and Nielsen, O. V. (1975). The Mallory–Weiss syndrome. *Acta Chir. Scand.*, **141**, 532
73 Hoerr, S. O. (1973). Prognosis for carcinoma of the stomach. *Surg. Gynecol. Obstet.*, **137**, 205
74 Morrissey, J. F. (1976). The diagnosis of early gastric cancer. A survey of experience in the United States. *Gastrointest. Endosc.*, **23**, 13
75 Cooley, R. N. (1961). The diagnostic accuracy of upper gastrointestinal radiologic studies. *Am. J. Med. Sci.*, **242**, 628
76 Witzel, L., Halter, R. A., Gretillat, P. A. *et al.* (1976). Evaluation of specific value of endoscopic biopsies and brush cytology for malignancies of the esophagus and stomach. *Gut*, **17**, 375.
77 Winawer, S. J., Posner, G., Lightdale, C. J. *et al.* (1975). Endoscopic diagnosis of advanced gastric cancer. Factors influencing yield. *Gastroenterology*, **69**, 1183
78 Hirschowitz, B. (1976). Early gastric cancer. *Gastrointest. Endosc.*, **23**, 45
79 Johansen, A. A. (1976). Early gastric cancer. In Morson, B. C. (ed.). *Current Topics in Pathology*, pp. 1–47. (New York: Springer-Verlag)
80 Danzi, J. T., Farmer, R. G., Sullivan, B. H. Jr *et al.* (1976). Endoscopic features of gastroduodenal Crohn's disease. *Gastroenterology*, **70**, 9
81 Bone, G. E. and McClelland, R. N. (1976). Management of gastric polyps – a review. *Rev. Surg.*, **33**, 211
82 Brand, B. and Bernstein, L. H. (1973). Emergency gastroscopic polypectomy for control of hemorrhage. *Gastroenterology*, **65**, 956
83 Siefert, E. and Elster, K. (1972). Endoscopic polypectomy in the stomach: indication technique and results. *Dtsch. Med. Wochenschr.*, **97**, 1199
84 Classen, J. and Demling, L. (1971). Operative gastroscopy: removal of gastric polyps through a fibre-optic gastroscope. *Dtsch. Med. Wochenschr.*, **96**, 1466
85 Gaisford, W. D. (1973). Gastrointestinal polypectomy via the fiber-endoscope. *Arch. Surg.*, **106**, 453
86 Jacobs, W. H. and Bruns, D. (1977). Endoscopic electrosurgical polypectomies of the upper gastrointestinal tract. *Am. J. Gastroenterol.* **68**, 241
87 Papp, J. P. (1973). Electrosurgical gastric polypectomy via the Olympus GIF endoscope. *Gastrointest. Endosc.*, **20**, 70
88 Rachail, M., Corallo, J. and Pellet, D. (1974). Electro-résection des polypes du tractus digestif sous contrôle fibroscopique. *Nouv. Presse Méd.*, **3**, 1375
89 Tsumeoka, K. and Uchida, T. (1964). Our techniques of gastric polyp resection under endoscopy. *Gastroint. Endosc.*, **11**, 174
90 Braasch, J. W. and Denbo, H. E. (1964). Tumors of the small intestine. *Surg. Clin. N. Am.*, **44**, 791

91 Fuller, J. W., Cruse, C. W., Williams, J. N. *et al.* (1976) Primary surgical lesions of the duodenum. *Rev. Surg.* **33**, 284

92 Chodak, G. W. and Passaro, E. Jr. (1978). Acid ingestion: need for gastric resection. *J. Am. Med. Assoc.*, **239**, 225

93 Lowe, J. E., Graham, D. Y., Boisaubin, E. V. Jr *et al.* (1979). Corrosive injury to the stomach: the natural history and role of fiberoptic endoscopy. *Am. J. Surg.*, **137**, 803

94 Haller, J. A. Jr, Andrews, H. G., White, J. J. *et al.* (1971). Pathology and management of acute corrosive burns of the esophagus: results of treatment in 285 children. *J. Pediat. Surg.*, **6**, 578

95 Carter, M. G. and Zamcheck, N. (1950). Esophagoscopy in upper gastrointestinal bleeding. *N. Engl. J. Med.*, **242**, 280

96 Palmer, E. D. (1952). Observations on the vigorous diagnostic approach to severe upper gastroduodenal hemorrhage. *Ann. Int. Med.*, **36**, 1484

97 Palmer, E. D. (1969). The vigorous diagnostic approach to upper-gastrointestinal tract hemorrhage. *J. Am. Med. Assoc.*, **207**, 1477

98 Hirschowitz, B. I., Luketic, G. C., Balint, J. A. *et al.* (1963). Early fiberscope endoscopy for upper gastrointestinal bleeding. *Am. J. Dig. Dis.*, **8**, 816

99 Allen, A. W. (1937). Acute massive hemorrhage from the upper gastrointestinal tract. *Surgery*, **2**, 713

100 Welch, C. E. (1949). Treatment of massive gastroduodenal hemorrhage. *J. Am. Med. Assoc.*, **141**, 1113

101 Crohn, B. B., Marshak, R. N. and Galinsky, D. (1948). Repeated gastroduodenal hemorrhages without discoverable explanation. *Gastroenterology*, **10**, 120

102 Halmagyi, A. (1970). Critical review of 425 patients with upper gastrointestinal hemorrhage. *Surg. Gynecol. Obstet.*, **130**, 419

103 Hoare, A. M. (1975). Comparative study between endoscopy and radiology in acute upper gastrointestinal hemorrhage. *Br. Med. J.*, **1**, 27

104 McCray, R. S., Martin, F., Amir-Ahmadi, H. *et al.* (1969). Erroneous diagnosis of hemorrhage from esophageal varices. *Am. J. Dig. Dis.*, **14**, 755

105 Sugawa, C., Werner, M. H., Hayes, D. F. *et al.* (1973). Early endoscopy. A guide to therapy for acute hemorrhage in the upper gastrointestinal tract. *Arch. Surg.*, **107**, 133

106 Gabrielson, N. (1970). Gastrophotography in upper gastrointestinal hemorrhage without roentgenographically demonstrable source of bleeding. *Endoscopy*, **2**, 174

107 Eastwood, G. L. (1977). Does early endoscopy benefit the patient with active upper gastrointestinal bleeding? *Gastroenterology*, **72**, 737

108 Novelline, R. A., Waltman, A. C., Athanasoulis, C. A. *et al.* (1976). Recent advances in abdominal angiography. In Stollerman, G. H. (ed.). *Advances in Internal Medicine.* Vol. 21, pp. 417–449.

109 Sniderman, K. W., Sos, T. A. and Casarella, W. A. (1979). Transcatheter alternatives to vasopressin infusion in colonic hemorrhage. *Contemp. Surg.*, **15**, 11

110 Todd, G. J. and Forde, K. A. (1979). Lower gastrointestinal bleeding with negative or inconclusive radiographic studies; the role of colonoscopy. *Am. J. Surg.*, **138**, 627

111 Wolff, W. I., Grossman, M. B. and Shinya, H. (1977). Angiodysplasia of the colon: diagnosis and treatment. *Gastroenterology*, **72**, 329

112 Geboes, K., Brökgert, L. and Vontrappen, C. (1975). Varices of the colon: diagnosis by colonoscopy. *Gastrointest. Endosc.*, **22**, 43

113 Pickens, C. A. and Tedesco, F. J. (1980). Colonic varices: an unusual cause of rectal bleeding. *Am. J. Gastroenterol.*, **73**, 73

114 Folkman, M. J. (1973). In discussion of paper by Wolff and Shinya, *Ann. Surg.*, **178**, 377

115 Martin, P. J. and Forde, K. A. (1979). Intraoperative colonoscopy: preliminary report. *Dis. Colon Rectum*, **22**, 234

116   Ogoshi, K., Niwa, M., Hara, Y. *et al.* (1973). Endoscopic pancreato-cholangiography in the evaluation of pancreatic and biliary disease. *Gastroenterology*, **64**, 210

117   Oi, I., Kobayashi, S. and Kondo, T. (1970). Endoscopic pancreato-cholangiography. *Endoscopy*, **2**, 103

118   Watson, W. C. (1966). Direct vision of the ampulla of Vater through the gastroduodenal fiberscope. *Lancet*, **1**, 902

119   McCune, W. S., Shore, P. E. and Moscovitz, H. (1968). Endoscopic cannulation of the ampulla of Vater. *Ann. Surg.*, **167**, 752

120   Takagi, K., Ikeda, S., Nakagawa, Y. *et al.* (1970). Endoscopic cannulation of the ampulla of Vater. *Endoscopy*, **2**, 107

121   Cotton, P. B., Blumgart, L. H., Davies, G. T. *et al.* (1972). Cannulation of papilla of Vater via fiber duodenoscope. *Lancet*, **1**, 53

122   Cotton, P. B., Salmon, P. R., Beales, J. S. M. *et al.* (1972). Endoscopic transpapillary radiographs of pancreatic and bile ducts. *Gastrointest. Endosc.*, **19**, 60

123   Blumgart, L. H., Cotton, P. B., Burwood, R. *et al.* (1972). Endoscopy and retrograde choledocho-pancreatography in the diagnosis of the jaundiced patient. *Lancet*, **2**, 1269

124   Vennes, J. A. and Silvis, J. E. (1972). Endoscopic visualization of the bile and pancreas ducts. *Gastrointest. Endosc.*, **18**, 149

125   Classen, M., Frühmorgan, P., Kozu, T *et al.* (1971). Endoscopic–radiologic demonstration of bilio-digestive fistulas. *Endoscopy*, **3**, 138

126   Shinya, H. and Wolff, W. (1975). Ampullary cannulation and endoscopic pancreatography. *Diagnostica*, **33**, 16

127   Block, M. A., Schuman, B. M. and Weckstein, M. L. (1975). Interpretative problems in endoscopic retrograde cholangiopancreatography. *Am. J. Surg.*, **129**, 29

128   Tsuchiya, R., Henmi, T., Kondo, N. *et al.* (1977). Endoscopic aspiration biopsy of the pancreas. *Gastroenterology*, **73**, 1050

129   Cooperman, A. M., Haaga, J. R., Reich, N. *et al.* (1978). Computed tomography: an aid to the abdominal surgeon. In Nyhus, L. M. (ed.). *Surgery Annual*. Vol. 10, pp. 73–104. (New York: Appleton-Century-Crofts)

130   Haaga, J. R. and Alfidi, R. J. (1976). Precise biopsy localization by computed tomography. *Radiology*, **119**, 603

131   Blumgart, L. H. (1978). Biliary tract obstruction: new approaches to old problems. *Am. J. Surg.*, **135**, 19

132   Fischer, M., Wolff, W. I., Gaffen, A. *et al.* (1973). Antegrade and retrograde visualization of the biliary tree. *Am. J. Gastroenterol.*, **60**, 6

133   Wolff, W. I. (1973). In discussion of paper by Longmire, McArthur, Bastounis and Hiatt. *Ann. Surg.*, **178**, 345

134   Hall, T. J., Blackstone, M. D., Cooper, M. J. *et al.* (1978). Prospective evaluation of endoscopic retrograde cholangiopancreatography in the diagnosis of periampullary cancers. *Ann. Surg.*, **187**, 313

135   Braasch, J. W. and Gregg, J. A. (1973). Surgical uses of pecoral retrograde pancreatography and cholangiography. *Am. J. Surg.*, **125**, 432

136   Silvis, S. E., Rohrmann, C. A. and Vennes, J. A. (1973). Diagnostic criteria for the evaluation of the endoscopic pancreatography. *Gastrointest. Endosc.*, **20**, 51

137   Smith, R. (1973). Progress in surgical treatment of pancreatic disease. *Am. J. Surg.*, **125**, 143

138   Warren, K. W. and Hoffman, G. (1976). Changing patterns in surgery of the pancreas. *Surg. Clin. N. Am.*, **56**, 3

139   Takemoto, T. (1979). *Endoscopic Retrograde Cholangiopancreatography*. (Tokyo/New York: Igaku-Shoin Medical Publishers)

140   Belohlavek, D., Koch, H., Rösch, W. *et al.* (1976). Five years experience in endoscopic retrograde cholangiopancreatography (ERCP). *Endoscopy*, **8**, 115

141 White, T. T. and Silverstein, F. E. (1976). Operative and endoscopic pancreatography in the diagnosis of pancreatic cancer. *Cancer*, **37**, 449

142 Zimmon, D. S. (1979). Endoscopic diagnoses and management of biliary and pancreatic disease. In Ravitch, M. M. (ed.). *Current Problems in Surgery*, **16**, 3. (Chicago: Year Book Publishers, Inc.)

143 Siegel, J. H. (1978). Endoscopic retrograde cholangiopancreatography and endoscopic papillotomy. *Curr. Con. Gastroenterol.*, **3**, 8

144 Classen, M. and Demling, L. (1974). Endoskopische Sphinkterotomie der Papilla Vateri und Steinextraktion aus dem Ductus choledochus. *Dtsch. Med. Wochenschr.* **99**, 496

145 Reiter, J. J., Bayer, H. P., Mennicken, M. D. *et al.* (1978). Results of endoscopic papillotomy: a collective experience from nine endoscopic centers in West Germany. *World J. Surg.*, **2**, 505

146 Safrany, L. (1978). Transduodenal endoscopic sphincterotomy and extraction of bile duct stones. *World J. Surg.* **2**, 457

147 Koch, H. (1977). Operative endoscopy. *Gastrointest. Endosc.*, **24**, 65

148 Zimmon, D. S., Falkenstein, D. B. and Kessler, R. E. (1975). Endoscopic papillotomy for choledocholithiasis. *N. Engl. J. Med.*, **293**, 1181

149 Orloff, M. J. (1978). Retained and recurrent bile duct stones – introduction. *World J. Surg.*, **2**, 401

150 Orloff, M. J. (1978). Importance of surgical technique in prevention of retained and recurrent bile duct stones. *World J. Surg.*, **2**, 403

151 Bakes, J. (1923). Die Choledochopapilloskopic nebst Bemerkungen über Hepaticus-drainage und Dilation der Papille. *Arch. Klin. Chir.*, **126**, 473

152 Nora, P. F., Berci, G., Dorazio, R. A. *et al.* (1977). Operative choledochoscopy. Results of a prospective study in several institutions. *Am. J. Surg.*, **133**, 105

153 Ottinger, L. W., Warshaw, A. L. and Bartlett, M. K. (1974). Intraoperative evaluation of the bile ducts. *Am. J. Surg.*, **127**, 465

154 Schein, C. J. (1969). Biliary endoscopy. *Surgery*, **65**, 1004

155 Schein, C. J. (1975). Influence of choledochoscopy on the choice of surgical procedure. *Am. J. Surg.*, **130**, 74

156 Shore, J. M. and Shore, E. (1970). Operative biliary endoscopy: experience with the flexible choledochoscope in 100 consecutive cholelithotomies. *Ann. Surg.*, **171**, 269

157 Warshaw, A. L. and Bartlett, M. K. (1974). Technique for finding and removing stones from intrahepatic bile ducts. *Am. J. Surg.*, **127**, 353

158 Berci, G., Shore, J. M., Morgenstern, L. and Hamlin, J. A. (1978). Choledochoscopy and operative fluorocholangiography in the prevention of retained bile duct stones. *World J. Surg.*, **2**, 411

159 Schein, C. J. (1978). 'Invited commentary' on paper by Berci, *et al. World J. Surg.*

160 Warshaw, A. L. (1978). 'Invited commentary' on paper by Berci, *et al. World J. Surg.*

161 Clarke, E. S. (1969). History of gastroenterology. In Paulson, M. (ed.). *Gastroenterologic Medicine* (Philadelphia: Lea & Febiger)

162 Milne, J. S. (1907). *Surgical Instruments in Greek and Roman Times*, pp. 149–50. (Oxford: Clarendon Press)

163 Kanazawa, T. and Tanaka, M. (1965). Endoscopy of colon. *Gastroenterol. Endosc.*, **7**, 398

164 Matsunaga, F., Tsushima, H. and Kuboto, T. (1959). Photography of the colon. *Gastroenterol. Endosc.*, **1**, 58

165 Niwa, H., Utsumi, Y., Kaneko, E. *et al.* (1969). Clinical experiences of colonic fiberscope. *Gastroenterol. Endosc.*, **2**, 163

166 Oshiba, S. and Watanabe, A. (1965). Endoscopy of the colon. *Gastroenterol. Endosc.*, **7**, 400

167 Turell, R. (1963). Fiberoptic coloscope and sigmoidoscope. *Am. J. Surg.*, **105**, 133

168 Turell, R. (1967). Fiberoptic sigmoidoscopes. *Am. J. Surg.*, **113,** 305
169 Overholt, B. F. (1969). Flexible fiberoptic sigmoidoscope. *CA – A Cancer Journal for Clinicians*, **19,** 81
170 Wolff, W. and Shinya, H. (1979). Kolonoskopie (Koloscopie) – historischen Hintergrund. In Ottenjann, R. and Classen, M. (eds.). *Gastroenterologische Endoskopie.* (Stuttgart: Ferdinand Enke)
171 Bohlman, T. W., Katon, R. M., Lipshutz, G. R. *et al.* (1977). Fiber-optic pansigmoidoscopy. *Gastroenterology,* **72,** 644
172 Cronstedt, J., Deurell, S. I. and Vestergaard, P. (1977). Total and subtotal colonoscopy with short instrument and without fluoroscopy. *Acta Med. Scand.*, **202,** 265
173 Marks, G. and Moses, M. L. (1973). The clinical application of flexible fiberoptic colonoscopy. *Surg. Clin. N. Am.*, **53,** 735
174 Winawer, J. J. (1977). A pioneer in flexible sigmoidoscopy. *Gastroenterology,* **73,** 1190
175 Belinsky, I., Shinya, H. and Wolff, W. I. (1973). Colonofibroscopy: technique in colon examination. *Am. J. Nurs.*, **73,** 306
176 Shinya, H. and Wolff, W. I. (1976). Colonoscopy. In Nyhus, L. M. (ed.). *Surgery Annual.* Vol. 8. (New York: Appleton-Century-Crofts)
177 Wolff, W. I., Shinya, H., Geffen, A. *et al.* (1972). Colonfiberoscopy. *Am. J. Surg.*, **123,** 180
178 Sivak, M. V. Jr., Sullivan, B. H. Jr. and Rankin, G. B. (1974). Colonoscopy: a report of 644 cases and review of the literature. *Am. J. Surg.*, **128,** 351
179 Waye, J. D. (1975). Colonoscopy: a clinical view. *Mt Sinai J. Med.*, **42,** 1
180 Williams, C. B. and Teague, R. H. (1973). Progress report: colonoscopy. *Gut,* **14,** 990
181 Amberg, J. R., Berk, R. N., Burhenne, H. J. *et al.* (1977). Colonic polyp detection: role of roentgenography and colonoscopy. *Radiology,* **125,** 225
182 Thoeni, R. F. and Menuck, L. (1977). Comparison of barium enema and colonoscopy in the detection of small colonic polyps. *Radiology,* **124,** 631
183 Dukes, C. E. and Bussey, H. J. R. (1958). The spread of rectal cancer and its effect on prognosis. *Br. J. Cancer,* **12,** 309
184 Gilbertsen, V. A., Knatternd, G. I., Lober, P. H. *et al.* (1965). Invasive carcinoma of the large intestine – a preventable disease? *Surgery,* **57,** 363
185 Turnbull, R. B., Kyle, K., Watson, F. R. *et al.* (1967). Cancer of the colon: the influence of the no-touch isolation technique on survival rates. *Ann. Surg.*, **166,** 420
186 Shinya, H. and Wolff, W. I. (1979). Morphology, anatomic distribution and cancer potential of colonic polyps: an analysis of 7,000 polyps endoscopically removed. *Ann. Surg.* **190,** 679
187 Castleman, B. and Krickstein, H. (1962). Do adenomatous polyps of the colon become malignant? *N. Engl. J. Med.*, **267** 469
188 Rider, J. A., Kirsner, J. B., Moeller, H. C. and Palmer, W. L. (1959). Polyps of the colon and rectum. A 4-year to 9-year follow-up study of patients. *J. Am. Med. Assoc.*, **170,** 638
189 Spratt, J. S. Jr, Ackerman, L. V. and Moyer, C. A. (1958). Relationship of polyps of the colon to colonic cancer. *Ann. Surg.*, **148,** 682
190 Morson, B. C. (1974). Evolution of cancer of the colon and rectum. *Cancer,* **34,** 845
191 Morson, B. C. and Bussey, H. J. (1970). Predisposing causes of intestinal cancer. In *Current Problems in Surgery*, pp. 81–83. (Chicago: Year Book Publishers, Inc.)
192 Enterline, H. T., Evans, G. W., Mercado-Lugo, R. *et al.* (1962). Malignant potential of adenomas of the colon and rectum. *J. Am. Med. Assoc.*, **179,** 322
193 Fenoglio, C. M. and Lane, N. (1975). The anatomic precursor of colorectal carcinomas. *J. Am. Med. Assoc.*, **231,** 640
194a Berci, G. Panish, J. and Morgenstern, L. (1973). Diagnostic colonoscopy and colonoscopic polypectomy. *Arch. Surg.*, **106,** 818
194b Grinnell, R. S. and Lane, H. (1958). Benign and malignant adenomatous polyps and

papillary adenomas of the colon and rectum. An analysis of 1856 tumors in 1335 patients. *Int. Abstr. Surg.*, **106**, 519

195 Ottenjann, R. (1972). Colonic polyps and colonoscopic polypectomy. *Endoscopy*, **4**, 212

196 Testas, P., Chary, A., Liquori, C. *et al.* (1975). L'Exploration du colon par fibroendoscopie et la polypectomie endoscopique. *Chirurgie*, **99**, 485

197a Williams, C., Muto, T., Rutter, K. R. P. (1973). Removal of polyps with fibreoptic colonoscope. *Br. Med. J.*, **1**, 451

197b Wolff, W. I. (1979). Colonoscopy updated. In Jordan, G. L. Jr. (ed.). *Advances in Surgery*. Vol. 13 (Chicago: Year Book Medical Publishers, Inc.)

198 Ghazi, A., Shinya, H. and Wolff, W. I. (1976). Treatment of volvulus of the colon by colonoscopy. *Ann. Surg.*, **183**, 263

199 Sanner, C. J. and Saltzman, D. A. (1977). Detorsion of sigmoid volvulus by colonoscopy. *Gastrointest. Endosc.*, **23**, 212

200 Montori, A., Viceconte, G., Miscusi, G. *et al.* (1976). Therapeutic colonoscopy. *Endoscopy*, **8**, 81

201 Kukora, J. S. and Dent, T. L. (1977). Colonoscopic decompression of massive non-obstructive cecal dilatation. *Arch. Surg.*, **112**, 512

202 Bachulis, B. L. and Smith, P. E. (1978). Pseudo-obstruction of the colon. *Am. J. Surg.*, **136**, 66

203 Hunt, R. H., Teague, R. H., Swarbrick, E. T. *et al.* (1975). Colonoscopy in management of colonic strictures. *Br. Med. J.*, **3**, 360

204 Wilson, S. M., Poisson, J., Gamache, A. *et al.* (1976). Intraoperative fiberoptic colonoscopy: 'The difficult polypectomy'. *Dis. Colon Rectum*, **19**, 136

205 Bolt, R. J. (1971). Sigmoidoscopy in detection and diagnosis in the asymptomatic individual. *Cancer*, **28**, 121

206 Gilbertsen, V. A. (1974). Proctosigmoidoscopy and polypectomy in reducing the incidence of rectal cancer. *Cancer*, **34**, 936

207 Borrie, J. and Goldwater, L. (1976). Columnar cell-lined esophagus: assessment of etiology and treatment. *J. Thorac. Cardiovasc. Surg.*, **71**, 825

208 Naef, A. P., Savary, M., Ozzello, L. *et al.* (1975). Columnar lined lower esophagus: an acquired lesion with malignant pre-disposition. *J. Thorac. Cardiovasc. Surg.*, **70**, 826

209 Teague, R. H. and Read, A. E. (1975). Polyposis in ulcerative colitis. *Gut*, **16**, 792

210 Waye, J. D. (1977). The role of colonoscopy in the differential diagnosis of inflammatory bowel disease. *Gastrointest. Endosc.*, **23**, 150

211 Geboes, K., Desmet, V. J., De Wolf-Peters, C. *et al.* (1978). The value of endoscopic biopsies in the diagnosis of Crohn's disease. *Am. J. Proctol. Gastroenterol. Col. Rest. Surg.*, **29**, 21

212 Goldsmith, O., Frankel, H., Gerety, D. *et al.* (1977). Fiberoptic sigmoidoscopy in an asymptomatic population. *Gastrointest. Endosc.*, **4**, 228

213 Marks, G., Boggs, H. W., Castro, A. F. *et al.* (1979). Sigmoidoscopic examinations with rigid and flexible fiberoptic sigmoidoscopes in the surgeon's office. *Dis. Colon Rectum*, **22**, 162

214 Marino, A. W. M. (1977). Looking ahead: types of flexible sigmoidoscopes and preparation of the patient. *Dis. Colon Rectum*, **20**, 91

215 Talbott, T. M. (1977). Looking ahead: evaluation of the new flexible sigmoidoscopes. *Dis. Colon Rectum*, **20**, 89

216 Madigan, M. R. and Halls, J. M. (1968). The extent of sigmoidoscopy shown on radiographs with reference to the rectosigmoid junction. *Gut*, **9**, 355

217 Axtell, L. M. and Chiazzo, L. Jr (1966). Changing relative frequency of cancers of the colon and rectum in the U.S. *Cancer*, **19**, 750

218 Berg, J. W. and Howell, M. A. (1974). The geographic pathology of bowel cancer. *Cancer*, **34**, 807

219 Corman, M. L., Collier, J. A. and Vridenheimer, M. C. (1975). Proctosigmoidoscopy – age criteria for examination in the asymptomatic patient. *CA–A Cancer Journal for Clinicians*, **25**, 286

220 Morton, P. C. (1978). Proctosigmoidoscopy in asymptomatic men: a 24-month study. *CA–A Cancer Journal for Clinicians*, **28**, 211

221 Prager, E. D., Swinton, N. W., Young, J. L. *et al.* (1974). Follow-up study of patients with benign mucosal polyps discovered by proctosigmoidoscopy. *Dis. Colon Rectum*, **17**, 322

222 Christie, J. P. (1980). Flexible sigmoidoscopy – why, where, and when? *Am. J. Gastroenterol.*, **73**, 70

223 Friedman, I. H., Grossman, M. B. and Wolff, W. I. (1977). The value of laparoscopy in general surgical problems. *Surg. Gynecol. Obstet.*, **144**, 906

224 Friedman, I. and Wolff, W. (1977). Laparoscopy: a safer method for liver biopsy in the high risk patient. *Am. J. Gastroenterol.*, **67**, 319

225 Friedman, I. and Wolff, W. (1978). Laparoscopy: a valuable adjunct to the abdominal surgeon's armamentarium. *Am. J. Surg.*, **135**, 160

226 Berci, G., Shore, J. M., Parish, J. and Morgenstern, L. (1973). The evaluation of a new peritoneoscope as a diagnostic aid to the surgeon. *Am. Surg.*, **178**, 37

227 Sugarbaker, P. H. and Wilson, R. E. (1976). Using celioscopy to determine stages of intra-abdominal malignant neoplasms. *Arch. Surg.*, **111**, 41

228 Trujillo, N. P. (1973). Can peritoneoscopy prevent a laparotomy? *Gastroenterology*, **64**, 129

2
Diagnosis of intra-abdominal disease by computerized axial tomography

J. R. HAAGA, R. J. ALFIDI and J. M. SHUCK

During the past several years there has been remarkable progress in the development and refinement of radiological equipment and techniques. Computerized tomography (CT), one of the most significant developments of this period, has proven to be a valuable clinical tool[1-8]. In this chapter we will discuss the diagnostic role of CT in the different organ systems and the use of CT for interventional techniques.

PRINCIPLES

The computerized tomograph is an imaging system which uses a finely collimated X-ray beam and a detector system in conjunction with a computer system to reconstruct a cross-sectional image of the body. While the X-ray beam is moved around the patient, the detector systems record the variation in the X-ray beam produced by each portion of the anatomy. The variation in the beam is dependent upon the density of the material the beam traverses; a high-density material, such as bone, produces a different measurement on the detectors than a low-density material such as air. Thousands of such measurements are made and collected by the computer which then calculates the 'density' or attenuation of the small tissue volumes in the cross-sectional area being examined. The 'density' or attenuation values are then displaced as individual picture points or matrix points in different shades of grey on the video monitor. Each shade of grey corresponds to a different 'density' or attenuation number. The composite picture of these different 'picture points' or matrix points produces the CT image. This discussion is an obvious oversimplification of the principles of CT; those interested in technical specifics are referred to the large variety of references dealing with the various types of scanning configurations, reconstruction techniques, modulation functions and other more technical data.

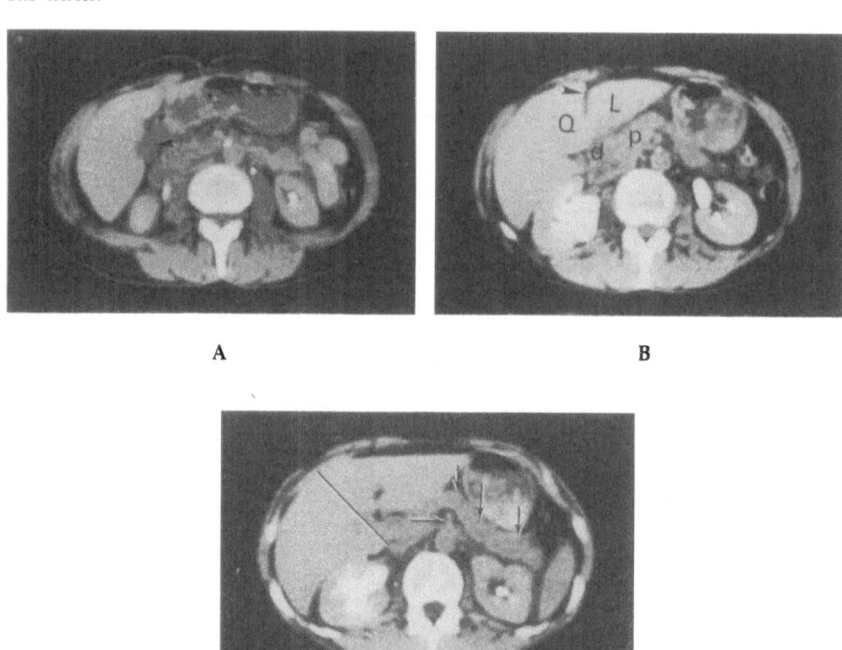

A   B

C

Figure 1 (**A**) CT scan through the liver at the level of the gallbladder. The gallbladder (arrow) appears as the low density, circular structure, medial to the liver. (**B**) Scan through the same patient demonstrates the falciform ligament (arrow) separating the anatomic left lobe (L) from the remainder of the liver. The quadrate lobe (Q) is immediately lateral to the falciform ligament. The head of the pancreas (p) is immediately medial to the duodenum (d). (**C**) Another section taken through the same patient at the level of the pancreas demonstrates the body and tail of the pancreas (vertical arrows); the superior mesenteric artery (horizontal arrow) is located immediately behind the body of the pancreas. The splenic vein runs directly posterior to the body and tail of the pancreas (arrow heads). The porta hepatis appears as the fat density structure centrally within the liver. This scan demonstrates an arbitrary line drawn right and left between arterial blood supply

LIVER

The normal, unenhanced liver has a uniform attenuation ranging between 40 and 70 attenuation units, except for low-density defects which represent the venous system. In those cases in which intravenous urographic contrast enhancement is utilized, the liver appears totally uniform and the venous structures are no longer visible. The individual lobes can be demonstrated consistently. The separation of the left lobe into the medial and lateral portions is demarcated by the fat density falciform ligament (Figure 1A, B, C). The separation of the right lobe from the right medial portion of the left lobe is not clearly defined, but this can be approximated by an imaginary vertical line drawn from the gallbladder to the vena cava. The caudate lobe is located between the vena cava and the porta hepatis. Within the porta hepatis is located the portal vein, hepatic artery and biliary system; the portal vein is usually clearly visualized because it is the largest structure within the porta hepatis. The unenhanced hepatic artery and undilated biliary system are only occasionally visualized without contrast material. With bolus intravenous injection of urographic contrast material and rapid sequence scanning, it is possible to visualize the intrahepatic portions of the artery and portal vein (Figure 2A,B).

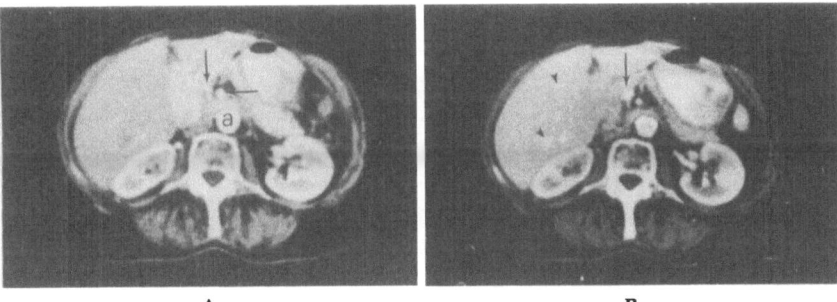

A   B

Figure 2   (A) This scan taken during the bolus injection of contrast material demonstrates the arterial phase of an injection. The aorta (a), superior mesenteric artery (horizontal arrow) and hepatic artery (vertical arrow) are opacified due to the contrast material. Small dense areas in the liver represent opacification of the intrahepatic arteries. The cortex of the kidney is much denser than the medullary region of the kidney.   (B) This scan taken 20 s after the initial scan demonstrates clearing of contrast from the arterial structures and opacification of the portal vein (arrow) and portal venous system within the liver (arrow heads). The differentiation of cortex and medulla is still apparent within the kidneys

The techniques for examining the liver may vary from one institution to another but most use intravenous urographic contrast to provide enhancement. There are several methods of contrast enhancement which may be used; these include bolus injection and continuous drip infusion. Definite advantages of any one of these types of contrast enhancement have not yet been proven, so there is still no method of choice.

Focal lesions

Benign and malignant focal lesions of the liver may produce alterations in its normal attenuation and contour. Most commonly, the attenuation values for all lesions are less dense than the normal parenchyma, but occasionally the density may be higher than normal. The margins of benign lesions are typically better-demarcated than those of malignant lesions; however, there may commonly be specific exceptions to this rule.

A variety of benign lesions can be visualized, and the appearance varies significantly depending upon the specific diagnosis. The most common benign abnormality demonstrated in the asymptomatic patient is the simple cyst. Such lesions are well-circumscribed and low in attenuation, being close to the density of water. Cysts may occur in asymptomatic patients or in patients with polycystic disease (Figure 3). The appearance of such cysts is so characteristic that no further evaluation or treatment is necessary unless there is antecedent history which might suggest that a cystic neoplasm or abscess should be considered.

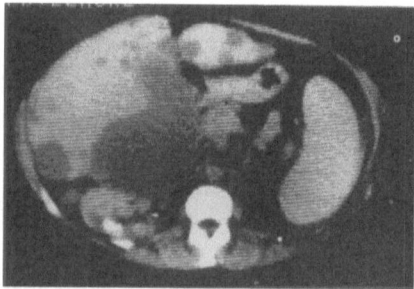

Figure 3 This scan demonstrates typical cystic disease of the liver. The cysts are low in density with a well-demarcated margin. Such cysts may be found in the asymptomatic patient as an incidental finding. This patient has polycystic disease of the liver

The second most common mass lesions of the liver are haemangiomas[9,10]. These vascular abnormalities appear as areas of low attenuation which have a characteristic appearance following a bolus injection of intravenous urographic contrast material. With such an injection, these vascular abnormalities go through a sequential change in their appearance. Initially, they are low in density. Immediately after the injection of contrast, the rim may be high in density. Approximately 10–15 min after an injection of contrast material, these lesions may be isodense in a normal liver (Figure 4A,B).

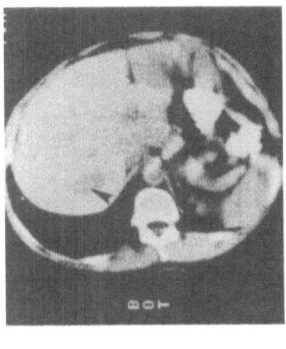 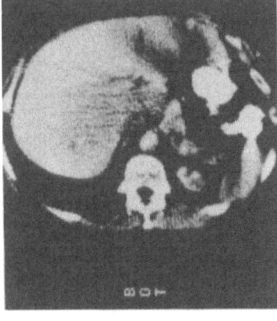

A   B

Figure 4 (A) This and Figure 4B demonstrate one of the typical appearances of a liver haemangioma. On the initial scan, without injection of contrast material, the haemangioma appears as an area of lesser density in the posterior right lobe (arrows). (B) After the injection of contrast material, the haemangioma now becomes isodense with the liver

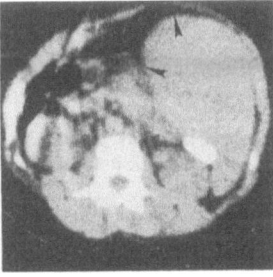

Figure 5 This scan demonstrates a hepatic adenoma which is isodense with the normal liver. There is a contour change anteriorly within the right lobe (arrows) which indicates the presence of a neoplasm

The final benign lesion we will discuss is the benign adenoma. Adenomas may be lower in density than the normal parenchyma; however, they quite commonly may be isodense with hepatic parenchyma. Thus, the only indication of an abnormality is a contour change (Figure 5). It is not surprising that these lesions are very similar in density to the

normal parenchyma because they are hamartomas of hepatic parenchymal elements.

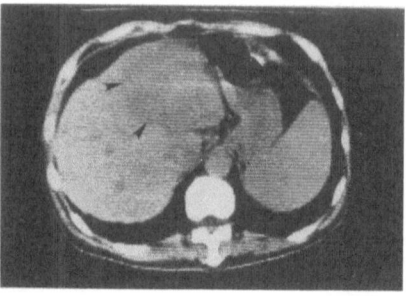

Figure 6 Hepatocellular carcinomas typically appear as areas of low density within the liver (arrows)

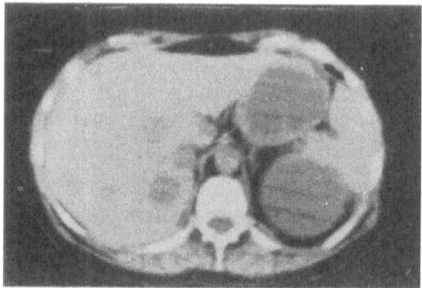

Figure 7 Scan taken through a patient with metastatic disease demonstrates multiple areas of lesser density scattered throughout the liver, characteristic of metastatic disease

Neoplastic focal disease in the liver may be either primary or metastatic. Hepatocellular carcinoma typically appears as an area of low attenuation (Figure 6), although occasionally such a lesion may be isodense
with normal hepatic parenchyma. In two series reported to date, CT
was successful in diagnosing 37 of 47 cases and 15 of 16 cases, respectively. In each of these series the detection accuracy was essentially
equivalent to that of a radionuclide scan in diagnostic accuracy. Such
metastatic disease is typically lower in density than the normal
parenchyma by approximately 20–30 numbers (Figure 7). Most types of
metastases are not specific in their appearance and cannot be distinguished from one another. However, there are certain tumours
which have characteristic areas of either very low density or very high

density; in such cases one can limit the differential possibilities. Metastatic tumours having very low attentuation, i.e. close to that of water, include mucinous tumours of the ovary, colon or stomach. Some very necrotic tumours, such as squamous cell carcinoma or transitional tumours, may also have a low attenuation characteristic (Figure 8). The mucinous tumours just mentioned may also occasionally have high-density areas which represent calcification; this phenomenon is relatively common in colonic metastases (Figure 9). The detection accuracy of CT for neoplastic disease, as reported in the literature, varies between 75 and 85%.

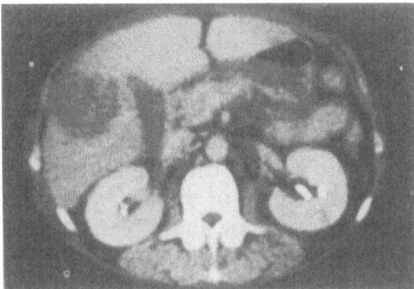

Figure 8 This scan is taken through a patient with very low density metastasis with squamous cell carcinoma. Such very low density lesions can be produced by mucinous or necrotic tumours

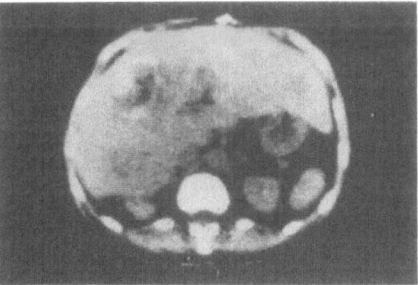

Figure 9 This scan demonstrates metastatic disease with calcification. Such calcification commonly occurs in metastases from mucinous neoplasms of the colon, stomach and ovary

Earlier reports did not demonstrate increased accuracy of CT over other modalities[9-22]; however, a recent report by Snow et al.[23] states that CT was more accurate than either radioisotope scanning or ultrasound.

In addition to the high diagnostic accuracy of CT, there are certain imaging advantages which result from technical aspects of the examination. In those patients in whom surgical resection of solitary metastasis is contemplated, CT can determine the extent of the neoplasm as it relates to the various lobes. For follow-up of chemotherapy or radiation therapy, CT is well-suited because it is reproducible from one examination to the next. Finally, in those instances in which other examinations are equivocal or confusing, CT can provide additional data which may consolidate a working diagnosis. For example, in patients in whom the left lobe is either absent or small, a radioisotope scan may be equivocal while the CT scan will demonstrate the presence of the normal right lobe and absence of the left lobe.

Diffuse hepatic disease

The CT appearance of diffuse parenchymal disease is quite variable. It depends on the aetiology of the disease and the severity of involvement. Cirrhosis in an early stage of development may not produce any change in the density, contour or shape of the liver. Later during the course of the disease when fatty infiltration occurs, the presence of fat is readily appreciated from the scan. In such cases, the venous system appears more dense relative to the fat density parenchyma (Figure 10). Although fat deposition is generally uniform, it may have a patchy or irregular distribution resembling that of a neoplasm[24]. In the late stages of cirrhosis the surface and contour of the lobes may be irregular and distorted by fibrotic bands and regenerating nodules (Figure 11). Finally, in cases of long-standing cirrhosis, there may be hypertrophy of the left and caudate lobes of the liver.

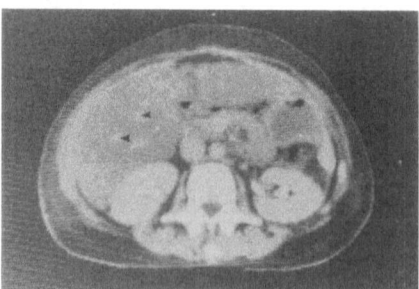

Figure 10   Typical appearance of fatty infiltration of the liver. The normal venous system (arrows) is higher in density than the liver. The liver is of fat density

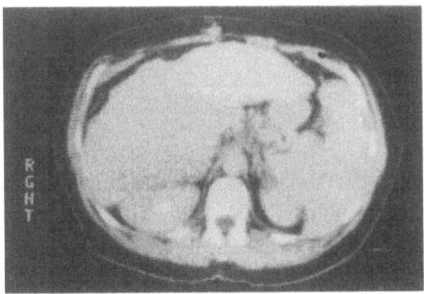

Figure 11 This patient with cirrhosis of the liver has irregularity of the margins produced by fibrosis and regenerating nodules

Fatty change in the liver is the most common diffuse disease; it is, however, non-specific and can result from a variety of disorders other than cirrhosis. We have observed such fatty changes from diabetes, obesity, endocrine disorders, infectious disease, toxic chemicals, medications or even trauma. Some storage diseases not involving lipid products produce an increase in the density of the liver.[25] Haemachromatosis, either primary or secondary, produces an increase in the density of the liver because of the presence of iron. Several authors have shown that the attenuation numbers increase linearly with iron content. Goldberg *et al.*[26] have shown that glycogen storage disease also produces an increase in the attenuation numbers of the liver (Figure 12).

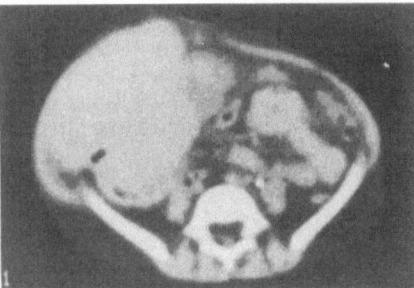

Figure 12 This scan taken through a patient with Von Giercke's disease shows areas of increased density produced by glycogen deposition

The role of CT in the detection of diffuse liver disease is dependent upon the nature of the clinical inquiry. If cirrhosis is being considered, there is unanimity in the literature: radioisotope scan is the investigative modality of choice. If the clinical question concerns the deposition of fat, iron or glycogen, CT is the modality of choice.

Hepatic trauma

We have found CT to be useful for the detection of haematomas in and around the liver; however, there are only limited numbers of cases reported in the literature. In such cases the haematoma may be accurately localized to the perihepatic or intrahepatic areas. Several hours after the formation of a haematoma the density of the blood is very close to that of the blood in the aorta (Figure 13). Later, the haematoma may become more dense than the blood contained in the vena cava or aorta; the cause of this has not been adequately explained[3]. As time progresses there is a breakdown of blood products and influx of body fluid so that the density of these areas decreases, approaching that of water (Figure 13).

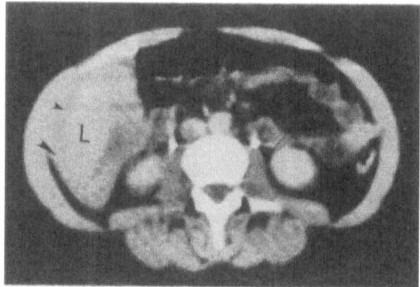

Figure 13 CT scan following a percutaneous liver biopsy demonstrating a haematoma around the liver. The liver (L) is contained within a large haematoma. The upper portion of the haematoma is fluid density (small arrow) while the lower portion is high density (larger arrow). This is produced by sedimentation of the blood products into the inferior portions of the cavity

BILIARY SYSTEM

The normal gallbladder and biliary system can be imaged by CT. The gallbladder appears as an oval, low-density structure on the undersurface of the right lobe of the liver (Figure 1A). The normal, unobstructed common bile duct and intrahepatic biliary radicals can be occasionally visualized with some high-resolution CT equipment, but they are not consistently visualized.

Biliary abnormalities can be consistently imaged with CT systems. Calculous disease of the gallbladder and biliary radicals without complete biliary obstruction is also detectable in many cases. In cases where a stone is high in density because of calcium or low in density because of cholesterol, the calculi are visible (Figure 14). Dilatation of the biliary system is apparent on a CT scan because the density of bile is significantly less than that of blood. Obstruction of the main biliary system appears as a branching, low-density structure in the porta hepatis region (Figure 15A,B). Segmental dilatation of the biliary system resulting from abnormalities such as sclerosing cholangitis, cholangiocarcinoma or neoplastic disease can also be seen and recognized because of this difference in the density of blood.

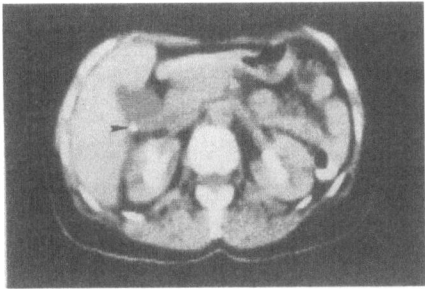

Figure 14 This scan taken through the gallbladder demonstrates a high-density calculus (arrow)

For evaluation of routine biliary problems, CT is not the modality of choice but it is indicated in selected cases. In the uncomplicated patient ultrasound study is efficacious and the modality of choice for the initial evaluation of either biliary dilatation or calculous disease. In those cases where ultrasound study is not technically satisfactory, CT is certainly indicated. Moreover, if biliary obstruction is present and the clinician suspects neoplasm, CT might be used as the initial examination because of its superior ability to define the presence and extent of neoplastic disease in the liver, porta hepatis and the pancreas. In these cases of suspected segmental biliary disease, CT is the modality of choice because it can demonstrate the segmental dilatations we have noted above. Ultrasound may not visualize such segmental dilatations because it cannot differentiate segmentally dilated areas of the biliary system from the normal venous system within the liver. Ultrasound cannot consistently differentiate between bile-containing spaces and blood in the venous system.

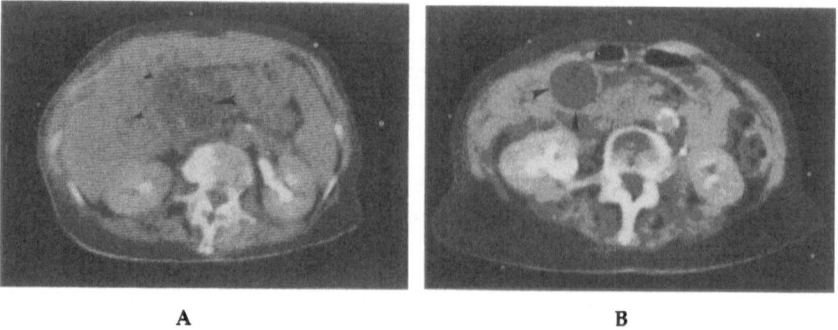

A   **B**

Figure 15 (A) This scan, taken through the level of the head of the pancreas and porta hepatis of the liver, demonstrates low-density structures which represent the dilated biliary tree (arrows). The circular, low-density structures centrally represent the dilated common bile duct (larger arrow). (B) Scan taken lower in the abdomen demonstrating the large 'Courvoisier gallbladder' (arrows)

PANCREAS

As a deep-seated organ in the anterior portion of the retroperitoneum, the pancreas has been difficult to image consistently with conventional modalities. With the advent of CT, which is unimpaired by visceral gas, the pancreas can now be routinely visualized[27-31].

Normal gland

The normal pancreas is located in the anterior pararenal space, immediately anterior and superior to the superior mesenteric artery. The body and tail of the pancreas are situated anterior to the splenic vein and are immediately caudad to the splenic artery (Figure 16A,B). The head of the pancreas is anterior to the superior mesenteric artery and the vena cava and immediately medial to the 2nd portion of the duodenum. The uncinate process of the pancreas is posterior to the superior mesenteric artery and vein. The texture of the normal gland is typically uniform but the margins may be somewhat irregularly interspersed with fat. The normal anteroposterior diameter of the pancreas ranges between 2.0 and 3.5 cm. We have formulated a relative measurement using the transverse diameter of the vertebral body as a 'yardstick'. The normal anteroposterior diameter of the pancreatic head should not exceed the full transverse diameter of the vertebral body; the anteroposterior diam-

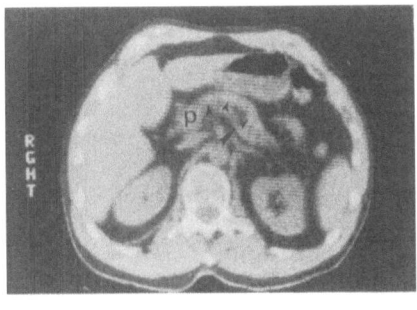 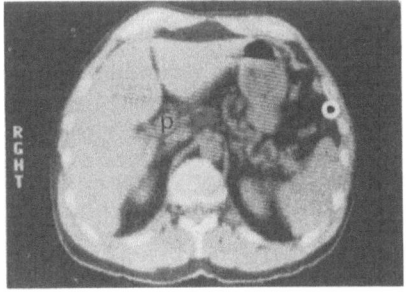

A   B

Figure 16 (**A**) This and Figure 16B demonstrate a normal pancreas. The normal pancreas (arrow heads) is located anterior to the splenic vein (arrow). The portal vein (p) is close to the upper margin of the head of the pancreas. The aorta and the superior mesenteric artery are posterior to the splenic vein and pancreas. (**B**) This scan, taken immediately above the head of the pancreas, demonstrates the tortuous splenic artery which borders on the superior margin of the pancreas. The portal vein (p) is in the porta hepatis of the liver prior to entry into the substance of the liver

eter of the body and tail should not exceed two-thirds of the transverse diameter of the vertebral body. These relative measurements correlate well with cadaver measurements (and have been noted as valid by several groups)[32]. In order to clearly define the head of the pancreas and to separate it from the antrum of the stomach and the duodenal bulb, oral contrast material should be administered. Moreover, in our experience, we have found that taking a scan of the patient in the lateral position with the right side down is also helpful in visualizing the pancreatic region[3,27].

Neoplasm

Adenocarcinoma of the pancreas produces enlargement of the gland and a contour change (Figure 17). The density of adenocarcinoma is the same as that of a normal gland. When neoplasm involves the head of the pancreas, there may be two changes noted distal to the mass. Early in the course of the disease there may be an obstructed pancreatic duct which appears as a radiolucent line in the central portion of the gland (Figure 18). In some cases the portion of the pancreas distal to the mass will be decreased in calibre, presumably secondary to parenchymal atrophy from obstruction of the duct. Lymph nodes in the immediate area of the gland may be enlarged where metastases have occurred. Extension of tumour beyond the confines of the pancreas into the retroperitoneum and perivascular areas can be clearly seen[3,27-34]. Because of the clear definition of such extension, one can logically hypothesize that CT should be useful for staging pancreatic carcinoma to determine inoperability[3]. For example, if involvement of the superior mesenteric vessels or portal veins can be demonstrated on CT, there is little hope for surgical cure. In such cases, intestinal or biliary diversion may be the most beneficial procedure to contemplate. This viewpoint is supported by several groups, although no prospective study has yet been conducted. Although most neoplasms can be easily diagnosed, it has not been possible to detect neoplasms confined to the gland itself. Those cases of ampullary carcinoma which are operable will demonstrate obstruction in the biliary system and in the pancreatic duct, indicating that the obstructing lesion is in the head; the margins of the lesion itself cannot be defined.

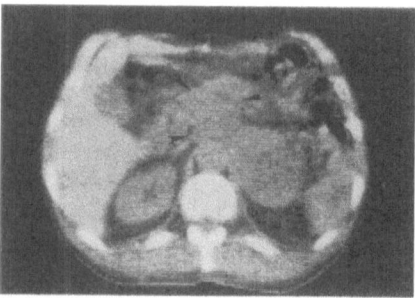

Figure 17 This scan demonstrates carcinoma of the pancreas. There is a large soft tissue mass in the head of the pancreas (arrows) which is extending into the retroperitoneum

Certain types of neoplasms in the pancreatic region have specific attenuation traits; others do not. Mucinous tumours may demonstrate areas of decreased density which are close to the density of water (Figure 19). Islet cell tumours and cystadenocarcinomas may contain calcium within the tumour masses[3]. Adenocarcinoma, apudomas, lymphomas and metastatic tumours in the pancreas appear as soft tissue density masses without any distinctive features.

The role of CT in evaluation for neoplasm has been defined differently by various groups[31-40], but there is a consensus that CT is the most accurate method for diagnosing normalcy, malignancy or inflammation. Some groups advocate CT as the initial examination in a patient suspected of neoplasm because it is consistently successful. Others have proposed a triage approach using ultrasound as the initial screening procedure followed by re-examination of the patient as needed. In those cases in which examination by ultrasound is not possible because of gas

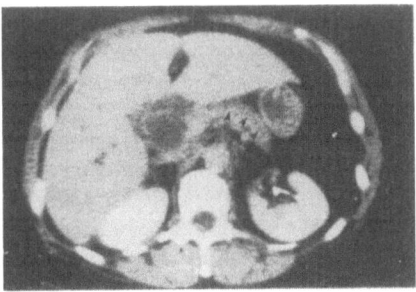

Figure 18 This scan is taken in a patient with carcinoma of the ampulla. The biliary system is dilated and appears as an area of low density scattered throughout the liver. The low-density area in the head of the pancreas represents the dilated common bile duct. The pancreatic duct is dilated and appears as a low-density line through the length of the pancreas (arrow heads)

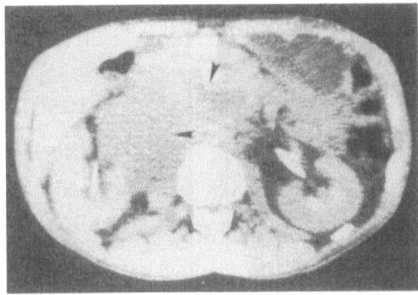

Figure 19 This scan demonstrates a mucinous carcinoma of the pancreas. The arrow heads point to the area of lower density which represent mucinous material within the tumour

or other technical factors, a CT scan will virtually always visualize the gland. In those cases where ultrasound is used as the initial examination and is positive, a CT examination can provide additional information with a high confidence level concerning the extent of the disease. For example, a CT scan can determine with greater accuracy the spread or extent of disease in the retroperitoneum and can give some estimate as to its resectability.

Pancreatitis

The diagnosis of pancreatitis is usually established by laboratory and clinical data, while imaging tests are utilized when complications are suspected. A simple, inflamed pancreas may have several appearances. In most instances of uncomplicated acute inflammation, the gland will be generally increased in size with a homogeneous density. In some instances there may be focal enlargement of the head, the appearance of which is indistinguishable from that of a neoplastic mass on the basis of image appearance alone. In either of these cases it is quite common to see enlargement or thickening of the anterior Gerota's fascia on the left side (Figure 20A,B). Most authors have explained this thickening in the fascia on the basis of spread of inflammatory exudate but the exact aetiology has not been determined[3]. This 'thickening' of Gerota's fascia is a very reliable differential sign to distinguish pancreatitis from neoplasm of the pancreas; however, the sign is applicable only to those cases which have not had surgery or radiation therapy.

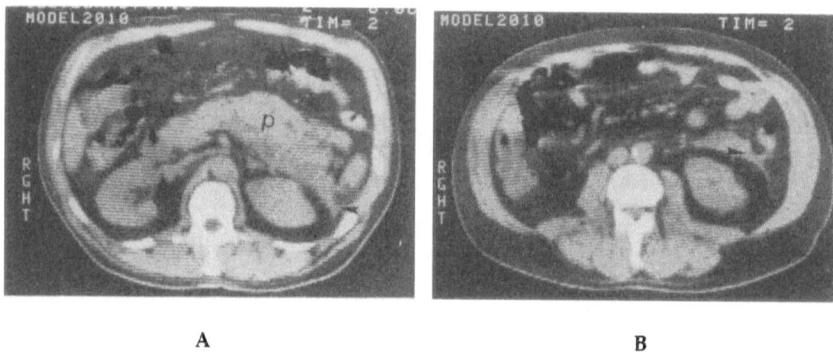

A   B

Figure 20 (**A**) This scan demonstrates enlargement of the pancreas (P). There is also thickening of Gerota's fascia (arrow). (**B**) Scan at a lower level than Figure 20(A) demonstrating thickening of Gerota's fascia inferiorly (arrow)

Haemorrhagic pancreatitis causes diffuse enlargement of the gland, although there may be fluid in the peripancreatic region in the anterior pararenal space. This inflammatory fluid may have a poorly defined margin, obscuring the margin of pancreas and spreading inferiorly within the anterior pararenal space. In many cases inflammatory exudate may be the precursor of a pseudocyst: as the inflammatory process matures, fibrous tissue may form a margin surrounding the inflammatory exudate, producing a pseudocyst.

The development of a pseudocyst is a most common complication of pancreatitis. Pseudocysts appear as fluid density masses with walls of variable thickness, located within or adjacent to the pancreas[3,37]. In those instances in which pseudocysts dissect into various anatomical spaces or cross fascial planes, the extent and spread of the inflammation can be accurately imaged. Such pseudocysts can dissect into the perinephric region, subdiaphragmatic space, mediastinum or lower abdomen (Figure 21).

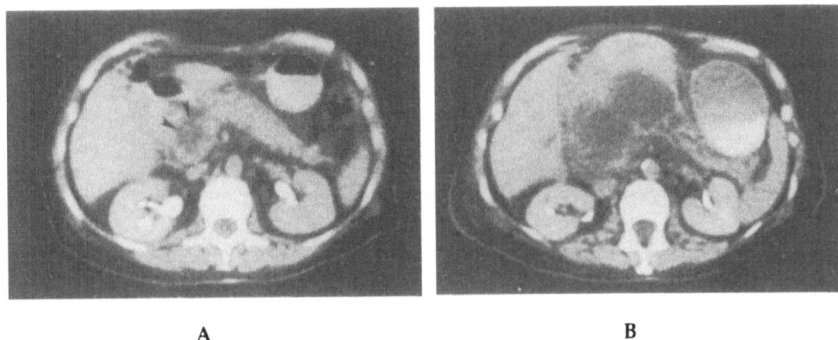

A   B

Figure 21   (A) This scan and Figure 21B demonstrate the evolution of a pseudocyst. This scan demonstrates a small cystic area (arrows) localized at the head of the pancreas.   (B) Several weeks later a second scan was taken at the same level, demonstrating a large cystic mass in the head of the pancreas. The pseudocyst has increased in size from the previous examination

Inflammatory phlegmons and pseudocysts can become superinfected by bacterial organisms; if such organisms are gas-producing ones, emphysematous pancreatitis may result. In such cases, CT demonstrates minute gas bubbles confined to the pancreas[8,39]; these may not be discernible on either ultrasound study or plain film radiographs (Figure 22).

When chronic pancreatitis occurs there may be deposition of calcium which is easily detectable on CT scan. The usual case of calcific pancreatitis has multiple calcifications of different sizes scattered throughout the parenchyma of the gland (Figure 23). In other cases, the calculi may occur within the duct system. When such calculi obstruct the pancreatic duct, dilatation of the duct may occur distal to the obstruction[40]. Moreover, when there is dilatation of the pancreatic duct, small calcifications may occur peripherally within the small, secondary radicals of the duct system (Figure 24). Accurate diagnosis of the presence of a single calculus in the pancreatic duct is important because if the obstruction is not relieved complete autolysis of the gland may occur. Resultant pancreatic insufficiency or even sepsis may develop from an unrelieved obstruction.

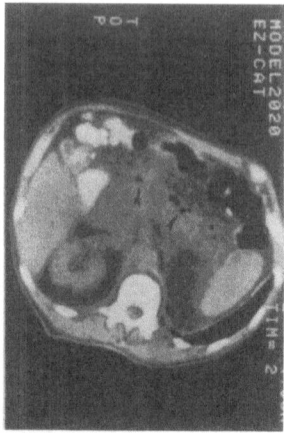

Figure 22 This patient with emphysematous pancreatitis demonstrates small gas bubbles (arrows) in the body and tail of the pancreas

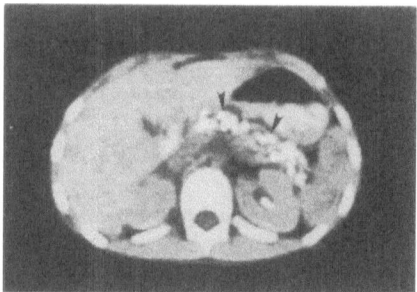

Figure 23 This scan taken through the area of the pancreas demonstrates multiple calcifications (arrows) scattered throughout the body and tail of the pancreas

An unusual change in the pancreas, reported previously in the pathology literature but not confirmed until recently in the radiological literature, is fatty replacement of the pancreas. In some instances fatty replacement may occur as a result of a total autolysis of the pancreas. In other instances this may be a benign occurrence resulting from diabetes, obesity or even senile atrophy and it may be of no clinical concern.

The role of different imaging systems for evaluation of the complications of pancreatitis is still disputed in the literature. Advocates of CT believe that CT is the modality of choice because of its reproducible image and ability accurately to identify both air and calcium. This ability

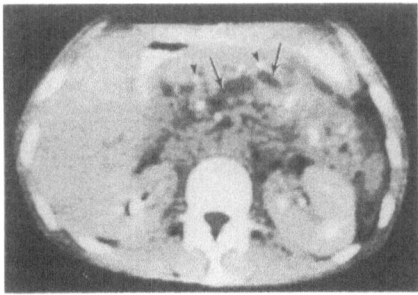

Figure 24 This scan taken through the level of the pancreas demonstrates a dilated common duct which appears as an area of lesser density (arrows). Within some of the dilated radicals there are small calcifications (arrow heads)

accurately to image 'gas' without artifacts means that CT can reliably detect the 'gas' in emphysematous pancreatitis, and CT study is unimpaired when an adynamic intestinal ileus occurs adjacent to the inflamed pancreas. Moreover, the full extent of any pseudocyst, whether confined to pancreas or extrapancreatic, can be well defined. With CT it is possible to characterize calcific densities in various locations as noted above. Advocates of ultrasound study correctly propose that most common and important complications of pancreatitis are pseudocysts confined to the pancreas, and that ultrasound is accurate in detecting such abnormalities. Most ultrasonographers will concede, however, that ultrasound is not satisfactory for accurately localizing calcium or for detecting gas in emphysematous pancreatitis and there may be problems with imaging the pancreas in patients with inflammation and adynamic ileus.

KIDNEYS

The normal kidneys characteristically appear as 'U-shaped' structures with homogeneous parenchyma. Centrally, the pelvocalyceal system has the density of soft tissue surrounded by low-density parapelvic fat (Figure 2A,B). With intravenous injection of urographic contrast material, the parenchyma enhances significantly and the excreted contrast material highlights the pelvocalyceal system. Distinction among the cortex, medullary region and papilla can be made after rapid injection of contrast material. Because of the ease of visualization of the kidneys, identification of ectopic locations or congenital fusion is quite simple (Figure 25). The normal fascial boundaries in the perinephric region and retroperitoneum can be seen. Anterior Gerota's fascia forms the anterior border of the perinephric space and the posterior boundary of the anterior pararenal space. The posterior Gerota's fascia forms the anterior boundary of the posterior pararenal space (Figure 26).

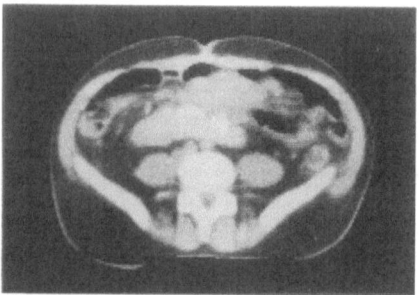

Figure 25 Scan taken through the level of the renal pelvis demonstrating a mass anterior to the vessels. Contrast material is located anteriorly. This is the typical appearance for an ectopic horseshoe kidney

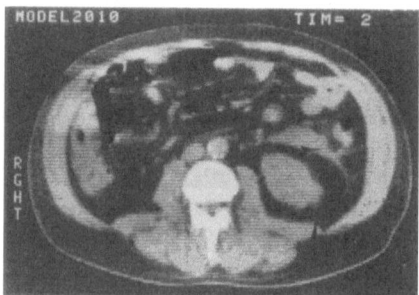

Figure 26 In this scan of a patient with pancreatitis, Gerota's fascia has been thickened, so it is quite obvious on the image. The anterior Gerota's fascia (horizontal arrow) forms the anterior boundary of the perinephric space. Posterior Gerota's fascia (vertical arrow) forms the posterior boundary of the perinephric space. The space anterior to anterior Gerota's fascia is the anterior pararenal space and that space posterior to posterior Gerota's fascia is the posterior pararenal space

The detection and differentiation of renal masses has been thoroughly investigated and discussed in the literature[41-55]. The typical renal cyst appears as a round, thin-walled, sharply marginated mass which is significantly lower in density than normal renal parenchyma (Figure 27). On the other hand, a typical renal neoplasm appears as a mass which is higher in density than a cyst but less dense than renal parenchyma (Figure 28). Occasionally, a small renal cell carcinoma may be isodense, both with and without injection of contrast material. Most institutions employ intravenous urographic contrast material to enhance the normal parenchyma, making abnormalities more clearly visible. When the typical appearance of either a simple cyst or a neoplasm is noted, one can be sufficiently confident of the diagnosis that no further investigation is required.

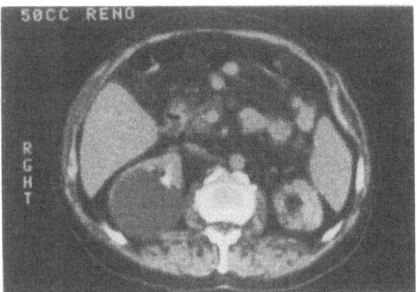

Figure 27 This scan demonstrates a typical simple renal cyst. A renal cyst is low in density and has a well-defined margin

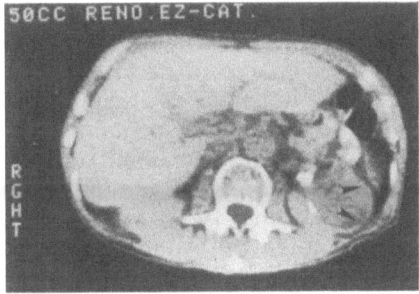

Figure 28 This scan demonstrates a carcinoma in the lateral portion of the left kidney. The mass is higher in density than the typical cyst and the margin is somewhat thick (arrows)

When a neoplasm is present CT has been quite accurate in determining its full extent[43]. Any invasion of the tumour into the retroperitoneum, fascial planes or renal veins can be noted (Figure 29). Metastatic disease in the liver is also clearly discernible. After resection of a renal tumour, CT has also proved effective for detecting recurrence in the surgical site or in the retroperitoneum and most investigators now consider that CT is the modality of choice for follow-up of post-nephrectomy patients.

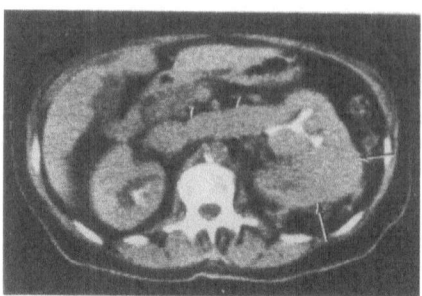

Figure 29 CT scan of a patient with a renal cell carcinoma (arrows). The tumour has invaded into the renal vein which crosses anterior to the aorta (arrow heads)

There are some instances, however, when a renal cyst will appear intermediate in density between that of a cyst and a carcinoma. In such cases other investigations, such as ultrasonography or diagnostic aspiration, should be employed. If either of those suggests the diagnosis of carcinoma, an angiogram should be performed to assess the vascular supply to the tumour and the vascular status of the opposite kidney.

The CT appearance of an angiomyolipoma is pathognomonic[46]. Angiomyolipomas characteristically contain fat, which is quite low in density, and present a very characteristic image. If such fat is noted, there is no question as to the diagnosis of angiomyolipoma (Figure 30).

Some mass lesions of the kidney may contain significant amounts of calcium: we have observed calcium in renal cell carcinomas, haematomas and haemorrhagic cysts. Using CT and ultrasound it has been difficult to distinguish among the three since neither may provide adequate information and angiography may be required. Technically speaking, the presence of calcium creates diagnostic problems for both CT and ultrasound examination. With CT, technical error is produced because of hardening of the X-ray beam which makes assessment of the density inaccurate. With ultrasound there may be 'acoustic shadowing' which again precludes adequate examination of the structures adjacent to the calcium.

Unusual lesions of the kidney, such as xanthrogranulomatous pyelonephritis, tuberculomas, abscesses, haemorrhagic cysts, inflammatory cysts and lymphomas may appear as indeterminate masses which may require aspiration or other evaluation.

RETROPERITONEUM

Abnormalities of the retroperitoneum produce alterations of the normal anatomy including the fascial planes, psoas muscles, blood vessels and

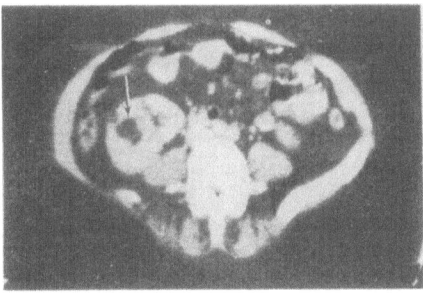

Figure 30 This scan demonstrates the typical appearance of an angiomyolipoma. In such cases, fat appears as very low density material within the kidney (arrows). This appearance is pathognomonic and no other evaluation is required

kidneys[56–69]. One of the most common findings with retroperitoneal tumours is the presence of a soft tissue mass which may obscure or displace normal structures. Tumours located around the major vessels may obscure the 'fat angle' around the aorta and the vena cava (Figures 31 and 32). Tumours located further from the major vessels may produce displacement or obstruction of the renal collecting system or displacement of the kidneys themselves. Another anatomical finding which may be noted is thickening of Gerota's fascia. This is, however, a non-specific sign which may be produced by both tumour and inflammation.

Both primary and metastatic tumours of the retroperitoneum produce soft tissue density mass lesions (Figure 33). Retroperitoneal tumours are relatively non-specific in their appearance except for some particular cell

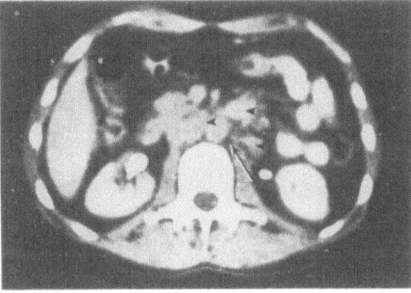

Figure 31 CT scan of a patient with retroperitoneal lymph node disease. The lymph nodes in the retroperitoneum are enlarged (small arrows). The fat angle behind the major vessel (arrow head) is still intact (arrow)

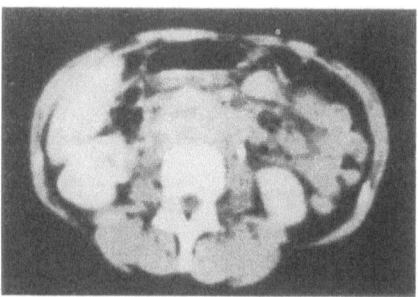

Figure 32 CT scan of a patient with enlarged retroperitoneal lymph nodes due to lymphoma. The 'fat angle' is obscured

types. Mucinous metastatic lesions either from stomach, colon, pancreas or ovary may be very low in density, i.e. close to that of water. Liposarcoma may also be quite low in density; characteristically it does not have the well-defined margins or septation as seen with mucinous tumours. Calcifications may occur in some tumours, including the mucinous tumours mentioned, chondrosarcomas, islet cell tumours and leiomyosarcomas.

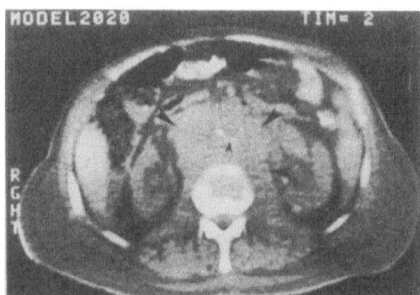

Figure 33 This scan demonstrates a fibrosarcoma of the retroperitoneum displacing the calcified aorta anteriorly. The aorta is noted by the arrow head and the arrows define the margins of the tumour

Assessment of para-aortic lymph node enlargement may be simple or difficult depending upon the degree of lymph node involvement. In cases where lymph nodes are not visible on CT scan, one may be confident that they are normal in size. In cases where the nodes are large enough to obscure the 'vascular angles', one may be sure of the diagnosis of neoplasm, either primary or metastatic. However, in cases where the lymph nodes measure between 5 and 15 mm in diameter, one cannot be certain if such enlargement is secondary to lymphadenitis or very early infiltration by lymphoma or carcinoma. Careful correlation with the clinical history is necessary.

Some comparisons of CT, ultrasound and lymphangiography have been made but conclusive results have not yet been published[58, 61, 63, 68, 69]. Certain comments may be made about the role of CT from the data available. Most authors agree that for non-Hodgkin's lymphomas, CT is the investigative modality of choice because of its accurate detection of soft tissue tumour involvement since non-Hodgkin's lymphomas may involve extranodal areas such as solid parenchymal organs and mesentery or psoas muscles. For Hodgkin's lymphoma and metastatic disease, it is possible for CT to miss very early intranodal involvement; in these instances lymphography is probably the most valuable early investigation.

ADRENAL GLANDS

CT has produced a revolutionary change in the diagnostic approach to adrenal abnormalities[55, 56]. Prior to the use of CT, the adrenal gland was a very difficult organ to evaluate accurately. The most effective methods of evaluation – adrenal arteriography and venography – were technically difficult, time-consuming and fraught with interpretive problems. Because of its ability to image the normal and abnormal adrenal gland, CT has emerged as the imaging system of choice for the adrenal gland.

The normal adrenal glands are located superior and anterior to the right and left kidney (Figure 34A,B). The right gland is usually linear in shape and located behind the vena cava at a level just below the point where the vena cava becomes intrahepatic in its course. The left adrenal gland is usually V-shaped and is located behind the splenic pedicle.

CT is effective for diagnosing all types of adrenal tumours, including pheochromocytomas, aldosterone-producing tumours and adrenocortical carcinomas. The pheochromocytomas we have observed have varied in size from 2 cm to greater than 15 cm in diameter (Figure 35). Although most of these are homogeneous in density, some are necrotic or have cystic areas scattered throughout. The effectiveness of CT in finding such tumours has been reported by several groups; all have confirmed that CT is as accurate as arteriography or venography for the evaluation of mass lesions.

Although aldosterone-producing tumours are generally smaller in size than pheochromocytomas, significant success has also been reported[3] in locating this type of tumour with CT. The density of such

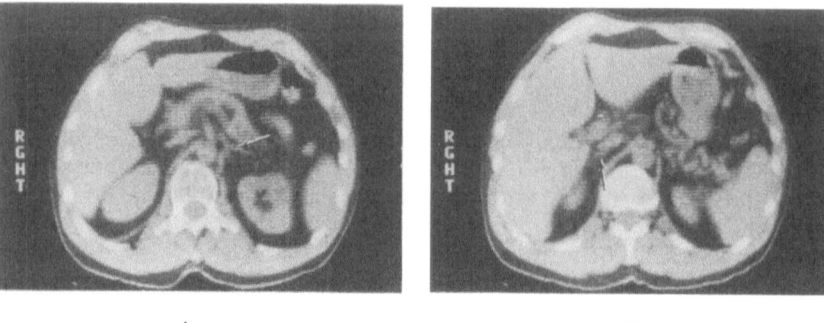

Figure 34 These two scans demonstrate the normal right and left adrenal glands. (**A**) The normal left adrenal gland is usually V-shaped (arrow) and located immediately behind the splenic vein and pancreas. (**B**) The right adrenal gland located behind the vena cava (arrows). The shape of the right adrenal gland is usually linear

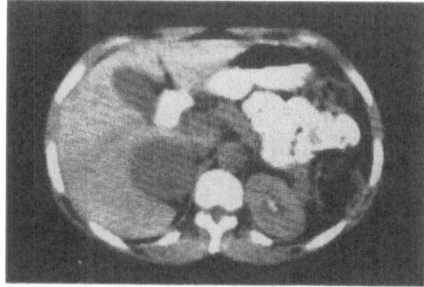

Figure 35 CT scan demonstrating a mass lesion in the area of the right adrenal gland which was diagnosed and proved to be a pheochromocytoma

tumours is variable and a significant number may appear 'fatty' in density. Adrenocortical carcinomas, on the other hand, appear as homogeneous dense masses located in the area of the adrenal glands. This tumour appears somewhat larger in size than either the pheochromocytomas or the aldosterone-producing tumours; it may also possess a 'fat density' in some instances.

Several benign tumours commonly involve the adrenal gland. Adrenal cysts are quite common. They appear as well-circumscribed, low-density masses similar to renal cysts; they are so characteristic in appearance that they do not require further investigation for diagnosis in the asymptomatic patient. Sometimes the cyst wall contains calcium. (Figure 36). Either adenomas or hyperplasia can produce a soft tissue mass in the area of the adrenal gland which is visible on CT scan. In

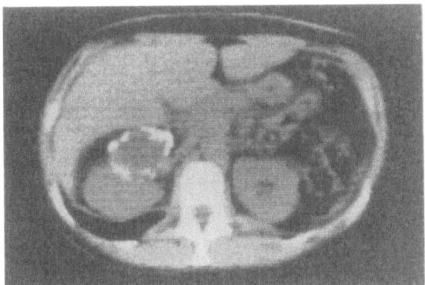

Figure 36 This scan demonstrates a calcified adrenal cyst of the areas anterior to the right kidney

certain cases of these abnormalities, the glands may be so large that they are indistinguishable from the above-mentioned adrenal tumours (Figure 37A,B). Hyperplasia typically can be identified because the shape of the gland is preserved and it may simply be increased in size. Finally, an uncommon tumour which may also involve the adrenal gland is a myolipoma; this tumour is of fat density (Figure 38).

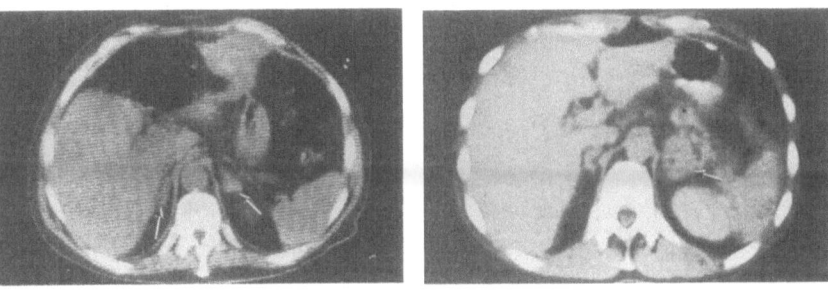

A   B

Figure 37 (A) CT scan demonstrating the typical adrenal hyperplasia in which the glands have retained their normal configuration, but are increased in size (arrows). (B) This scan demonstrates a patient with hyperplasia so significant that there is an apparent mass in the left adrenal gland (arrow)

INTRA-ABDOMINAL ABSCESSES

Intra-abdominal abscesses can be accurately detected and localized in parenchymal organs such as liver, kidney, pancreas or in the peritoneal spaces. Abscesses within solid parenchymal organs appear as well-

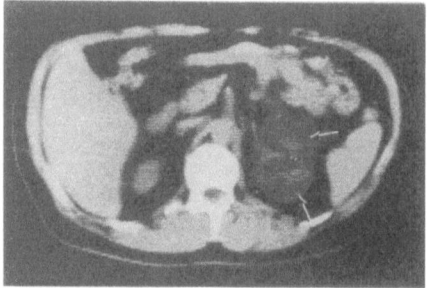

Figure 38 There is a fat density mass in the area of the left adrenal gland which proved to be a myolipoma (arrows)

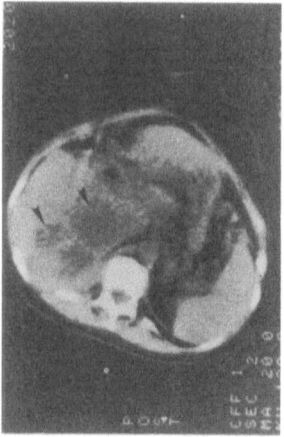

Figure 39 This scan of a patient lying at an angle demonstrates an abscess in the right lobe of the liver (arrows). The abscess appears as several round areas of lower density than the normal liver.

circumscribed fluid densities (Figure 39). Localization of abscesses in the various anatomical areas of the solid organs such as liver is quite simple since the lobar anatomy of the liver is clearly defined. A liver abscess is well-delineated as an area of low density which can be easily localized in the appropriate lobe. If a fistulous tract exists with an abscess, or if gas-forming organisms are present, such collections may contain gas visible on CT scan. A distinct advantage of CT is that, unimpaired by intestinal gas or bone, one can determine the exact extent of an abscess and its involvement in different portions of an organ or the various peritoneal spaces. For example, if an inflammatory process begins within the pelvis, one can trace on CT scan the spread of the abscess along the right paracolic gutter into the right subdiaphragmatic space (Figure 40A–D). In addition to tracing the exact pathways of inflammatory processes, one can locate small abscesses which are well-defined in various peritoneal regions. In this manner, exact localization of abscesses in the paracolic spaces, right and left subhepatic spaces, right and left subdiaphragmatic space and the omental bursa is possible (Figure 41). This simplifies the planning of surgical drainage procedures because one can identify which abscess collections require surgical exploration and others amenable to percutaneous drainage. In the left upper quadrant, for example, one can clearly distinguish between an abscess of the inferior or superior recess of the lesser sac and one in the left subhepatic space. When an abscess is localized to the left subhepatic space, at times a limited drainage procedure may be effective, rather than the larger surgical procedure which might be required for a lesser sac abscess. When abscesses occur in the retroperitoneum, CT examination permits precise localization in various anatomical spaces such as the perinephric, anterior pararenal and posterior pararenal space. Moreover, such examination can determine when an abscess is confined to the kidney or tracks along fascial planes (Figure 42).

The high accuracy of CT for detecting intra-abdominal abscesses has been repeatedly documented. In the first report from our group[70], the accuracy of detection was 91%; in subsequent papers, similar detection accuracies have been noted[71-84]. The only shortcoming of CT in this regard is that it is unable to differentiate various types of fluid collections including abscess, lymphocele and haematoma and it may be necessary to aspirate a specimen for culture or biochemical evaluation. CT-guided aspiration is a valuable diagnostic adjunct and will be discussed in the next section.

BIOPSIES AND ASPIRATIONS

In addition to diagnosis, CT has proved useful for guiding a variety of percutaneous interventional procedures. Because of its unique imaging properties, CT procedures permit applications which are not possible with other interventional techniques[85-92]. Interventional procedures include the recovery of material for cytology, histology or bacteriology and therapeutic drainage. A wide variety of instruments and equipment may be necessary and useful.

CT offers numerous technical advantages over other imaging modalities. It provides direct visualization of the biopsy instrument in the

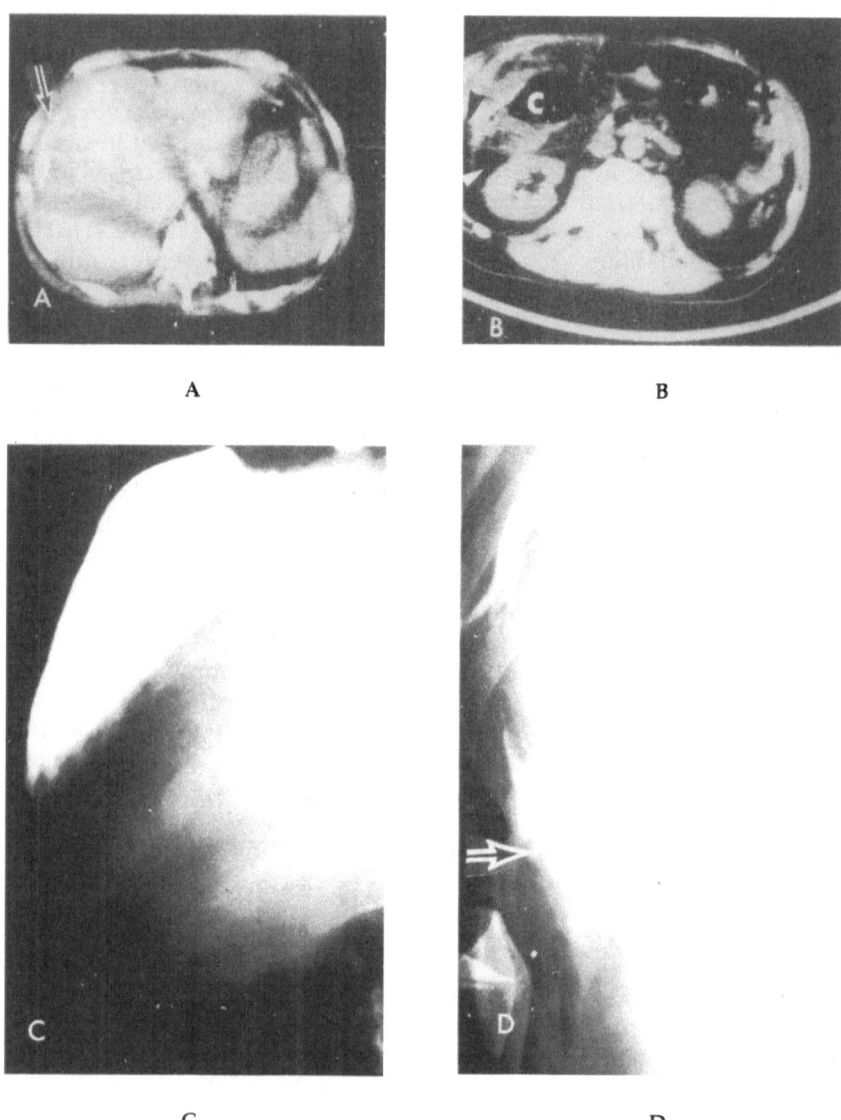

Figure 40 (**A**) This scan demonstrates contrast material injected into a right subdiaphragmatic abscess (arrow). (**B**) This scan shows a fluid collection (black arrow) immediately adjacent to the colon (C). It represents a paracolic abscess. (**C**) Radiograph demonstrating a sinogram of a subdiaphragmatic abscess. (**D**) Radiograph showing injection of the paracolic abscess which was noted in Figure 40B

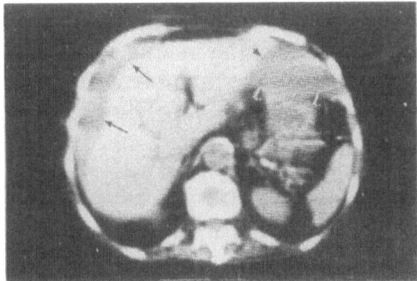

Figure 41 CT scan demonstrating an abscess in the right subdiaphragmatic space (arrows). There is also an abscess which has spread to the anterior left subdiaphragmatic space (arrow heads)

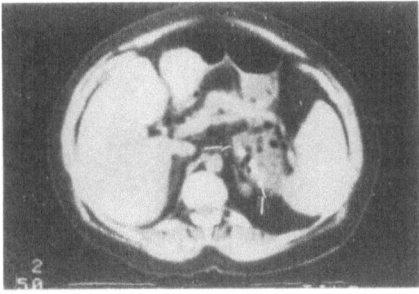

Figure 42 There is an abscess (arrows) in the retroperitoneum posterior to the pancreas

cross-sectional dimension, it is unimpaired by gas or bone, and CT images provide complete detail of both normal and abnormal anatomy. Because the system has an air interface around the patient, no coupling material is required, and alterations of the skin surface, such as wounds or sinuses, do not interfere with CT-guided procedures.

In those instances in which a cytological result will aid clinical inquiry, a 22-gauge needle may be used to obtain specimen tissue. Because of the small needle calibre there is a high safety factor. The needle may penetrate bowel or solid parenchymal organs with only a minimal chance of bacterial contamination or bleeding. Furthermore, we have found that the 'skinny' needle is well-suited for aspiration of vascular lesions or lesions close to major vessels. The 'skinny' needle is quite commonly used to biopsy pancreas, para-aortic tumours and vascular lesions of the liver and the kidney. (Figures 43A,B and 44).

Although the possibility of complication is small, bleeding, pneumo-peritoneum and infection have been reported[67]. The only disadvantage of 'skinny'-needle aspiration biopsy is that a cytological specimen alone is provided and the information available is not always as complete as that provided by a larger histological specimen.

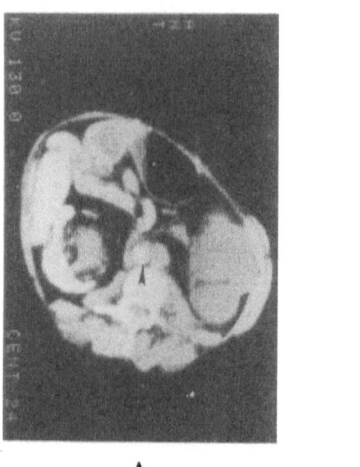
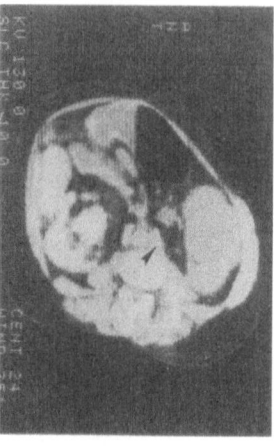

A   B

Figure 43 (A) This scan demonstrates an intravenous bolus injection of contrast material which opacifies the aorta (arrow). The round mass next to the aorta represents a lymph node. (B) This scan demonstrates a needle (arrow) aspiration of a para-aortic node (arrow)

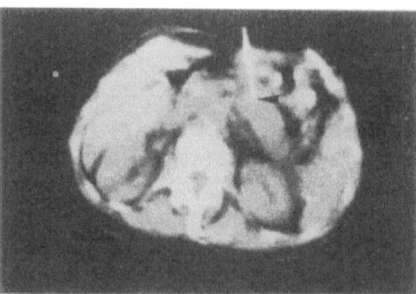

Figure 44 'Skinny' needle aspiration of a pancreatic carcinoma. Arrow points to the tip of the needle in the pancreas

When the clinical situation warrants a larger histological specimen and anatomical factors are appropriate, a cutting type of needle such as a Menghini or a 'true-cut' needle can be used (Figure 45). This type of needle is useful when the tissue for biopsy is accessible from the skin without requiring penetration of a viscus or another organ. The lesion should be avascular; the 'vascularity' of a lesion may be assessed by rapid-sequence CT scanning and bolus injection of contrast material (Figure 46). This bolus technique is especially useful when biopsy of an 'unknown lesion' is planned, since vascular abnormality may be distinguished from an avascular mass. In vascular lesions, use of the cutting needle is deferred and a 'skinny' needle aspiration will be obtained[92]. For example, a haemangioma of the liver may appear as a mass lesion on routine scan but this has a characteristic appearance on CT scan. In such vascular lesions, 'skinny' needle aspiration is safe; if the lesion is avascular, a cutting needle may be safely used. Since instituting the bolus technique for assessing vascularity of lesions, we have had no complications from bleeding and have had good recovery of tissue specimens (Table 1 and Table 2).

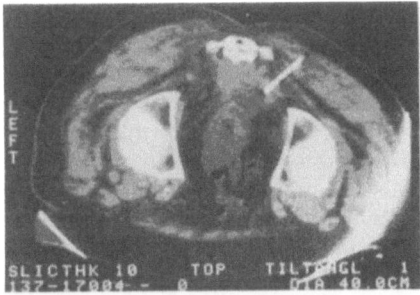

Figure 45 Needle biopsy of a presacral mass between the rectum and the sacrum. Biopsy was positive for adenocarcinoma

The merit of CT-guided biopsy procedures has been confirmed in numerous published articles[85-90]. In our preliminary article we were successful in 75% of our procedures. Subsequent experience and improvement of the technique have increased the recovery of diagnostic tissue to 86%. Other authors have reported similarly good recovery rates. As further testimony to its usefulness, a small report from our group discussed three cases of biopsies of recurring rectal cancer which were negative by surgical biopsy, but positive by CT biopsies.

The role of interventional CT procedures relative to other interventional procedures has been defined differently by different groups. Some groups have used CT-guided procedures as secondary, indicated on those occasions when other interventional procedures such as fluoroscopic- or ultrasonic-guided procedures do not provide a satisfac-

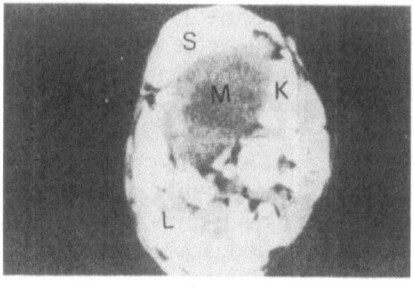 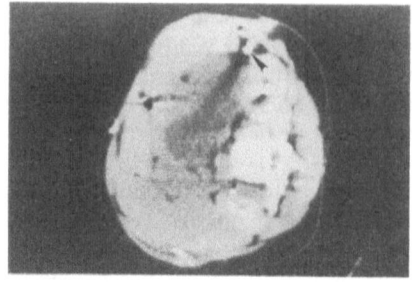

A   B

Figure 46 (A) This scan demonstrates bolus injection of contrast material in a patient lying on the right side. Note the high density of the normal spleen (S), kidneys (K) and liver (L). The mass (M) is avascular and does not demonstrate much enhancement with the injection of contrast. (B) This scan demonstrates biopsy of a retroperitoneal tumour. Arrow points to the Menghini needle. The biopsy was positive for adrenal cortical carcinoma

tory result. Other groups have triaged the abnormalities to either ultrasound or CT-guided procedures depending on the size of the lesion. Ferrucci *et al.* preferred to biopsy lesions less than 5 cm in diameter with CT guidance. In our practice we have tailored our interventional procedures to the individual patient, taking into consideration the information required, the location and size of the abnormality and patient clinical status. For example, in the patient with a known malignancy in whom a metastasis is suspected, a cytological specimen will often suffice to confirm the presence of a malignancy. In those instances in which a suspicious area has been found and there is no established diagnosis, we prefer to use a large, cutting-type needle which can provide a histological rather than a cytological specimen. We have found that in undiagnosed malignancy, one obviously cannot anticipate cell type. If the malignancy is a lymphoma, liposarcoma or other, less common type of neoplasm, or even a benign abnormality, the larger core specimen can provide a definitive diagnosis rather than a simple cytological confirmation of malignancy (Figure 47). If a large core biopsy is indicated, we have erred on the side of using CT guidance because of the additional safety factor that it provides. Firstly, one can be confident that a normal structure, such as intestine, gallbladder, etc. is not inappropriately biopsied by the large needle. Secondly, using the bolus injection technique, one can identify those neoplastic abnormalities and some benign abnormalities which are highly vascular. For vascular lesions we defer large-needle biopsy, but instead perform an aspiration type of procedure. Our group and others have found that the bolus injection technique can not only assess vascularity, but may at times confirm the diagnosis of a vascular, benign abnormality such as a cavernous haemangioma of the liver. Moreover, there are certain instances in which a

Table 1 Menghini needle biopsy results*

Region: final diagnosis	Success rate
Retroperitoneum	
metastatic disease	5/5
lymphoma	2/4
subtotal	7/9
Liver	
metastatic disease	7/7
hepatitis	1/1
haemangioma	1/3†
subtotal	9/11
Kidney	
papillary adenoma	1/1
infarct	1/1
subtotal	2/2
Adrenal	
metastatic disease	2/2
primary adenocarcinoma	1/1
subtotal	3/3
Other (pelvis, bone)	
metastatic disease	3/3
ovarian	1/1
subtotal	4/4
TOTAL	25/29

* Reproduced with permission, from Ref. 87.
† One haemangioma was diagnosed by biopsy; one by surgery; and one by laparoscopy

vessel may be totally surrounded by tumour. The margins of the vessel cannot be seen except by bolus injection; in such cases, one can success-fully obtain a large core biopsy specimen without inadvertently perfo-rating the vessel. Finally, in those instances in which the patient has a propensity for bleeding or some immunological deficiency, we believe that it is important to provide accurate placement of the biopsy instru-ment in order to avoid inadvertent penetration of parenchymal organs and also inadvertent contamination of sterile spaces by penetration of bowel. No matter what criteria various groups have used for the appli-cation of CT-guided procedures, all agree that it is the most precise and accurate method for recovery of a diagnostic specimen.

For aspirations and drainage of fluid collections suspected of being abscesses, CT has also proved quite useful. After fluid collections are ac-curately localized, as discussed previously, CT guidance can position a

Table 2 Aspiration biopsy results*

Region: final diagnosis	Success rate
Retroperitoneum	
metastatic disease	4/4
lymphoma	0/3
normal	1/1
abscess	1/1
subtotal	5/11
Kidney	
renal carcinoma	1/2
cyst	1/1
subtotal	2/3
Liver	
cyst	1/1
abscess	1/1
subtotal	2/2
Spleen: lymphoma	1/1
Pelvis: normal	0/1
TOTAL†	10/14

* Reproduced, with permission, from Ref. 87.
† Total was 18 cases, but four normal cases with negative biopsies were not tabulated

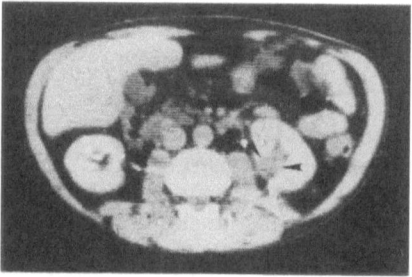

Figure 47 This scan demonstrates a Menghini biopsy of a focal area (arrows) of the kidneys suspected of being a mass lesion. This proved to be a haemorrhagic infarct. Reprinted by permission of the authors, Haaga, J. R. and Morrison, S. C., 'CT Appearance of renal infarct', *Journal of Computerized Axial Tomography*, **4**(2), 246–247 (April 1980)

needle in a suspect area. Because all structures and anatomical spaces can be seen and avoided if necessary, inadvertent contamination of a sterile space by intestinal or colonic material is unlikely. It is important to avoid inadvertent contamination because a sterile fluid collection which contains protein-rich material, such as ascitic fluid, haematoma or pseudocyst, is fertile ground for bacterial growth. Moreover, cultures of material recovered after a needle has penetrated bowel may prove spurious. Obviously, valid cultures obtained by careful aseptic techniques are invaluable as conclusive proof of an abscess and are very useful in selecting proper antibiotic therapy.

We believe that the key for effective percutaneous drainage of intra-abdominal abscesses is the clear anatomical detail provided by CT. CT is capable of visualizing the complete extent of an abscess in various anatomical spaces. Although the number of articles appearing in the literature proposing percutaneous drainage are few, there is a consensus of opinion that CT is the modality of choice for determining and selecting the mode of percutaneous drainage[70,81,92].

Our method and rationale for performing percutaneous drainage procedures are as follows. We believe that, depending upon the clinical status of the patient, the character and anatomical location of the abscess and the nature of its purulent material, percutaneous drainage may be attempted (Figure 48A–C). In those patients who are not good operative candidates or who are so critically ill that anaesthesia represents a significant risk, we believe that percutaneous drainage should be attempted in virtually all. On the other hand, patients who are good surgical candidates should be selected for percutaneous drainage procedures depending upon the anatomical location and nature of the abscess. We believe that it is prudent to attempt to drain those abscesses which are confined to no more than two anatomical spaces and are unilocular. Further, these should be lesions which can be approached percutaneously without penetrating an uninvolved organ. At the time of placement of the drainage catheter the radiologist must be sure that the material to be drained is not too viscous. When the abscess material is extremely viscous, surgical drainage is probably the procedure of choice because of its high success rate and low mortality and morbidity. The rationale we have outlined is somewhat conservative and is not adhered to by other individuals who drain abscesses percutaneously; others believe that a percutaneous trial is warranted in every case.

In performing drainage procedures, two methods are used: a modified Seldinger technique and a Trochar technique[70,81,92]. In those abscesses which are small, centrally located and require accurate placement of a catheter, a modified Seldinger technique utilizing an 8-French angiographic catheter is employed. In such cases puncture of the abscess is performed with a needle. Following successful puncture of an abscess, an angiographic guide wire is placed into the cavity, the needle removed and the angiographic catheter is placed in the abscess cavity over the wire guide. In those abscesses which are large, superficial and accessible, a 12- to 16-French trochar catheter may be used. A variety of

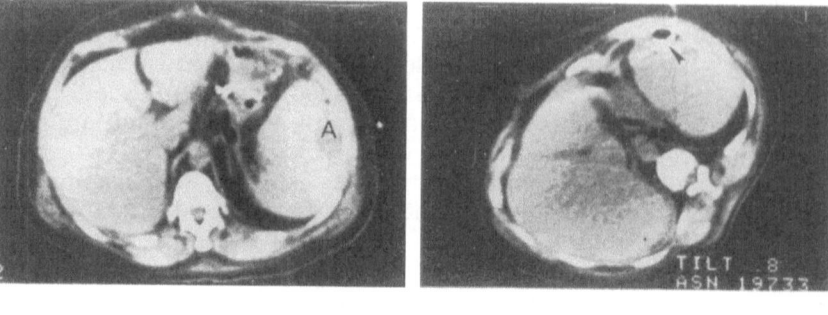

A   B

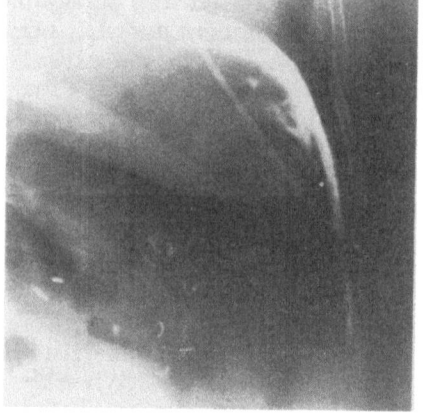

C

Figure 48   (A) This scan demonstrates a left subdiaphragmatic abscess (A).   (B) The same abscess after insertion of catheter (arrow).   (C) Sinogram injection of contrast material into the subdiaphragmatic cavity. Drainage of the abscess was accomplished by percutaneous catheter placement

trochars are now available; all are somewhat similar in that a central sharp cannula is covered by a plastic catheter.

We have been quite successful in obtaining specimens using CT guidance. In our last report we were successful in obtaining specimens from 63 of 70 fluid collections suspected of being abscesses. Furthermore, in a second group of 33 suspected abscesses in which we attempted drainage, we were successful in accomplishing drainage in 28 patients[92].

CONCLUSION

Computerized tomography is an effective imaging modality which has been used in virtually every organ system within the abdomen. As has been discussed throughout the chapter, there are certain areas within the abdomen for which CT investigation has now become the modality of choice over other available imaging modalities. From the present data it would appear that CT is already the modality of choice in assessment of the adrenal gland and pancreas, the evaluation of abscesses and the retroperitoneum. In certain other areas such as the liver, kidneys and biliary system, CT is generally used as an adjunctive modality, to clarify or more completely evaluate abnormalities after other tests have been performed. As an interventional tool, CT has proven to be a very accurate and useful modality; in our experience CT biopsies have not superseded other interventional procedures but have added a new dimension to interventional radiology.

References

1   Alfidi, R. J., Haaga, J. R., Meaney, T. F., *et al.* (1975). Computed tomography of the thorax and abdomen: a preliminary report. *Radiology*, **117**, 257–64

2   Alfidi, R. J. and Haaga, J. R. (1976). Computed body tomography, *Radiol. Clin. N. Am.*, **14**, 563–70

3   Haaga, J. R. and Reich, N. E. (1978). *Computed Tomography of Abdominal Abnormalities.* (St. Louis: Mosby)

4   Stanley, R. J., Sagel, S. S. and Levitt, R. G. (1976). Computed tomography of the body: early trends in application and accuracy of the method. *Am. J. Radiol.*, **127**, 53–67

5   Sheedy, P. F., Stephens, D. H., Hattery, R. R., Muhm, J. R. and Hartman, G. W. (1976). Computed tomography of the body: initial clinical trial with the EMI prototype. *Am. J. Radiol.*, **127**, 23–51

6   Stephens, D. H., Hattery, R. R. and Sheedy, P. F. (1976). Computed tomography of the abdomen: early experience with the EMI body scanner. *Radiology*, **119**, 331–5

7   Sagel, S., Stanley, R. J. and Evens, R. G. (1976). Early clinical experience with motionless whole-body computed tomography. *Radiology*, **119**, 321–30

8   Stephens, D. H., Sheedy, P. F., Hattery, R. R. and Hartman, G. W. (1976). Initial clinical experience with computerized tomography of the body. *Radiol. Clin. N. Am.*, **14**, 149–58

9   Barnett, P. H., Zerhouni, E. A., White, R. I. Jr. and Siegelman, S. S. (1980). Computed tomography in the diagnosis of cavernous hemangioma of the liver. *Am. J. Radiol.*, **134**, 439–47

10 Freeny, P. C., Vimont, T. R. and Barnett, D. C. (1979). Cavernous hemangioma of the liver: ultrasonography, arteriography and computed tomography. *Radiology*, **132**, 143

11 Stephens, D. H., Sheedy, P. F. II, Hattery, R. R., *et al.* (1977). Computed tomography of the liver. *Am. J. Radiol.*, **128**, 579–90

12 Alfidi, R. J., Haaga, J. R., Havrilla, T. R., Pepe, R. G. and Cook, S. A. (1976). Computed tomography of the liver. *Am. J. Radiol.*, **127**, 69–74

13   Levitt, R. G., Sagel, S. S., Stanley, R. J. and Jost, R. G. (1977). Accuracy of computed tomography of the liver and biliary tract. *Radiology*, **124**, 123–8
14   Itai, Y., Nishikawa, J. and Tasaka, A. (1979). Computed tomography in the evaluation of hepatocellular carcinoma. *Radiology*, **131**, 165
15   Kunstlinger, F., Federle, M. P., Moss, A. A. and Marks, W. (1980). Computed tomography of hepatocellular carcinoma. *Am. J. Radiol.*, **134**, 431–7
16   Moss, A. A., Schrumpf, J. D., Schnyder, P., Korobkin, M. and Shimshak, R. R. (1979). Computed tomography of focal hepatic lesions: blind clinical evaluation of the effect of contrast enhancement. *Radiology*, **131**, 427
17   Wooten, W. B., Bernardino, M. E. and Goldstein, H. M. (1978). Computed tomography of necrotic hepatic metastases. *Am. J. Radiol.*, **131**, 839
18   Scherer, U., Santos, M. and Lissner, J. (1979). CT studies of the liver *in vitro*: a report on 82 cases with pathological correlation. *J. Comput. Assist. Tomogr.*, **3**, 589–95
19   MacCarty, R. L., Stephens, D. H., Hattery, R. R. and Sheedy, P. F. II (1979). Hepatic imaging by computed tomography: comparison with ⁹⁹ᵐTc-sulfur colloid, ultrasonography and angiography. *Radiol. Clin. N. Am.*, **17**, 137
20   Bryan, P. J., Dinn, W. M., Gross, Z. D., Wistow, B. W., McAfee, J. G. and Kieffer, S. A. (1977). Correlation of computed tomography, gray scale ultrasonography, and radionuclide imaging of the liver in detecting space-occupying processes. *Radiology*, **124**, 387–93
21   Stephens, D. H., Sheedy, P. F., Hattery, R. R. and MacCarty, R. L. (1977). Computed tomography of the liver. *Am. J. Radiol.*, **128**, 579–90
22   Friedman, M. L., Esposito, F. J., Ostrum, B. J., Cantor, R. E. and Sherman, B. P. (1979). Computerized tomography and radionuclide scanning in hepatic disease: retrospective study. *Radiology*, **130**, 575
23   Snow, J. R., Judson, H., Goldstein, H. M. and Wallace, S. (1979). Comparison of scintigraphy, sonography and computed tomography in the evaluation of hepatic neoplasms. *Am. J. Radiol.*, **132**, 915
24   Mulhern, C. B. Jr., Arger, P. H., Coleman, B. G. and Stein, G. N. (1979). Nonuniform attenuation in computed tomography study of the cirrhotic liver. *Radiology*, **132**, 399
25   Long, J. A. Jr., Doppman, J. L., Nienhus, A. W. and Mills, S. R. (1979). Computed tomographic analysis of beta-thalassemic syndromes with hemochromatosis: pathologic findings with clinical and laboratory correlations. *J. Comput. Assist. Tomogr.*, **4**, 159–65
26   Royal, S. A., Beiderman, B., Goldberg, H. I., Koerper, M. and Thaler, M. M. (1979). Detection and estimation of iron, glycogen and fat in liver of children with hepatomegaly using computed tomography (CT). *Ped. Res.*, 493
27   Haaga, J. R., Alfidi, R. J., Zelch, M. G., Meaney, T. F., Boller, M., Gonzalez, L. and Jeldon, G. I. (1976). Computed tomography of pancreas. *Radiology*, **120**, 289–95
28   Haaga, J. R., Alfidi, R. J., Havrilla, T. R., Tubbs, R., Gonzalez, L. and Meaney, T. F. (1977). Definitive role of CT scanning of the pancreas. *Radiology*, **124**, 723–30
29   Haaga, J. R. and Alfidi, R. J. (1976). CT scanning of the pancreas. *J. Belg. Radiol.*, **59**, 281–6
30   Levitt, R. G., Jost, R. G., Trachtman, J., *et al.* (1977). A computer assisted method to determine the diagnostic efficacy of computed tomography of the body. *Radiology*, **123**, 97–101
31   Petasnick, J. R. and Clark, J. (1976). Computed tomography of the abdomen: initial experience. *Gastrointest. Radiol.*, **1**, 201–8
32   Sheedy, P. F. II, Stephens, D. H., Hattery, R. R., MacCarty, R. L. and Williamson, B. Jr. (1977). Computed tomography of the pancreas. *Radiol. Clin. N. Am.*, **15**, 3
33   Haaga, J. R. and Alfidi, R. J. (1977). Computed tomographic scanning of the pancreas. *Radiol. Clin. N. Am.*, **15**, 3

34 Joseph, K. T., Stanley, R. J., Melson, G. L. and Sagel, S. S. (1979). Computed tomography: general review. *Radiol. Clin. N. Am.*, **17**, 105

35 Callen, P. W., Breiman, R. S., Korobkin, M., Mani, J. R. and DeMartini, W. J. (1979). Carcinoma of the tail of the pancreas: unusual CT appearance. *Am. J. Radiol.*, **133**, 135

36 Dembner, A. G., Jaffe, C. C., Simeone, J. and Walsh, J. (1979). New computed tomographic sign of pancreatitis. *Am. J. Radiol.*, **133**, 477

37 Ferrucci, J. T. Jr., Wittenberg, J., Black, E. B., Kirkpatrick, R. H. and Hall, D. A. (1979). Computed body tomography in chronic pancreatitis. *Radiology*, **130**, 175

38 Shirkhoda, A. and Mittelstaedt, C. A. (1978). Demonstration of pancreatic cysts in adult polycystic disease by computed tomography and ultrasound. *Radiology*, **131**, 1074

39 Mendez, G. Jr. and Isikoff, M. B. (1979). Significance of intrapancreatic gas demonstrated by CT: review of nine cases. *Am. J. Radiol.*, **132**, 59

40 Fishman, A., Isikoff, B. M., Barkin, J. S. and Friedland, J. T. (1979). Significance of a dilated pancreatic duct on CT examination. *Am. J. Radiol.*, **133**, 225

41 Williamson, B. Jr., Hattery, R. R., Stephens, D. H. and Sheedy, P. F. (1978). Computed tomography of the kidneys. *Semin. Roentgenol.*, **13**, 249–55

42 Magilner, A. D. and Ostrum, B. J. (1978). Computed tomography of the diagnosis of renal masses. *Radiology*, **126**, 215–8

43 Stewart, B. H., Straffon, R. A., Haaga, J. R. and Seidelman, F. E. (1978). Urological applications of computerized axial tomography. *Trans. Am. Assoc. Genitourin, Surg.*, **70**, 119–30

44 Harris, R. D. and Seat, S. G. (1978). Value of computerized tomography in evaluation of kidney. *Urology*, **12**, 729–32

45 Rabinowitz, K., Segal, A. J., Rao, H. K. and Pathak, A. (1978). Computed tomography in diagnosis of infantile polycystic kidney disease. *J. Urol.*, **120**, 616–17

46 Hansen, G. C., Hoffman, R. B., Sample, W. F. and Becker, R. (1978). Computed tomography diagnosis of renal angiomyolipoma, *Radiology*, **128**, 789–91

47 Hadar, H. and Meiraz, D. (1980). Renal sinus lipomatosis: differentiation from space-occupying lesion with aid of computed tomography. *Urology*, **15**, 86–90

48 Levine, E., Lee, K. R. and Weigel, J. (1979). Preoperative determination of abdominal extent of renal cell carcinoma by computed tomography. *Radiology*, **132**, 395–8

49 Love, L., Reynes, C. J., Churchill, R. and Moncada, R. (1979). Third generation CT scanning in renal disease. *Radiol. Clin. N. Am.*, **17**, 77–90

50 Segal, A. J. and Spitzer, R. M. (1979). Pseudo thick-walled renal cyst by CT. *Am. J. Radiol.*, **132**, 827–8

51 Rubin, B. E. (1979). Computed tomography in the evaluation of renal lymphoma. *J. Comput. Assist. Tomog.*, **3**, 759–64

52 McClennan, B. L., Stanley, R. J., Nelson, G. L., Levitt, R. G. and Sagel. S. S. (1979). CT of the renal cyst: is cyst aspiration necessary? *Am. J. Radiol.*, **133**, 671–5

53 Levine, E., Lee, K. R., Weigel, J. W. and Farber, B. (1979). Computed tomography in the diagnosis of renal carcinoma – complications Hippel–Lindau syndrome. *Radiology*, **130**, 703–6

54 McClennan, B. L. and Fair, W. R. (1979). CT scanning in urology. *Urol. Clin. N. Am.*, **6**, 342–74

55 McClennan, B. L. and Fair, W. (1979). Pursuit of the renal mass (Letter). *N. Engl. J. Med.*, **300**, 1118

56 Steward, B. H., Bravo, E. L., Haaga, J. R., Meaney, T. F. and Terazi, R. (1978). Localization of pheochromocytoma by computerized tomographic scan. *N. Engl. J. Med.*, **299**, 460

57 Stewart, B. H., James, R., Haaga, J. R. and Alfidi, R. J. (1978). Urological applications of computerized axial tomography: a preliminary report. *J. Urol.*, **120**, 198

58 Alcorn, F. S., Mategrano, V. C., Petasnick, J., *et al.* (1977). Contributions of compu-

ted tomography in staging and management of malignant lymphomas. *Radiology*, **125**, 7–17

59   Haaga, J. R. and Reich, N. E. (1978). *Computerized Tomography of Abdominal Abnormalities*. St. Louis: Mosby

60   Havrilla, T. R., Reich, N. E. and Haaga, J. R. (1977). The floating aorta in computerized tomography: a sign of retroperitoneal pathology. *Comput. Axial Tomogr.*, **1**, 2

61   Redman, H. C., Glatstein, E., Castellino, R. A., *et al.* (1977). Computed tomography as an adjunct in the staging of Hodgkin's disease and non-Hodgkin lymphomas. *Radiology*, **124**, 381–5

62   Stephens, D. H., Williamson, B., Sheedy, P. F., Hattery, R. R. and Miller, W. E. (1977). Computed tomography of the retroperitoneal space. *Radiol. Clin. N. Am.*, **15**, 3

63   Zelch, M. G. and Haaga, J. R. (1979). Clinical comparison of computed tomography and lymphangiography for detection of retroperitoneal lymphadenopathy. *Radiol. Clin. N. Am.*, **17**, 157

64   Burney, B. T. and Klatte, E. C. (1979). Ultrasound and computed tomography of the abdomen in the staging and management of testicular carcinoma. *Radiology*, **132**, 415

65   Korobkin, M., Callen, P. W. and Fisch, A. E. (1979). Computed tomography of the pelvis and retroperitoneum. *Radiol. Clin. N. Am.*, **17**, 301

66   Alter, A. J., Uehling, D. T. and Zwiebel, W. J. (1979). Computed tomography of retroperitoneum following nephrectomy. *Radiology*, **133**, 663

67   Havrilla, T. R., Reich, N. E., Seidelmann, F. E. and Haaga, J. R. (1979). Computed tomography of the kidneys and retroperitoneum: current status. *Radiology*, **131**, 569

68   Lee, J. K. T., Stanley, R. J., Sagel, S. S. and Levitt, R. G. (1978). Accuracy of computed tomography in detecting intraabdominal and pelvic adenopathy in lymphoma. *Am. J. Radiol.*, **131**, 311–15

69   Lee, J. K. T., Stanley, R. J., Sagel, S. S. and McClennan, B. L. (1978). Accuracy of CT in detecting intraabdominal and pelvic lymph node metastases from pelvic cancers. *Am. J. Radiol.*, **131**, 675–9

70   Haaga, J. R., Alfidi, R. J., Havrilla, T. R., *et al.* (1977). CT detection and aspiration of abdominal abscesses. *Am. J. Radiol.*, **128**, 465–74

71   Stephenson, T. F., Guzzetta, L. R. and Tagulinao, D. A. (1978). CT-guided seldinger catheter drainage of a hepatic abscess. *Am. J. Radiol.*, **131**, 323–4

72   Aronberg, D. J., Stanley, R. J., Levitt, R. G. and Sagel, S. S. (1978). Evaluation of abdominal abscess with computed tomography. *J. Comput. Assist. Tomogr.*, **2**, 384–7

73   Gerzof, S. G., Robbins, A. H. and Birkett, D. H. (1978). Computed tomography in the diagnosis and management of abdominal abscesses. *Gastrointest. Radiol.*, **3**, 287–94

74   Korobkin, M., Callen, P. W., Filly, R. A., Hoffer, P. B., Shimshak, R. R. and Kressel, H. Y. (1978). Comparison of computed tomography, ultrasonography and Gallium-67 scanning in the evaluation of suspected abdominal abscess. *Radiology*, **129**, 89–93

75   Daffner, R. H., Halber, M. D., Morgan, C. L., Trought, W. S., Thompson, W. M. and Rice, R. P. (1979). Computed tomography in the diagnosis of intra-abdominal abscesses. *Ann. Surg.*, **189**, 29–33

76   Biello, D. R., Levitt, R. G. and Melson, G. L. (1979). The roles of Gallium-67 scintigraphy, ultrasonography and computed tomography in the detection of abdominal abscesses. *Semin. Nucl. Med.*, **9**, 58–65

77   Levitt, R. G., Biello, D. R., Sagel, S. S. *et al.* (1979). Computed tomography and 67GA citrate radionuclide imaging for evaluating suspected abdominal abscess. *Am. J. Radiol.*, **132**, 529–34

78   Callen, P. W. (1979). Computed tomographic evaluation of abdominal and pelvic abscesses. *Radiology*, **131**, 171–5

79   Mendez, G. Jr., Isikoff, M. B. and Morillo, G. (1979). The role of computed tomo-

graphy in the diagnosis of renal and perirenal abscesses. *J. Urol.*, **122**, 582–6

80 Wolverson, M. K., Kagannadharao, B., Sundaram, M., Joyce, P. F., Riaz, M. A. and Shields, J. B. (1979). CT as a primary diagnostic method in evaluating intra-abdominal abscess. *Am. J. Radiol.*, **133**, 1089–95

81 Gerzof, S. G., Robbins, A. H., Birkett, D. H., Johnson, W. C., Pugatch, R. D. and Vincent, M. E. (1979). Percutaneous catheter drainage of abdominal abscesses guided by ultrasound and computed tomography. *Am. J. Radiol.*, **133**, 1–8

82 Filly, R. A. (1979). Annual oration. Detection of abdominal abscesses: a combined approach employing ultrasonography, computed tomography and Gallium-67 scanning. *J. Can. Assoc. Radiol.*, **30**, 202–10

83 Mendez, G. Jr., Isikoff, M. B. and Hill, M. C. (1980). Retroperitoneal processes involving the psoas demonstrated by computed tomography. *J. Comput. Assist. Tomogr.*, **4**, 78–82

84 Ralls, P. W., Boswell, W., Henderson, R., Rogers, W., Boger, D. and Halls, J. (1980). CT of inflammatory disease of the psoas muscle. *Am. J. Radiol.*, **134**, 767–70

85 Haaga, J. R., and Alfidi, R. J. (1976). Precise biopsy localization by computed tomography. *Radiology*, **118**, 603–7

86 Haaga, J. R., Reich, N. E., Havrilla, T. R. and Alfidi, R. (1977). Interventional CT scanning. *Radiol. Clin. N. Am.*, **15**, 449–456

87 Haaga, J. R. (1979). New techniques for CT-guided biopsies. *Am. J. Radiol.*, **133**, 633–41

88 Haaga, J. R. and Vanek, J. (1979). Computed tomographic guided liver biopsy using the menghini needle. *Radiology*, **133**, 405–8

89 Haaga, J. R., Highman, L. M., Cooperman, A. V. and Owens, F. J. (1979). Percutaneous CT-guided pancreatography and pseudocystography. *Am. J. Radiol.*, **132**, 829–30

90 Ferrucci, J. T., Wittenberg, J., and Mueller, P. R. (1980). Diagnosis of abdominal malignancy by radiologic fine-needle aspiration biopsy. *Am. J. Radiol.*, **134**, 323–30

91 Haaga, J. R., Alfidi, R. J., Cooperman, A. M., Havrilla, T. R. and Meaney, T. F. (1976). 'Definitive treatment of a large pyogenic liver abscess with CT guidance'. *Cleve. Clin. Q.*, **43**, 85–8

92 Haaga, J. R., George, C., Weinstein, A. J. and Cooperman, A. M. (1979). New interventional techniques in the diagnosis and management of inflammatory disease within the abdomen. *Radiol. Clin. N. Am.*, **17**, 485–513

3
Angiography in diagnosis and control of bleeding

T. E. GALLANT, A. J. GREENFIELD AND
C. A. ATHANASOULIS

INTRODUCTION

Angiography for localization of bleeding sites in the gastrointestinal tract was initially introduced by Baum *et al.*[1] in 1965. Subsequent reports of vasopressin infusions in the superior mesenteric artery to control haemorrhage opened a new era in radiology, that of therapeutic angiography. In addition to vasopressin infusions and following the lead of the neurosurgeons, angiographers over the past 10 years have come to routinely employ embolization with particulate matter to control haemorrhage.

Patients referred for angiographic control of haemorrhage may be haemodynamically unstable: the angiography suite must thus be equipped and staffed as an intensive care unit. Appropriate devices for constant electrocardiographic and pressure monitoring are mandatory. Resuscitative materials, including equipment for DC cardioversion, must be at hand as well as a variety of fluids for resuscitation including crystalloids and albumin. Close proximity to a well-stocked and fully staffed blood bank is mandatory. In addition to the vascular radiologist and his assistant, our emergency on-call team includes a specially trained radiological technologist and a nurse trained in intensive care, both available within 45 min notice. Radiographic and fluoroscopic equipment must be optimal. We have found the 105 mm camera coupled to our image-intensifier to be indispensable in emergency arteriographic procedures. Because scout films are unnecessary for cine fluorophotography, the camera considerably shortens the procedure and provides adequate documentation of pertinent findings.

METHODS AND MATERIALS

Vasopressin

Nusbaum[2,3] first reported the use of selective arterial infusion of vasopressin (Surgical Pituitrin, Parke Davis) to decrease portal hypertension and control bleeding gastro-oesophageal varices. Since then, intra-arterial and intravenous vasopressin infusions have been widely used to control gastrointestinal haemorrhage. Pitressin decreases mesenteric blood flow by 60% when introduced directly into the superior mesenteric artery and 40% when given intravenously[4]. The decrease in mesenteric blood flow results from arterial constriction and bowel wall contraction[5]. Intra-arterial vasopressin infusions are effective in the control of gastric mucosal and colonic diverticular bleeding[5]. Intravenous vasopressin is as effective as intra-arterial infusion in the acute control of haemorrhage from gastro-oesophageal varices[6,7].

Vasopressin is administered intra-arterially through an angiographically positioned catheter by a constant infusion pump. Following demonstration of contrast extravasation, a trial infusion of 0.2 U/min is undertaken for 20 min after which repeat arteriography is performed. If extravasation is not demonstrated on repeat study, the catheter is secured in position and the patient is transferred to an intensive care unit with the pump running. If extravasation continues, the infusion rate is increased to 0.3 U/min and arteriography is repeated 20 min later. The infusion rate may be increased to 0.4 U/min if necessary to control haemorrhage. Should contrast extravasation be demonstrated at the 0.4 U/min infusion rate, the bleeding artery is embolized. Patients who have received selective pitressin infusion must be monitored in an intensive care unit for signs of further haemorrhage and require observation for the water retention and hyponatraemia associated with pitressin infusion. Our usual schedule consists of 24 h of infusion at the dose rate which initially controlled the haemorrhage, followed by gradual weaning by 0.1 U/min until the patient has been free of haemorrhage without pitressin infusion for 24 h. During the last 12 h period, catheter patency is maintained with 5% dextrose and water running at 30 cc/h. The catheter may then be removed if bleeding does not recur.

Intravenous pitressin may be infused through a large-bore peripheral line at the same dose rate as is used for intra-arterial infusion[7]. However, infusion through a centrally placed line is preferable because extravasation may result in skin necrosis. After haemorrhage is controlled, intravenous pitressin should also be gradually weaned. Should upper gastrointestinal haemorrhage in a patient with portal hypertension fail to resolve on maximal intravenous pitressin infusion while clotting factors are within the normal range, selective celiac and superior mesenteric arteriography may be performed to rule out non-variceal bleeding sources. If arterial contrast extravasation is not seen, selective superior mesenteric arterial pitressin infusion may be tried, to obviate emergency portacaval shunting. Occasionally, variceal bleeders are controlled only with intra-arterial pitressin infusion.

Embolic materials

Autologous clot

Transcatheter embolization of a spinal arteriovenous malformation was reported by Doppman in 1969[8]. Subsequently, others[9,10] utilized autologous clot to control haemorrhage from various sites. A sample of the patient's blood is drawn and allowed to clot. The thrombus is then cut into cubes and injected through the catheter. Treatment with heat, epsilon-aminocaproic acid (Amicar) and thrombin improve clot stability but intravascular thrombus is lysed within 24 h of embolization[10]. Despite ready availability, thrombus is now seldom used because of its rapid dissolution.

Surgical gelatin

Surgical gelatin (Gelfoam, Upjohn, Kalamazoo, MI) is the most commonly employed particulate embolic material today. Intravascular Gelfoam particles are engulfed by giant cells and phagocytized within 40 days[11], so that embolized vessels may recanalize[11]. Surgical gelatin is available as a sterile sponge or in a prepared powder, but we use only the sponge for embolization.

At the time of embolization, sterile gelatin sponges are cut into 4 mm strips which are subsequently broken into cubes. The cubes are suspended in a bowl of dextrose and water with or without added antibiotics. Using a needle and/or forceps the wetted Gelfoam pledgets are loaded singly or in pairs into the open barrels of 1 cc syringes. The syringe plungers are then replaced with the emboli resuspended in flush solution. While fluoroscopically monitoring catheter tip stability, the particles are briskly injected into the catheter. Once the Gelfoam is lodged within the catheter, it is flushed into the desired vessel using 1 cc syringes of flush solution. Frequent test injections of contrast are made under fluoroscopy during embolization to assess flow. Embolization is complete when flow in the target vessel is nearly ablated. Follow-up arteriography is generally performed from a site proximal to the site of embolization so that embolic particles are not dislodged. Balloon occlusion catheters are used whenever possible to prevent distal embolization[12]. We do not generally render Gelfoam radiopaque. Small surgical clips may be attached to the pledgets prior to embolization, but we have not found this clinically helpful.

Polyvinyl alcohol

Polyvinyl alcohol (Ivalon, Unipoint Industries, Highpoint, NC) has been used for intravascular occlusion for about 5 years[13]. It is a permanently occlusive agent[14] which expands longitudinally from the compressed state after embolization, forming a firm vascular plug. The Ivalon sponge as obtained from the manufacturer is moistened, packed firmly in a 50 cc syringe barrel and dried under vacuum. The compressed sponge is then removed from the syringe and cold gas sterilized. Particles for embolization are obtained by punching out suitably sized pieces with a hole punch. These particles are handled in much the same fashion as Gelfoam except that they are not soaked for a prolonged period in flush solution.

Steel coils

Gianturco-Anderson coils (Cook Inc., Bloomington, IN) are helical segments of coiled guidewire with attached Dacron fibres[15]. They have been used extensively for over 5 years to occlude medium-sized and large vessels[15-17]. New mini-coils are also available for embolization of small to medium-sized vessels. The coils are pushed through non-tapered angiographic catheters with a special guidewire system. Under fluoroscopic guidance the coils are expelled from the catheter into the desired vessel. Coil occlusion is permanent.

Detachable balloons

White[18] has reported considerable experience with the use of detachable silicone balloons (Becton-Dickinson, Rutherford, NJ) for transcatheter embolization; 4 mm balloons are currently available and 8 mm balloons will soon be marketed. They afford permanent occlusion but prior to release may be inflated and deflated to achieve optimal placement. The balloons are injected coaxially through 5- or 7-French polyethylene catheters. Because the silicon membrane is semipermeable, balloons must be inflated with an isotonic solution. We use Metrizamide (Sterling Winthrop Research Institute, Rensselar, NY) to fill and opacify the balloons. The delivery system is somewhat cumbersome and the cost of each balloon is considerable, limiting their use.

Isobutyl-2-cyanoacrylate

Bucrylate (Ethicon Inc., Somerille, NJ) is a tissue adhesive which affords instant, permanent vascular occlusion[19]. It may be rendered radiopaque with tantalum powder (2 g/ml) (Fansteel Metals, North Chicago, IL) or iophendylate (1 cc : 1 cc) (Pantopaque, Lafayette Pharmacal Inc., Lafayette, Indiana)[20]. Because Bucrylate polymerizes instantly on contact with ionic media, it is best injected through a coaxial catheter system (Cook Inc., Bloomington, Indiana). The 3-French Teflon inner catheter is positioned through a standard selective angiographic catheter. The coaxial catheter is flushed immediately before and after embolization with 5% dextrose and water. Immediately upon completion of injection the inner catheter is withdrawn to prevent it from being glued in place. Polymerization is somewhat delayed by the addition of iophendylate. In a 1 : 1 mix, polymerization occurs in 3.5 s compared to 1 s for the undiluted monomer.

Complications

The most frequently reported complication of transcatheter therapy is embolization of non-target organs[21-24]. Visceral infarction following embolization has also been reported[25-26]. The stiff steel coils may dissect the target artery upon emerging from the catheter, creating a pseudoaneurysm at the embolization site[16]. Intrapancreatic pseudoaneurysms are particularly delicate. Lina *et al.*[27] reported rupture of three such aneurysms in patients during attempted embolization. In addition to these complications, there are those of general angiography including arterial injury in the groin, renal failure from high contrast doses and injury to the vessels under study.

GASTROINTESTINAL TRACT HAEMORRHAGE

Arteriography to delineate the source of gastrointestinal haemorrhage is reserved for those patients who do not respond to standard conservative therapeutic measures. The presence or absence of blood in the nasogastric tube aspirate, and the results of emergency endoscopy, are most helpful in directing the angiographer toward a region of haemorrhage. Radionuclide bleed scans may also be helpful[28].

If a prosthetic vascular graft is present, or if there has been penetrating trauma, biplane aortography should be performed to rule out an arterioenteric fistula or a pseudoaneurysm[29]. Contrast extravasation into

the gastrointestinal tract may be seen radiographically[1] if the rate of haemorrhage equals or exceeds 0.5 cc/min.

Upper gastrointestinal haemorrhage

Celiac arteriography is performed to rule out pancreatic or duodenal
ulcer haemorrhage. A left gastric artery injection is necessary to assess
gastric mucosal haemorrhage. If no extravasation is seen from these
sites, the superior mesenteric artery is injected. Replaced right hepatic
artery branches and duodenal collateral vessels arising from the superior mesenteric artery are occasional sources of haemorrhage. Small
bowel sources of bleeding, including arteriovenous malformations[30],
tumours, and embryological malformations may also be visualized.

Not infrequently, these injections will demonstrate no site of bleeding. If gastro-oesophageal varices have been demonstrated endoscopically or angiographically, they may be considered to be the source of
haemorrhage in the absence of arterial extravasation. One is unlikely to
see frank contrast extravasation from bleeding varices[31]. It must be
remembered, however, that cirrhotic patients frequently bleed from
extravariceal sources, such as ulcers and gastritis. Rarely arterioportal
shunts may result in portal hypertension; these may be opacified from
celiac or superior mesenteric artery injections[32].

Haemorrhage from Mallory–Weiss tears or erosive oesophagitis is
controlled with selective vasopressin injection into the left gastric
artery[33]. Of patients with haemorrhagic gastritis, 84% are controlled
with selective pitressin infusion[34], but 16% experience rebleeding
(Figure 1). Only about 50–60% of patients with haemorrhagic gastric
ulcers are controlled with pitressin infusion. Patients who continue to
bleed on pitressin may undergo Gelfoam embolization[35] (Figure 2).

Bleeding from duodenal ulcers is controlled with pitressin infusion in
only about one-third of cases[36]. Massively bleeding duodenal ulcers
may be successfully treated with embolization of the gastroduodenal
artery with Gelfoam or cyanoacrylate[37] (Figure 3). There is less experience with the angiographic control of small bowel bleeding although
Baum et al.[31] have found that anastomotic ulcers frequently respond to
pitressin infusions. Tod et al.[38] have found that such ulcers may be successfully embolized. Angiography and methylene blue injections via
selectively placed catheters are helpful for the pre- and intra-operative
localization of small bowel arteriovenous malformations[30] (Figure 4).

Variceal haemorrhage is as successfully treated with intravenous
vasopressin as it is with intra-arterial infusion[6,7]. Complication rates are
comparable with either infusion method[39]. About 50% of acute variceal
bleeders may be expected to stop bleeding on pitressin therapy[6,7].
Widrich has transhepatically embolized gastro-oesophageal varices with

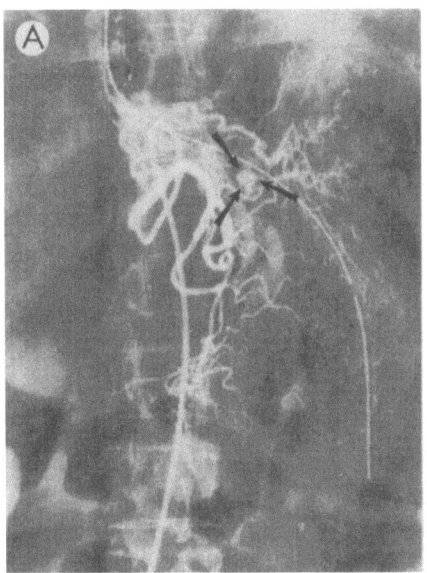

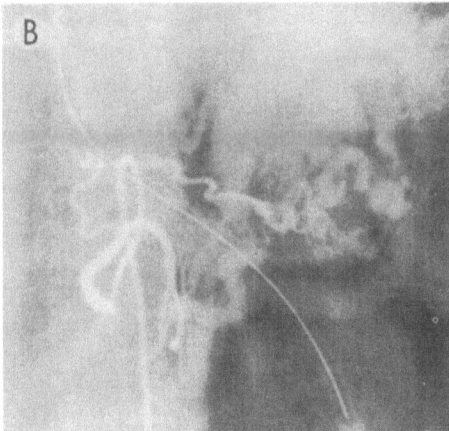

Figure 1 Stress bleeding from the stomach controlled with intra-arterial vasopressin. **(A)** Left gastric arteriogram shows extravasation in the area of the gastric fundus (arrows). **(B)** Left gastric arteriogram after 20 min of vasopressin infusion into the left gastric artery at 0.2 U/min. There is no extravasation and the bleeding was clinically controlled

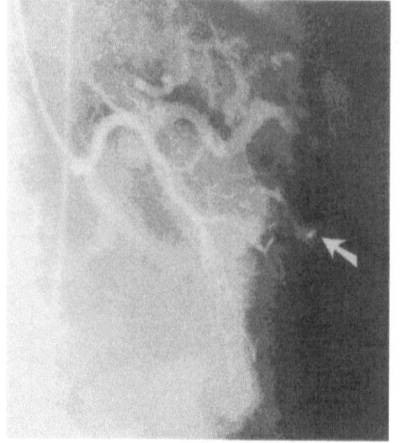

A

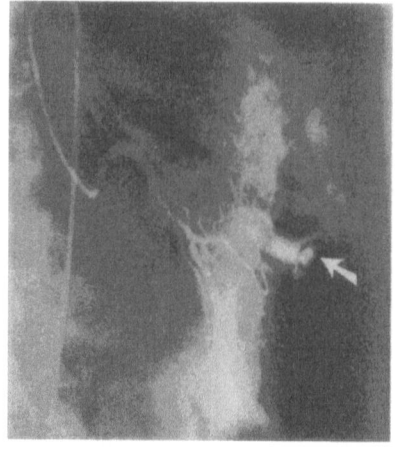

B

C

Figure 2 Gastric bleeding controlled with embolization. **(A)** Left gastric arteriogram shows extravasation in the stomach (arrow). **(B)** During the later phase of the arteriogram, the site of bleeding is clearly delineated (arrow). **(C)** The bleeding branch of the left gastric artery has been occluded (arrow) with two plugs of surgical gelatin. There is no further extravasation

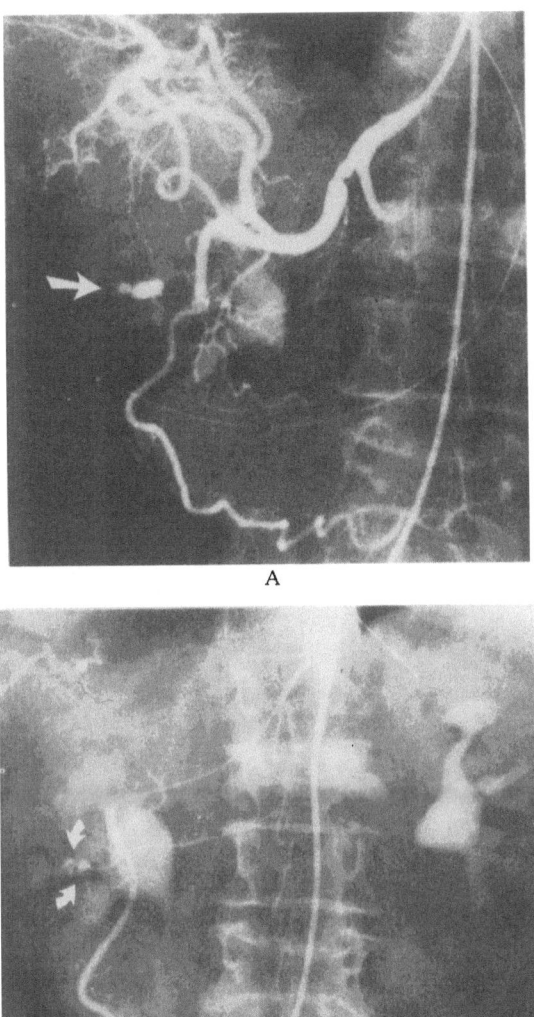

A

B

Figure 3 Bleeding from a duodenal ulcer controlled with transcatheter embolization.
(**A**) The arrow points to contrast extravasation from a branch of the gastroduodenal
artery. (**B**) A small catheter has been selectively advanced into the gastroduodenal artery
and the bleeding branch was embolized with plugs of surgical gelatin. Arrows point to
contrast extravasation retained from previous injections. Following embolization, there
was no extravasation and the bleeding was clinically controlled

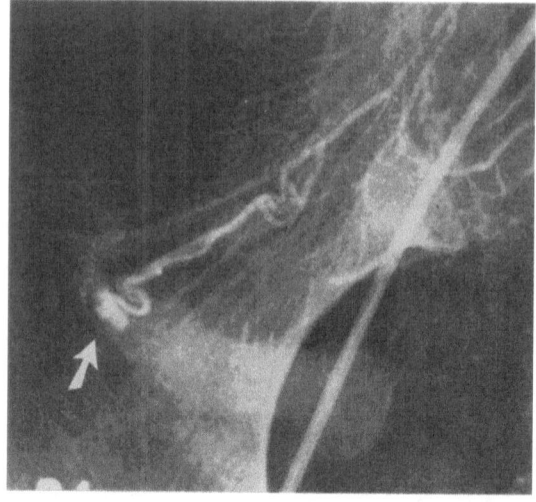

A

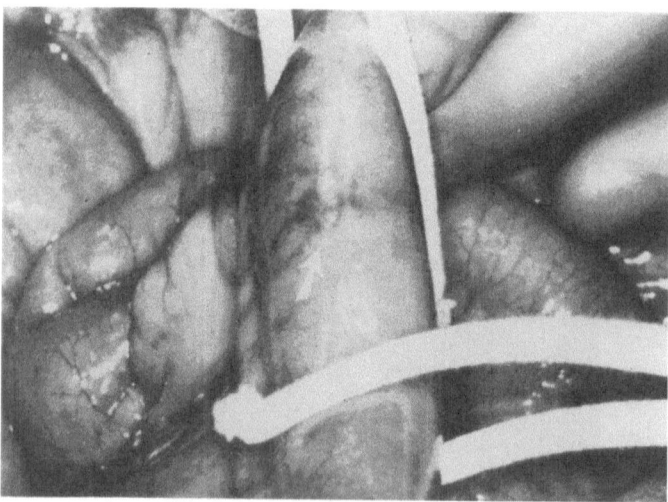

B

Figure 4 Angiographic localization of an arteriovenous malformation of the small bowel. **(A)** Magnification arteriogram shows arteriovenous malformation of the small bowel (arrow). **(B)** At laparotomy methylene blue has been injected via a catheter selectively positioned prior to operation in the mesenteric arterial branch supplying the malformation. This facilitated intra-operative localization and excision of the lesion (arrow)

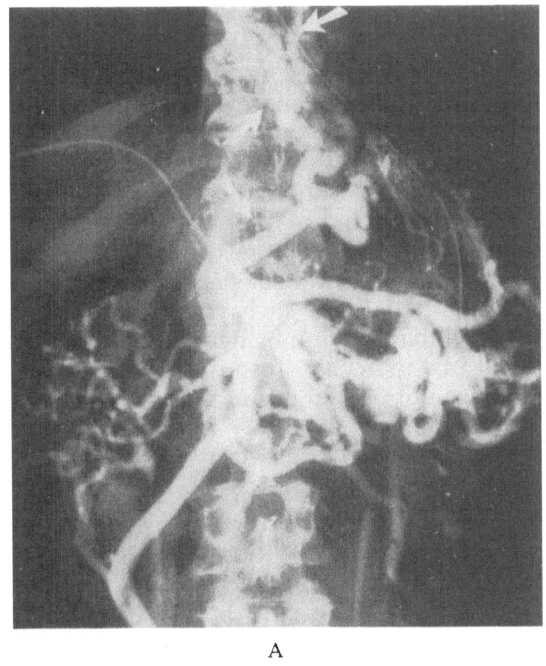

A

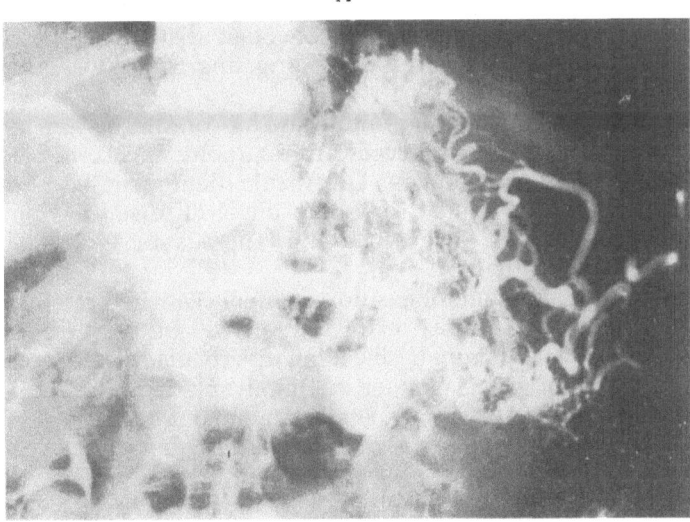

B

Figure 5 Transhepatic obliteration of gastro-oesophageal varices. **(A)** Arrows point to coronary vein and massive gastro-oesophageal varices. **(B)** The coronary vein has been occluded with Gelfoam soaked in Sotradecol and Bucrylate. Varices no longer opacify

Gelfoam pledgets soaked in sodium tetradecyl sulphate (Sotradecol), to control haemorrhage in 81% of actively bleeding cirrhotics[40] (Figure 5). Lunderquist et al.[41] found that many embolized coronary veins will recanalize, but they did not use Sotradecol as a sclerosing agent. Such variceal occlusion increases portal venous pressures and probably opens other collateral pathways to systemic veins[40]. One must occlude all tributaries to the oesophageal varices in order to prevent recanalization and rebleeding[40]. Bucrylate has not been used in a sufficient number of cases for assessment[40]. Bleeding from the hepatic puncture site is the most severe complication of transhepatic coronary vein obliteration. Widrich et al.[40] reported three such episodes in 38 patients. These workers routinely embolize the transhepatic needle tract with Gelfoam upon withdrawal of the needle. In our hands, transhepatic coronary vein obliteration has not proved useful in controlling variceal bleeding. Portal venous hypertension secondary to arteriovenous fistula may be treated by embolic occlusion of the artery supplying the fistula.

Lower gastrointestinal haemorrhage

We use the Tc99m labelled red cell bleeding scan[28] to assess the activity of bleeding and to direct us towards a probable site of haemorrhage. Should bleeding recur within 24 h of isotope administration, the patient may be rescanned without reinjection of technetium. Delay in obtaining a follow-up scan may suggest an erroneously distal bleeding point. In patients with acute massive rectal bleeding, angiography should be performed on an urgent basis.

Other modalities, including routine and air contrast barium studies as well as endoscopy, should precede arteriography in chronic bleeders to rule out bleeding carcinomas. Diverticula demonstrated on barium enema may not be assumed to be the source of lower gastrointestinal haemorrhage because diverticula and angiodysplastic lesions may coexist in elderly patients[42].

The diagnostic angiographic study commences with superior mesenteric arteriography. Contrast extravasation will be seen from actively bleeding diverticula (Figure 6). Bleeding diverticula are most commonly encountered in the right colon, as is angiodysplasia[42]. The angiographic findings of angiodysplasia are subtle and may require magnification views for confirmation. The vascular malformation itself may be seen as a small tuft of abnormal vessels on the antimesenteric bowel border. The vein draining an angiodysplastic lesion opacifies early in the arteriographic sequence and it remains densely opaque throughout the venous phase (Figure 7)[43]. Occasionally, areas of neovascularity denote the presence of unsuspected caecal carcinomas[42]. In patients with episodic lower gastrointestinal bleeding, one must carefully look for the vitelline

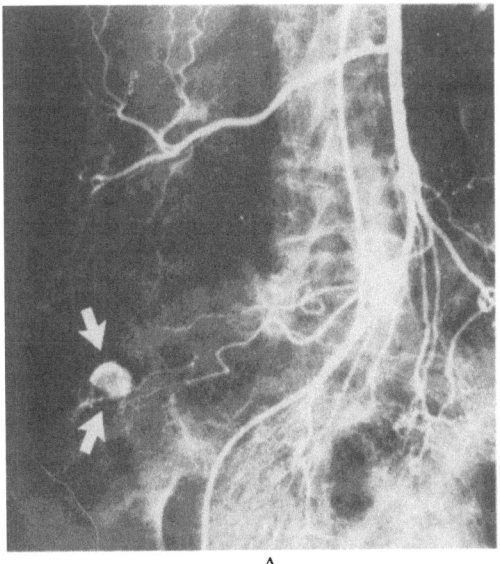

A

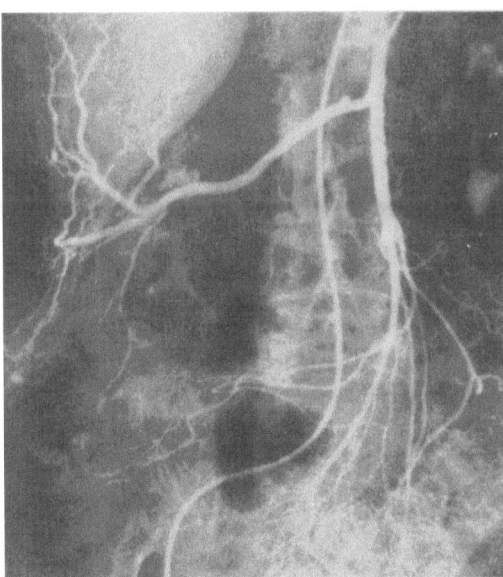

B

Figure 6 Colonic diverticular bleeding controlled with intra-arterial vasopressin. **(A)** Mesenteric arteriogram shows extravasation of contrast in a bleeding diverticulum of the right colon (arrows). **(B)** Arteriogram repeated after the intra-arterial infusion of vasopressin at 0.2 U/min shows no further extravasation

artery suppling a Meckel's diverticulum. The vitelline artery, when present, arises as the terminal branch of the superior mesenteric artery. It is generally untapered and without side branches. Most Meckel's diverticula are supplied by short and undistinguishable ileal arterial branches, however[44].

If the superior mesenteric arteriogram is negative, selective inferior mesenteric arteriography is performed. Films should include views of the entire rectum. Should both superior and inferior mesenteric arteriography fail to demonstrate a bleeding source, selective celiac arteriography should be undertaken to rule out an upper gastrointestinal source of haemorrhage, since celiac arterial branches may also supply the transverse colon.

Approximately 11% of patients with haematochezia studied by Boley et al.[45] were discharged without a definitive diagnosis. Of the patients in his study, 39% were found to have bleeding diverticula while 10% had angiodysplasia. The true incidence of angiodysplasia is probably higher than he reported, however[43].

Having demonstrated diverticular haemorrhage angiographically, one can usually control it with pitressin infusion into the corresponding mesenteric artery: bleeding was controlled with pitressin in 22 of 24

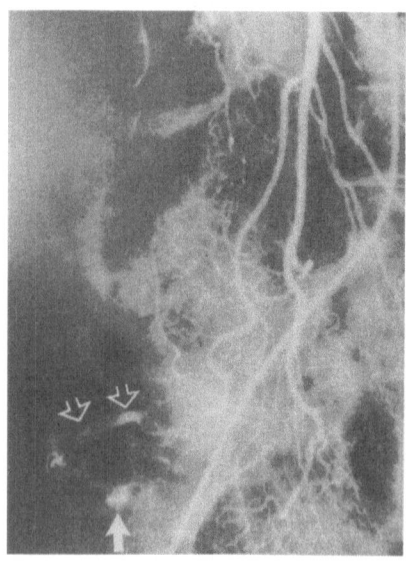

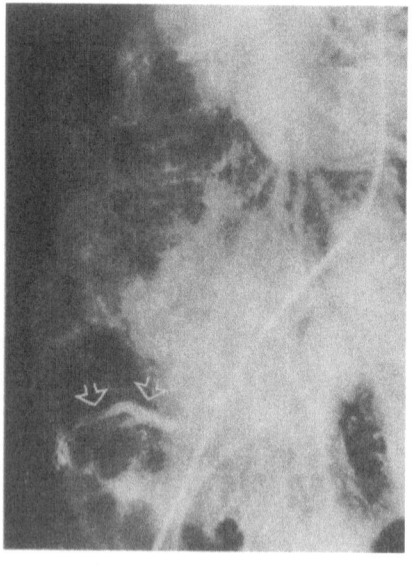

A   B

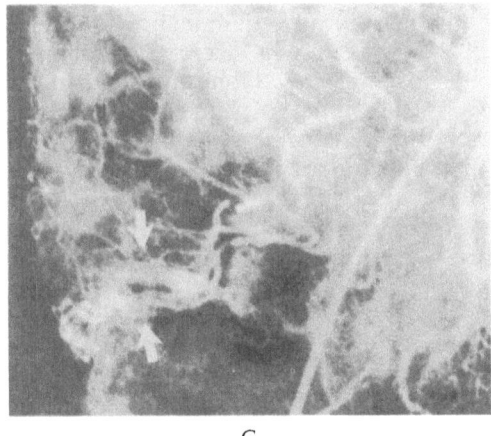

C

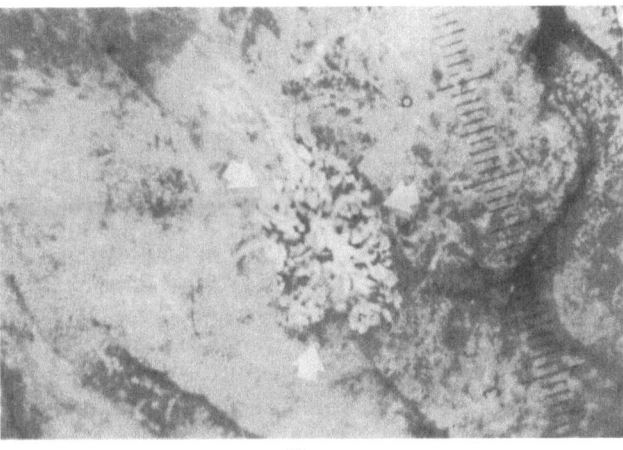

D

Figure 7 Colonic angiodysplasia. **(A)** Mesenteric arteriogram shows a vascular tuft (arrow) and early opacification of a draining vein (arrowheads) of the caecum. **(B)** During the late phase of the arteriogram there is intense opacification of the draining vein (arrowheads). **(C)** Magnification arteriography shows simultaneous opacification of arteries and a vein in the caecum at the site of angiodysplasia (arrows). **(D)** Angiodysplasia (arrows) as seen under the dissecting microscope. The vessels have been injected with silicone rubber

patients with angiographically demonstrated diverticular haemorrhage[46]. Nine of 12 patients who were not operated upon did not rebleed after initial haemostasis. None of the 10 patients who subsequently underwent segmental or subtotal colonic resection rebled. Bookstein et al. reported transcatheter embolization of five active bleeders, three with diverticula, one with a colonic ulcer and one with ischaemic colitis. None of his patients rebled[47] but on subsequent studies, embolization was complicated by bowel infarction in one patient.

The importance of angiodysplasia as a cause of chronic blood loss in the elderly is generally underestimated[42]. Meticulous angiography is necessary to demonstrate the lesion, including high-dose magnification superior mesenteric arteriography. Most angiodysplastic lesions are found in the right or proximal transverse colon. Of 38 patients reported by Welch, 31 underwent right colectomy. Six of these patients continued to bleed postoperatively, although two were subsequently found to have an extracolonic bleeding source. Right hemicolectomy is the suggested mode of therapy[42]. Bookstein et al.[47] embolized two caecal angiodysplastic lesions with Gelfoam. Both patients subsequently rebled and underwent partial colectomy.

HEPATIC HAEMORRHAGE

Hepatic haemorrhage is usually so massive that hepatic arteriography demonstrates extravasation of contrast into the peritoneum or biliary tract. Because of the high incidence of anomalous vessels supplying the liver, meticulous arteriography must be performed to adequately opacify all hepatic branches, including those arising from the superior mesenteric or from the left gastric artery[48]. Only after all hepatic arteries have been opacified can one be assured that active haemorrhage is not arising from the liver. One should carefully assess the films for portal venous or bile ductal filling from the arterial injections. Both arterioportal and arteriobiliary fistulas are amenable to transcatheter embolization.

The dual blood supply to the liver enables one to treat massive haemorrhage by dearterialization[48]. Surgical ligation of the hepatic artery has been advocated by a number of authors for treatment of massive bleeding from hepatic lacerations, tumours or aneurysms[48-52]. Selective preoperative hepatic arteriography is essential to delineate hepatic arterial anatomy prior to ligation and to establish the precise source of haemorrhage[49,50,52]. In their series of 108 cases, Aldrete et al.[53] found that 19% of patients admitted with hepatic trauma suffered severe hepatic lacerations with major blood loss requiring partial hepatectomy. Such patients are potential candidates for hepatic artery ligation and/or embolization (Figure 8).

Embolization of a discrete bleeding source in the liver has been utilized by a number of angiographers over the past 5 years[54-57]. Gelfoam has been the most frequently employed embolic material. It may be soaked in an antibiotic solution prior to use, especially when embolizing a potentially contaminated field[57]. Superior mesenteric arteriography with venous folow-through should be performed before hepatic arterial embolization to assess portal venous patency and the direction of blood flow. Patients with severe portal hypertension and reversal of flow may fare poorly following arterial embolization. As suggested with surgical hepatic artery ligation, the gastrointestinal tract should be rested for approximately a week following embolization with parenteral nutrition used as necessary. Because hepatocytes derive oxygenation from portal venous blood following arterial obliteration, administration of oxygen over the first week is recommended to raise the oxygen concentration of portal venous blood[48]. We administer intravenous broad-spectrum antibiotics to patients who have undergone extensive hepatic dearterialization to prevent abscess formation. Ischaemic injuries may follow transcatheter hepatic embolization and gangrenous cholecystitis has been reported[48]. Hepatic failure may occur with dearterialization of a liver which is more than 70% compromised by injury or trauma[37].

PANCREATIC HAEMORRHAGE

Pseudoaneurysms of intrapancreatic or peripancreatic arteries may develop as a complication of pancreatitis[58-60]. These pseudoaneurysms may rupture into the pancreatic duct and cause massive haemorrhage[60]. Such bleeding may be extremely difficult to control surgically as anatomical planes are disrupted by pancreatitis and the aneurysms are difficult to localize. Preoperative celiac and superior mesenteric arteriograms are necessary to precisely define pancreatic vascular anatomy and to delineate the source of haemorrhage. Actively bleeding pseudoaneurysms opacify the pancreatic and common ducts on selective arteriography.

Selective transcatheter embolization of pancreatic pseudoaneurysms has been performed but rupture into the pancreatic duct has been reported as a complication[27]; fortunately arterioductal fistulas are themselves amenable to transcatheter obliteration. Exacerbation of pancreatitis has not been reported following such embolization. Transcatheter embolization with cyanoacrylate has been life-saving in patients with massive bleeding related to pancreatic surgery, pancreatic abscess, etc. (Figure 9).

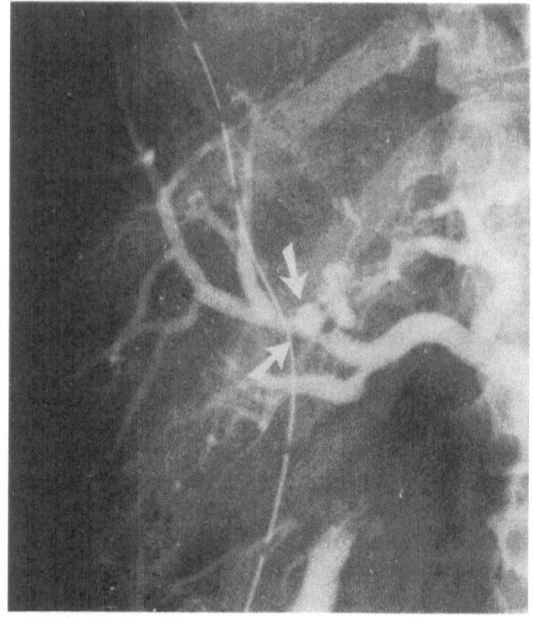

A

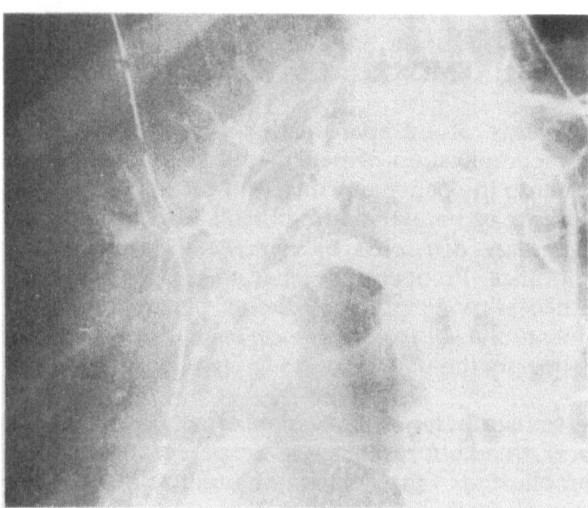

B

Figure 8 Transcatheter occlusion of a bleeding aneurysm of the heptic artery. **(A)** Hepatic arteriogram shows a false aneurysm of the hepatic artery (arrows). · **(B)** The hepatic artery and the aneurysm were occluded with cyanoacrylate (arrow). There has been no rebleeding and no ill effects within 2 years of follow-up

GENITOURINARY TRACT HAEMORRHAGE

With widespread deployment of new and non-invasive diagnostic studies, angiography is less important in the aetiological diagnosis of genitourinary tract haemorrhage than it was 5 years ago. Ultrasound and computed tomography with or without percutaneous needle biopsy can accurately diagnose most renal masses. The declining importance of angiography in the diagnosis of genitourinary tract haemorrhage has been more than balanced by the increasing importance of angiographic therapy. We are frequently called upon to control haemorrhage following trauma or to palliate patients with unresectable neoplasms. Since pharmacological agents are not effective in the control of genitourinary tract bleeding, particulate embolization is our primary mode of therapy[5].

Diagnostic arteriography is necessary in patients with active haemorrhage or absent renal function following trauma. Patients with both blunt and penetrating trauma should be worked up with a midstream aortogram prior to selective injections. Penetrating midline trauma requires an initial biplane aortogram to rule out an aortic pseudo-aneurysm or fistula. Arterial interruptions in the renal pedicle, including intimal injuries and transections, are best studied without selective arteriography. When assessing the source of haemorrhage following needle biopsy or from a known tumour, one may proceed directly with magnification views of all renal arteries to rule out small arteriovenous malformations, arterial pseudoaneurysms, and small hypovascular masses. Occasionally renal and gonadal venography are necessary in such patients to rule out venous angiomas. Bilateral hypogastric arteriography is necessary to diagnose and treat haemorrhage from the lower genitourinary tract.

Renal haemorrhage

Surgical therapy of post-traumatic haematuria results in a nephrectomy rate of nearly 50%[61]. Because transcatheter embolization controls bleeding with a smaller loss of renal tissue, angiographic control of haemorrhage has been widely employed since the first case report of Rizk *et al.* in 1973[62]. Segmental renal infarctions resulting from therapeutic emboli have not resulted in hypertension, although collaterals supplying relatively ischaemic areas of kidney may stimulate the juxtaglomerular apparatus[63]. Follow-up studies on embolized patients have revealed good renal function.

Percutaneous needle renal biopsy may cause a transient arteriovenous fistula in up to 20% of patients[64] but most of these fistulas resolve

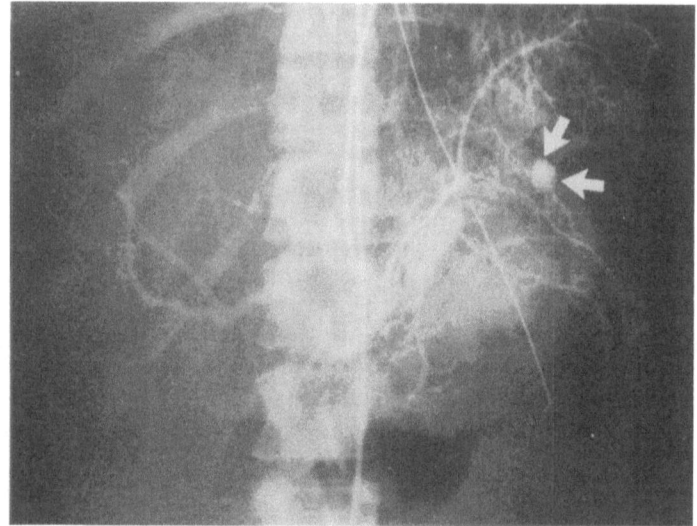

A

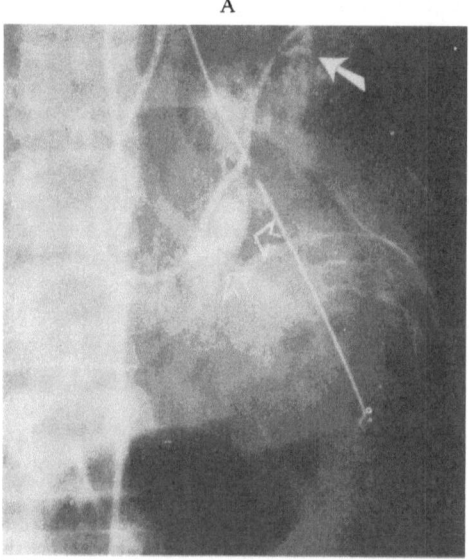

B

Figure 9 Bleeding following pancreatic surgery controlled with embolization. (A) Contrast extravasation (arrows) is noted from branches of the left inferior phrenic artery in the retroperitoneum. Retroperitoneal bleeding in this patient occurred a few hours following pancreatic resection for benign disease. (B) The bleeding branch from the inferior phrenic artery has been occluded with Gelfoam and cyanoacrylate (arrow). The arrowheads point to opacification of the left adrenal gland which is a normal finding

spontaneously. Surgical treatment results in a relatively high nephrectomy rate[64] and numerous authors have reported successful transcatheter embolization without aggravation or creation of hypertension[62-70]. Similar success has been reported following transcatheter embolization of either surgical or accidental penetrating renal injuries[63,71-73]

Persistent renal haemorrhage may be treated with therapeutic embolization in patients who have suffered blunt trauma if aortic and renal pedicular injuries are absent. Angiographically one may see pseudoaneurysms or contrast extravasation from fractured kidneys. A number of patients have been successfully treated[74,75], although nephrectomy may be necessary at a later date if extensive renal injury has resulted in a significant urine leak[63].

Autologous blood clot treated with Amicar has a number of theoretical advantages over other embolic materials for the treatment of traumatic renal haemorrhage. Blood clot is more rapidly lysed from normal vessels than from injured ones and results in good preservation of renal parenchyma[63]. Since bleeding may occur relatively frequently[63], we employ Gelfoam routinely and have a low incidence of complications (Figure 10). If large vessels are disrupted, steel coils or detachable balloons may be used to control bleeding. Tissue cements are less frequently used.

Chronic haemorrhage from renal neoplasms, either benign or malignant, may be easily controlled with embolization. One need not see active contrast extravasation prior to therapy in such circumstances. Chronic debilitating haemorrhage from renal angiomyolipomas has been controlled by embolization[76,77] and troublesome haemorrhage from unresectable renal carcinoma is also readily amenable to embolotherapy. Permanent occlusive agents such as Ivalon and Bucrylate should be employed to avoid rebleeding: Goldstein et al.[78] reported that Gelfoam-embolized arteries in four of six renal cell carcinomas were recanalized at follow-up. After renal embolization, one should expect considerable flank pain which may require narcotic analgesia over the ensuing 48 h[78-80]. Haematuria caused by metastases to the kidneys has also been successfully treated by arterial occlusion[81].

Vesicular and ureteric haemorrhage

Lower urinary tract haemorrhage is readily amenable to embolic control. Haemorrhage from an ileal loop must be assessed with selective superior mesenteric arteriography. If such haemorrhage is the result of portal hypertension with bleeding varices within the loop, transhepatic portography must be performed and the varices selectively embolized.

Vesicular haemorrhage must be assessed with selective bilateral internal iliac arteriography. Contrast extravasation may be seen, but if a

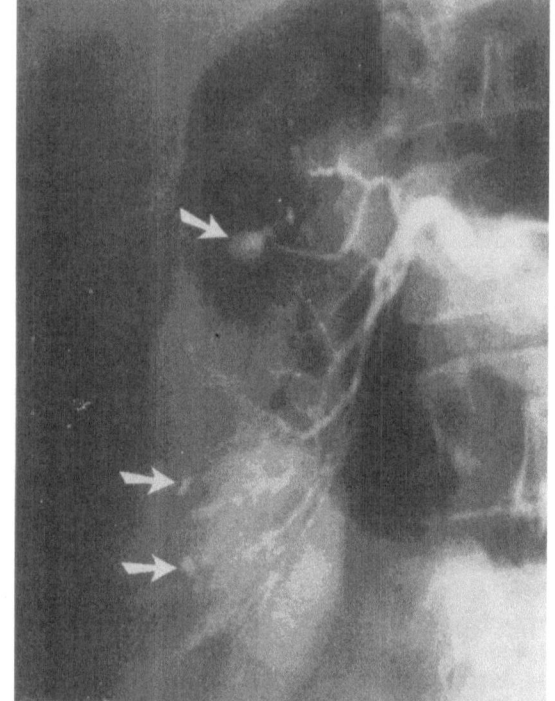

A

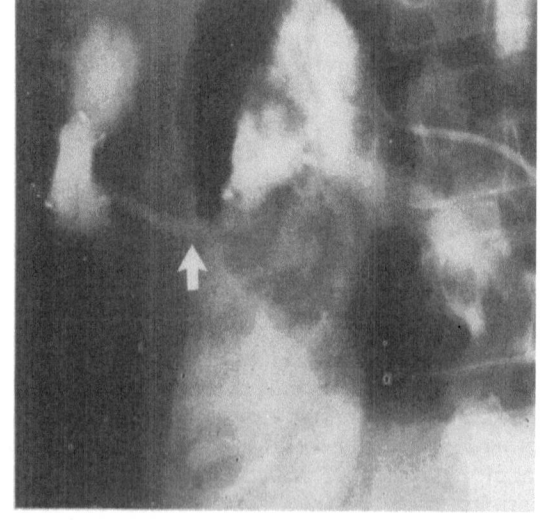

B

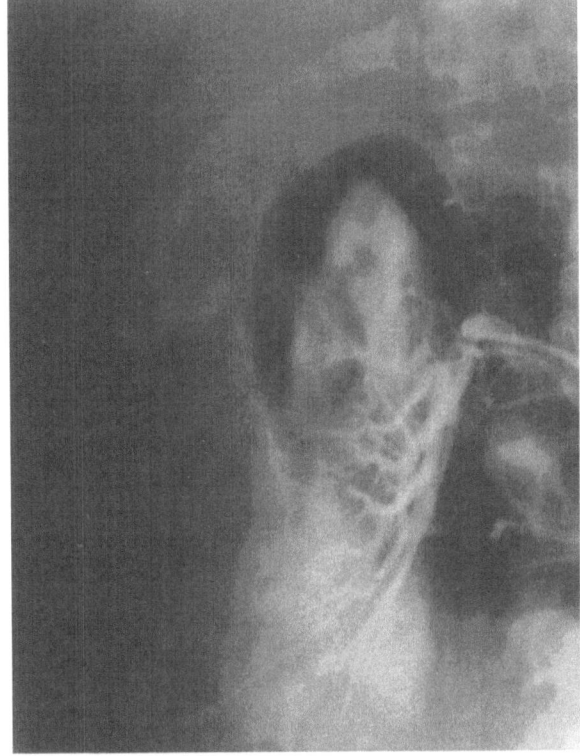

C

Figure 10 Intrarenal haemorrhage controlled with transcatheter embolization. **(A)** Right renal arteriogram shows aneurysms of the renal arterial branches in a patient with arteritis (arrows).   **(B)** One of the aneurysms has ruptured and there is massive bleeding into the subcapsular space (arrow).   **(C)** Selective embolization and occlusion of a bleeding branch with one plug of Gelfoam has controlled the bleeding

bladder source of haemorrhage has been accurately diagnosed by other modalities one may proceed with embolization, even if a discrete bleeding site was not demonstrated angiographically. Chronic haemorrhage from bladder tumours has been treated with a number of embolic agents[82–84]; permanently occlusive agents are obviously desirable.

Haemorrhage from the male reproductive system

Prostatic haemorrhage must be assessed with bilateral internal iliac arteriography because bleeding prostatic vessels frequently have a bilateral blood supply. Gross extravasation of contrast is frequently visualized.

Uncontrolled haemorrhage following prostatic surgery is uncommon. Haemostasis has been readily achieved, however, with hypogastric arterial Gelfoam embolization[85] (Figure 11). After embolization, bilateral selective hypogastric arteriography is necessary to assess completeness of haemostasis.

Gynaecological haemorrhage

Bilateral hypogastric arteriography will demonstrate contrast extravasation from the female genital tract in cases of active haemorrhage[86, 87]. In chronic bleeders one need not demonstrate extravasation prior to embolization[88].

Uterine haemorrhage from a number of sources has been amenable to embolotherapy. Olcott et al.[87] used Gelfoam and lead pellets to de-arterialize a large uterine arteriovenous malformation. Today, Bucrylate or steel coils are the agents of choice. Unrelenting postpartum haemorrhage may be successfully controlled with emboli. A number of chronically bleeding uterine tumours have been controlled with the use of permanent occlusive agents[87, 88–90]. Traumatic or neoplastic vaginal haemorrhage may be controlled in similar fashion[91] (Figure 12).

MUSCULOSKELETAL HAEMORRHAGE

Because patients with severe musculoskeletal haemorrhage frequently have other severe injuries, appropriate priorities for diagnosis and therapy must be established early[92]. Life-threatening injuries, including haemorrhage from major abdominal vessels must be assessed and treated first. Massive pelvic haemorrhage may be treated with transfusion and with a G-suit during initial evaluation. The overall mortality associated with such trauma is between 18 and 26%[93]. In their autopsy study, Patterson and Morton[92] found that 37 of 88 patients who died following pelvic fractures exsanguinated from their injuries. Arteriography may be required for the diagnosis of other injuries, including aortic lacerations and intra-abdominal visceral injuries. Iliac arteriography may be performed in conjunction with these studies to assess and treat pelvic haemorrhage as indicated.

The Massachusetts General Hospital experience has been reported[94–96] and summarized by Matalon et al.[97]. Twenty-eight patients underwent angiography for massive pelvic bleeding associated with fractures. Contrast extravasation from branches of the hypogastric artery was seen in 20 patients, of whom 18 underwent transcatheter embolization. Bleeding was controlled angiographically in 17 (Figures 13, 14). No patient with a negative arteriogram continued to bleed clinically. Half of the

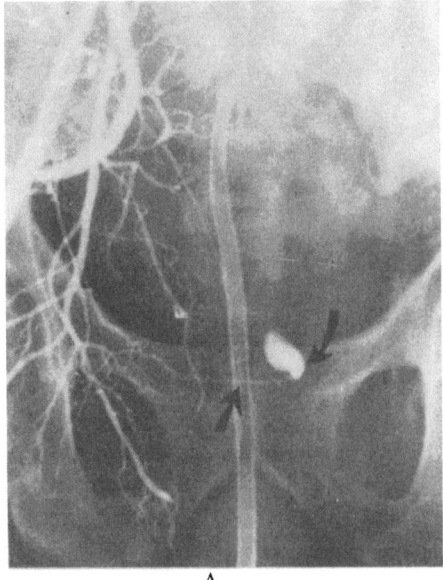

A

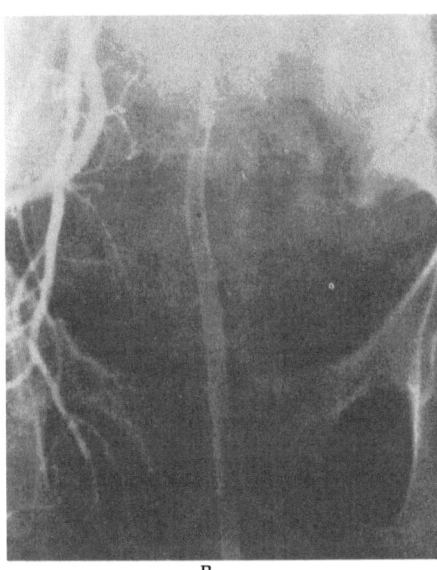

B

Figure 11 Bleeding in the prostatic bed controlled with embolization. **(A)** Hypogastric arteriogram shows contrast extravasation in the prostatic bed following biopsy and transurethral partial resection (arrows). **(B)** Following embolization of branches of the hypogastric artery there is no further extravasation

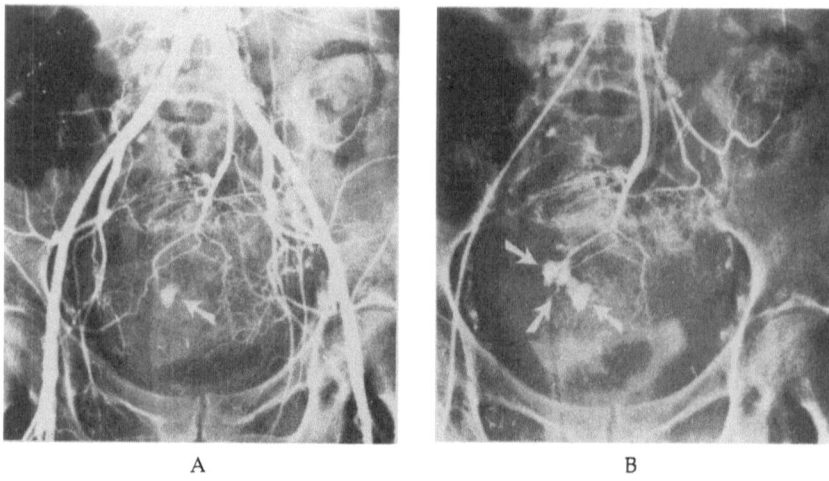

A   B

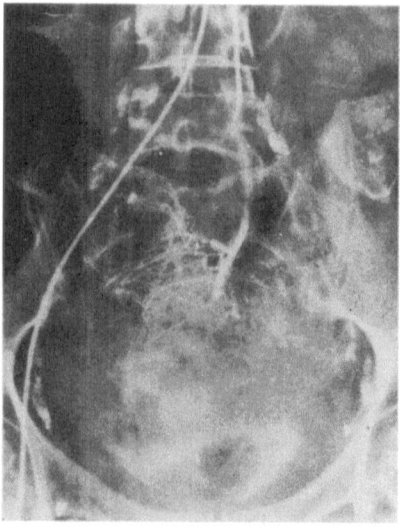

C

Figure 12 Vaginal bleeding in a patient with carcinoma of the cervix treated with radiation therapy.   (**A**) Pelvic arteriogram shows extravasation in the pelvis at a site of a rectovaginal fistula (arrow).   (**B**) Extravasation is noted to originate from branches of the inferior mesenteric artery (arrows).   (**C**) Extravasation and bleeding have been controlled with embolization of the superior haemorrhoidal artery with plugs of surgical gelatin

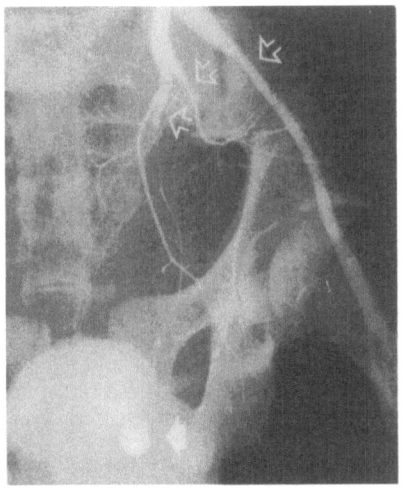
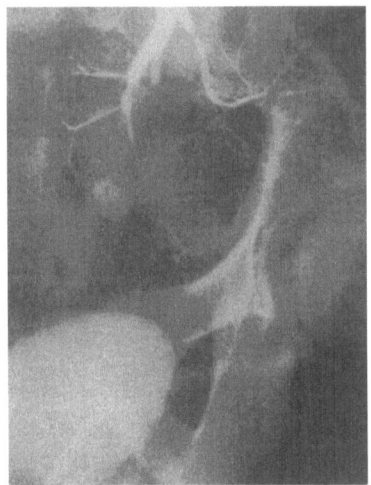

A   B

Figure 13   Bleeding from obturator artery controlled with surgical gelatin embolization. A 15-year-old boy sustained numerous injuries in an automobile accident. **(A)** Left common iliac arteriogram. Catheter from right femoral artery. Active bleeding from obturator artery (arrow). Arterial compression from massive pelvic haematoma evident (open arrows). **(B)** After embolization with surgical gelatin: occlusion of obturator artery and segmental occlusion of inferior gluteal artery without extravasation. Transfusion requirement subsided and the patient survived. (From Ref. 97, with permission)

patients who underwent pelvic arteriography and embolization subsequently died, compared with 38% of those who did not undergo arteriography. There was one complication in the embolized group of 18 patients; that of a peroneal artery embolus.

Surgical exploration of retroperitoneal and pelvic haematomas is not routinely carried out because the local tamponade effect of an intact peritoneum is thus lost[98]. Blind hypogastric artery ligation is not helpful in controlling haemorrhage[92] but embolization is effective since the emboli are deposited near the site of arterial injury and rebleeding from collaterals is unlikely[98]. An abdominal aortogram is not adequate to assess pelvic vascular injury: selective hypogastric arteriography will demonstrate contrast extravasation not seen at aortography[98]. Venous studies are not worthwhile, because low-pressure venous bleeding will tamponade with correction of clotting factors and replacement of intravascular volume[98]. Haemorrhage from the extremities is usually best handled by local surgical intervention, prior to which selective arteriography is frequently useful in the diagnosis of specific vascular injuries

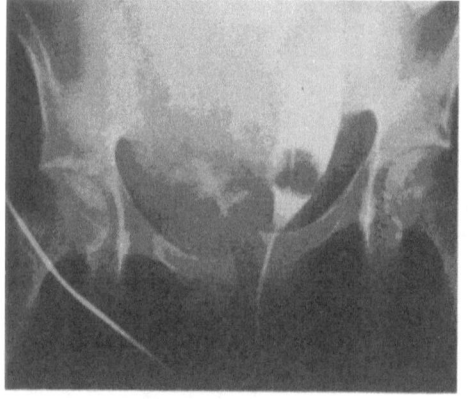

A

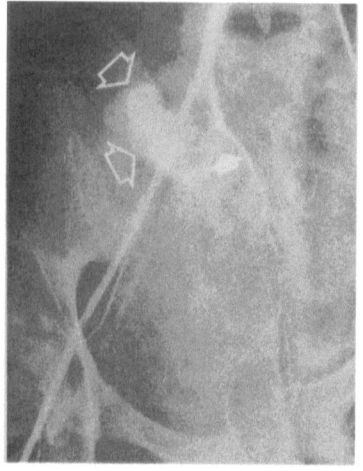

B

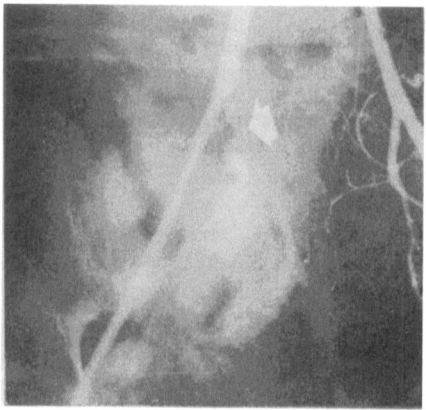

C

Figure 14 Bleeding from iliolumbar artery controlled with Gelfoam embolization in a 19-year-old girl with numerous injuries from an automobile accident. **(A)** Disruption of symphysis pubis, right sacroiliac joint and massive haematoma displacing the bladder. **(B)** Right common iliac arteriogram. Catheter from left. Massive extravasation from iliolumbar artery (open arrows). Catheter in right femoral vein (closed arrows). Injection through catheter showed iliac veins to be intact. **(C)** After occlusion of iliolumbar artery with Gelfoam. Note occlusion of proximal hypogastric artery (arrow). Contrast is retained in soft tissues from previous extravasation. Transfusion requirements: 33 units before embolization; 6 units after. Patient survived. (From Ref. 97, with permission)

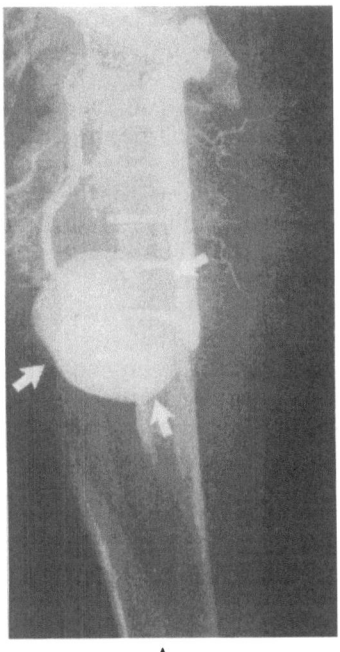
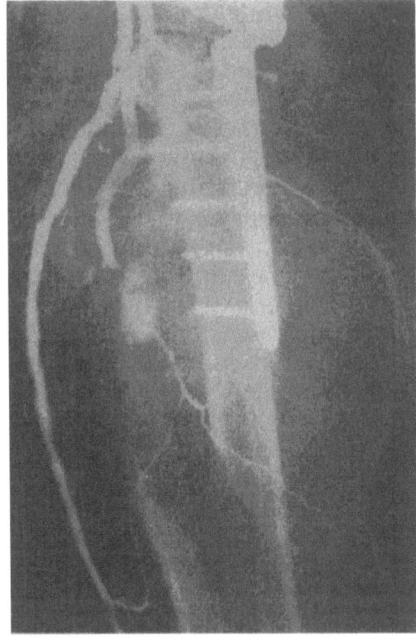

A   B

Figure 15 False aneurysm of the deep femoral artery occluded with Gelfoam. **(A)** Arrows point to a false aneurysm of the femoral artery, the result of a fracture of the femoral shaft. **(B)** The aneurysm has been occluded with embolization with surgical gelatin.

(Figure 15). Gelfoam is the embolic agent of choice for pelvic and retroperitoneal haemorrhage but other materials including tissue cements have been employed. Spontaneous retroperitoneal and pelvic haemorrhage from tumour or over-anticoagulation may be treated with embolization[99], but such patients infrequently require interventional therapy.

SPLENIC HAEMORRHAGE

Significant splenic injury frequently occurs as a part of multiple trauma[100]. The diagnosis of splenic rupture generally rests on clinical and scintigraphic findings. Patients in whom routine studies are equivocal may undergo arteriography or arteriography may be performed as part of a comprehensive examination in the trauma patient. Splenic contusion causes a mottled parenchymal pattern at arteriography. A local filling defect may reflect an early draining vein. Frank disruption of the spleen results in a peripheral avascular mass effect or other gross parenchymal defects with or without frank extravasation of contrast[101]. Multiple spleens or a single spleen with focal infarcts may cause confusion in the patient with significant abdominal trauma.

Because of the increased incidence of overwhelming sepsis following splenectomy there is considerable interest in non-surgical treatment of splenic injuries and in surgical splenic repair[102]. Some advocates of conservative management recommend angiographic follow-up in such patients before allowing them to resume normal activity. They find angiographic evidence of healing reassuring[103], but Sherman[103] has found that late splenic rupture is rare. Fisher and associates[104] have found follow-up scans to be adequate in this regard; in the absence of an expanding haematoma, patients were returned to normal activity.

The level of enthusiasm for splenic embolization has been considerably dampened by reports of post-embolic abscess formation[17,105]. Splenic embolization for traumatic haemorrhage is probably only an emergency procedure[106]. Under any circumstance, systemic broad-spectrum antibiotics should be administered for 10 days following splenic embolization. In this regard, prophylactic embolization of splenic artery aneurysms has been recommended by Probst et al., who reported limited success in two patients in whom steel coils were used for embolization[107].

HAEMOPTYSIS

Acute massive haemoptysis may complicate a number of respiratory diseases. An 80% mortality was reported by Thomas et al.[108]. Such haemorrhage usually arises from abnormal systemic arteries which have enlarged in response to chronic pulmonary disease[109,110]. Systemic, non-bronchial arteries may penetrate the lung through pleural adhesions and participate in the development of haemoptysis[111]. Selective bronchial artery catheterization and embolization with Gelfoam has controlled bleeding[110-112] (Figure 16). For patients with intermittent massive haemoptysis one need not demonstrate contrast extravasation from abnormal systemic arteries prior to embolization[112]. The arterial supply to the anterior spinal artery may arise from intercostal arteries, the intercostal–bronchial trunk or the cervico-intercostal trunk. Selective contrast injections into arteries supplying interspinal branches may cause transverse myelitis. Such contribution to spinal cord vascularity is an absolute contraindication to embolization[111,112].

Selective catheter embolization of systemicopulmonary arteries is an attractive alternative to surgery in patients who have severely compromised pulmonary function. Acute haemoptysis may be controlled in

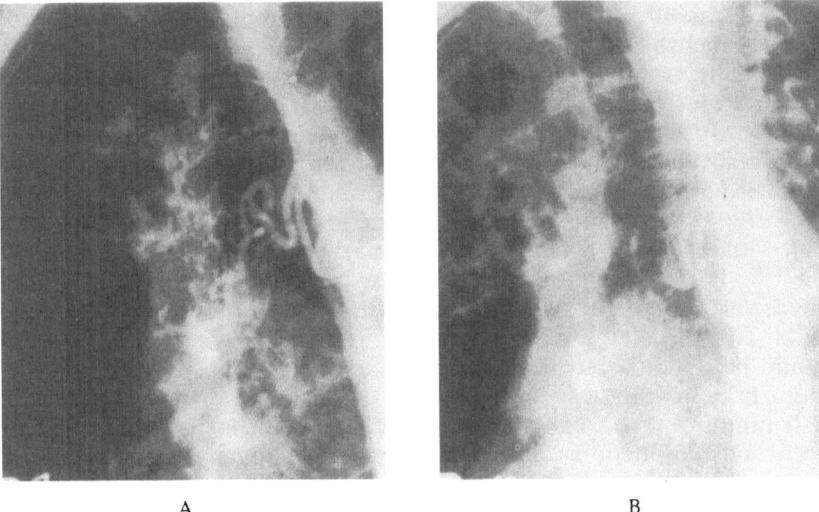

A   B

Figure 16 Bronchial artery embolization to control massive haemoptysis in a patient with cystic fibrosis. **(A)** The catheter has been selectively placed in the bronchial artery. **(B)** The distal branches of the bronchial artery have been occluded with pledgets of surgical gelatin

about 85% of patients by Gelfoam embolization[110, 111]. Recurrent haemorrhage may develop in a third of patients so treated, although the recurrent haemorrhage is usually less voluminous than the original episode[111, 112]. Embolic treatment of haemoptysis is especially advantageous in patients with cystic fibrosis because it allows vigorous and uninterrupted pulmonary toilet[112], but such treatment may also be required as a useful palliative procedure in patients with neoplasia[110].

HEAD AND NECK HAEMORRHAGE

A biplane aortic arch study is necessary prior to selective brachiocephalic arteriography in patients with penetrating trauma of the lower neck and upper chest. In the absence of trauma, selective carotid or subclavian arteriography may be undertaken directly. Active bleeding results in free contrast extravasation at arteriography. Subtle intimal irregularities and pseudoaneurysms may be seen following either blunt or penetrating trauma.

Severe recurrent epistaxis unresponsive to conservative therapy has been successfully treated by Gelfoam embolization of external carotid artery branches[113-115]. Recurrent haemorrhage develops in 10–20% of patients but, unlike surgical ligation, embolization may be repeated[115]. No significant neurological complications have been reported following this procedure but meticulous technique is necessary to avoid inadvertent embolization of the internal carotid circulation. Mild local pain in the embolized area develops in most patients but resolves within 72 h.

Massive haemorrhage from neoplastic erosion of major arteries has been successfully treated with temporary balloon catheter tamponade[116,117]. It may be necessary to place balloons both upstream and downstream from the site of erosion in order to prevent back bleeding[117]. The catheter may be removed in about a week. The balloon should be deflated but the catheter should be left in place for several hours prior to removal[116]. Permanent occlusion of arteries traversing such tumours using balloon catheters has not been reported but the recent development of 8 mm detachable balloons makes such an approach feasible.

SUMMARY

Over the past 10 years angiography has come to be routinely employed in the diagnosis and treatment of haemorrhage from nearly every organ system. Sources of both acute and chronic bleeding can be identified although arteriography is most useful acutely. In the patient with chronic haemorrhage, one must rely upon the identification of anatomical abnormalities such as arteriovenous malformations which are likely to be responsible for chronic blood loss. In such situations we are unlikely to demonstrate extravasation of contrast from the vascular tree. Vasoconstriction with vasopressin is useful in the gastrointestinal tract but elsewhere angiographic control of haemorrhage must rely upon physical occlusive agents, both particles and tissue cements, to afford either temporary or permanent vaso-occlusion, depending on clinical circumstance.

References

1 Baum, S., Nusbaum, M., Blakemore, W. S. and Finkelstein, A. K. (1965). The pre-operative radiographic demonstration of intra-abdominal bleeding from undetermined sites by percutaneous selective celiac and superior mesenteric arteriography. *Surgery*, **58**, 797

2 Nusbaum, M., Baum, S., Sakyalak, P. and Blakemore, W. S. (1967). Pharmacologic control of portal hypertension. *Surgery*, **62**, 299

3 Nusbaum, M., Baum, S., Kuroda, K. and Blakemore, W. S. (1968). Control of portal hypertension by selective arterial drug infusion. *Arch. Surg.*, **97**, 1005

4 Simmons, J. T., Baum, S., Sheehan, B. A., Ring, E. J., Athanasoulis, C. A., Waltman, A. C. and Coggins, P. C. (1977). The effect of vasopressin on hepatic arterial blood flow. *Radiology*, **124**, 637

5 Athanasoulis, C. A. (1980). Therapeutic applications of angiography. (First of two parts). *N. Engl. J. Med.*, **302**, 1117

6 Johnson, W. C., Widrich, W. C., Ansell, J. E., Robbins, A. H. and Nabseth, D. C. (1977). Control of bleeding varices by vasopressin: a prospective randomized study. *Ann. Surg.*, **186**, 369

7 Chojkier, M., Groszmann, R. J., Atterbury, C. E., Bar-Meir, S., Blei, A. T., Frankel, J., Glickman, M. G., Kniaz, J. C., Schade, R., Taggart, G. J. and Conn, H. O. (1979). A controlled comparison of intraarterial and intravenous infusions of vasopressin in hemorrhage from esophageal varices. *Gastroenterology*, **77**, 540

8 Doppmann, J. C., DiChiro, G. and Ommzaya, A. (1968). Obliteration of spinal arteriovenous malformation by percutaneous embolization. *Lancet*, **1**, 477

9 Rösch, J., Dotter, C. T. and Brown, M. J. (1972). Selective arterial embolization. A new method for control of acute gastrointestinal bleeding. *Radiology*, **102**, 303

10 Bookstein, J. J., Chlosta, E. M., Foley, D. and Walter, J. F. (1974). Transcatheter hemostasis of gastrointestinal bleeding using modified autogenous clot. *Radiology*, **113**, 277

11 Barth, K. H., Strandberg, J. D. and White, R. I. (1977). Long term follow-up of transcatheter embolization with autologous clot, oxycel and Gelfoam in domestic swine. *Invest. Radiol.*, **12**, 273

12 Greenfield, A. J., Athanasoulis, C. A., Waltman, A. C. and LeMoure, E. R. (1978). Transcatheter embolization: prevention of embolic reflux using balloon catheters. *Am. J. Roentgenol.*, **131**, 651

13 Tadavarthy, S. M., Moller, J. H. and Amplatz, K. (1975). Polyvinyl alcohol (Ivalon) – a new embolic material. *Am. J. Roentgenol.*, **125**, 609

14 Castaneda-Zuniga, W. R., Sanchez, R. and Amplatz, K. (1978). Experimental observations on short and long-term effects of arterial occlusion with Ivalon. *Radiology*, **126**, 783

15 Gianturco, C., Anderson, J. H. and Wallace, S. (1975). Mechanical devices for arterial occlusion. *Am. J. Roentgenol.*, **124**, 428

16 Anderson, J. H., Wallace, S., Gianturco, C. and Gerson, L. P. (1979). 'Mini' Gianturco stainless steel coils for transcatheter vascular occlusion. *Radiology*, **132**, 301

17 Wallace, S., Gianturco, C., Anderson, J. H., Goldstein, H. M., Davis, L. J. and Bree, R. L. (1976). Therapeutic vascular occlusion utilizing steel coil technique: Clinical applications. *Am. J. Roentgenol.*, **127**, 381

18 White, R. I., Jr, Kaufman, S. L., Barth, K. H., DeCaprio, V. and Strandbert, J. D. (1979). Embolotherapy with detachable silicone balloons: technique and clinical results. *Radiology*, **131**, 619

19 Dotter, C. T., Goldman, M. L. and Rösch, J. (1975). Instant selective arterial occlusion with isobutyl 2-cyanoacrylate. *Radiology*, **114**, 227

20 Freeny, P. C., Mennerger, R., Kidd, C. R. and Bush, W. H. (1979). Long term radiographic–pathologic follow-up of patients treated with visceral transcatheter occlusion using isobutyl 2-cyanoacrylate (Bucrylate). *Radiology*, **132**, 51

21 Chuang, V. P. (1979). Nonoperative retrieval of Gianturco coils from the abdominal aorta. *Am. J. Roentgenol.*, **132**, 996

22 Ganz, D. L., Dole, K. B. and Adelman, L. S. (1977). Spinal cord infarction following therapeutic renal artery embolization. *J. Am. Med. Assoc.*, **237**, 2841

23 Mukamel, E., Hadar, H., Nissenkorn, I. and Servadio, C. (1979). Widespread dissemination of Gelfoam particles complicating occlusion of renal circulation. *Urology*, **14**, 194

24 Tisnado, J., Beachley, M. C., Cho, S. R. and Amendola, M. (1979). Peripheral emboli-

zation of a stainless steel coil. *Am J. Roentgenol.*, **133**, 324

25   Jacob, E. T., Shapira, Z., Morag, B. and Rubenstein, Z. (1979). Hepatic infarction and gallbladder necrosis complicating arterial embolization for bleeding duodenal ulcer. *Dig. Dis. Sci.*, **24**, 482

26   Bradley, E. C., III and Goldman, M. L. (1976). Gastric infarction after therapeutic embolization. *Surgery*, **79**, 421

27   Lina, J. R., Jaques, P. and Mandell, V. (1979). Aneurysm rupture secondary to transcatheter embolization. *Am. J. Roentgenol.*, **132**, 553

28   Winzelberg, G. G., McKusick, K. A., Strauss, H. W., Waltman, A. C. and Greenfield, A. J. (1979). Evaluation of gastrointestinal bleeding by red blood cells labeled in vivo with Technetium-99m. *J. Nucl. Med.*, **20**, 1080

29   Athanasoulis, C. A., Waltman, A. C., Novelline, R. A., Krudy, A. G. and Sniderman, K. W. (1976). Angiography: its contribution to emergency management of gastrointestinal hemorrhage. *Radiol. Clin. N. Am.*, **14**, 265

30   Athanasoulis, C. A., Moncure, A. C., Greenfield, A. J., Ryan, J. A. and Dodson, T. F. (1980). Intraoperative localization of small bowel bleeding sites with combined use of angiographic methods and methylene blue injection. *Surgery*, **87**, 77

31   Baum, S., Athanasoulis, C. A. and Waltman, A. C. (1973). Gastrointestinal hemorrhage: angiographic diagnosis and control. *Adv. Surg.*, **7**, 149

32   Ponsky, J. L., Hoffman, M. and Rhodes, R. S. (1979). Arteriovenous fistula and portal hypertension secondary to islet-cell tumor of the pancreas. *Surgery*, **85**, 408

33   Baum, S. and Nusbaum, M. (1971). The control of gastrointestinal hemorrhage by selective mesenteric arterial infusion of vasopressin. *Radiology*, **98**, 497

34   Athanasoulis, C. A., Baum, S., Waltman, A. C., Ring, E. J., Imbembo, A. and VanderSalm, T. J. (1974). Control of acute gastric mucosal hemorrhage. *N. Engl. J. Med.*, **290**, 597

35   Filston, H. C., Jackson, D. C. and Johnsrude, I. S. (1979). Arteriographic embolization for control of recurrent severe gastric hemorrhage in a 10 year old boy. *J. Pediat. Surg.*, **14**, 276

36   Eisenberg, H. and Steer, M. (1976). The nonoperative treatment of massive pyloroduodenal hemorrhage by retracted autogenous clot embolization. *Surgery*, **79**, 414

37   Granmayeh, M., Wallace, S. and Schwarten, D. (1979). Transcatheter occlusion of the gastroduodenal artery. *Radiology*, **131**, 59

38   Todd, T. R., Weinman, G., McIntyre, D., Simon, J. B., Groll, A. and West, R. O. (1979). Selective superior mesenteric embolization for small intestinal hemorrhage. *Can. J. Surg.*, **22**, 283

39   Greenfield, A. J., Waltman, A. C., Athanasoulis, C. A., Novelline, R. A. and Dedrick, C. G. (1979). Vasopressin in control of gastrointestinal hemorrhage: complications of selective intraarterial vs. systemic infusions. *Gastroenterology*, **76**, 1144

40   Widrich, W. C., Johnson, M. C., Robbins, A. H. and Nabseth, D. C. (1978). Esophagogastric variceal hemorrhage: its treatment by percutaneous transhepatic coronary vein occlusion. *Arch. Surg.*, **113**, 1131

41   Lunderquist, A., Simert, G., Tylén, U. and Vang, J. (1977). Follow-up of patients with portal hypertension and esophageal varices treated with percutaneous obliteration of gastric coronary veins. *Radiology*, **122**, 59

42   Welch, C. E., Athanasoulis, C. A. and Galdabini, J. J. (1978). Hemorrhage from the large bowel with special reference to angiodysplasia and diverticular disease. *World J. Surg.*, **2**, 73

43   Athanasoulis, C. A., Galdabini, J. J., Waltman, A. C., Novelline, R. A., Greenfield, A. J. and Ezpeleta, M. L. (1978). Angiodysplasia of the colon: a cause of rectal bleeding. *Cardiovasc. Radiol.*, **1**, 3

44   Tubiana, J. M., Dana, A., Regent, D., Son, D. T. and Chermet, J. (1978). Etude critique de la valeur de l'artériographie mésentérique supérieure dans le diagnostic des

deverticules de Meckel. *Radiol. Electrol.*, **59**, 689

45   Boley, S. J., DiBiase, A., Brandt, L. J. and Sammartano, R. J. (1979). Lower intestinal bleeding in the elderly. *Am. J. Surg.*, **137**, 57

46   Athanasoulis, C. A., Baum, S., Rösch, J., Waltman, A. C., Ring, E. J., Smith, J. C., Jr, Sugarbaker, E. and Wood, W. (1975). Mesenteric arterial infusions of vasopressin for hemorrhage from colonic diverticulosis. *Am. J. Surg.*, **129**, 212

47   Bookstein, J. J., Noderi, M. J. and Walter, J. F. (1978). Transcatheter embolization for lower gastrointestinal bleeding. *Radiology*, **127**, 345

48   Mays, E. T., Conti, S., Fallahzadeh, H. and Rosenblatt, M. (1979). Hepatic artery ligation. *Surgery*, **86**, 536

49   Shi, E. C. and Ham, J. M. (1978). Traumatic haemobilia treated by hepatic artery ligation. *Aust. N.Z. J. Surg.*, **48**, 550

50   Lewis, R. T. (1979). Nontraumatic hematobilia: disparate episodes 7 years apart in the same patient. *Can. J. Surg.*, **22**, 175

51   Jona, J. Z. (1978). Ligation of the main hepatic artery for exsanguinating liver laceration in an adolescent. *J. Trauma*, **18**, 225

52   Floyd, W. N., Jr (1979). Traumatic hemobilia: coordination of roentgenographic, scintigraphic and angiographic findings. *South. Med. J.*, **72**, 420

53   Aldrete, J. S., Halpern, N. B., Ward, S. and Wright, J. O. (1979). Factors determining the mortality and morbidity in hepatic injuries. Analysis of 108 cases. *Ann. Surg.*, **189**, 466

54   Touloune, F., Meslout, A., Belyamani, K. and Benyahia, B. (1978). Embolisation de l'artère hépatique dans le cas de traumatisme du foie. *Maroc Med.*, **1**, 45

55   Parc, R., Legros, A., Huguet, C., Malafosse, M., Bloch, P., Gallot, D. and Loygue, J. (1979). Embolisations et désantérialisations hépatiques. A propos de 32 observations. *Ann. Chir.*, **32**, 713

56   Lambeth, W. and Rubin, B. E. (1979). Nonoperative management of intrahepatic hemorrhage and hematoma following blunt trauma. *Surg. Gynecol. Obstet.*, **148**, 507

57   Porter, L. L., III, Houston, M. C. and Kadir, S. (1979). Mycotic aneurysms of the hepatic artery. Treatment with arterial embolization. *Am. J. Med.*, **67**, 697

58   White, A., Baum, S. and Buranasiri, S. (1976). Aneurysms secondary to pancreatitis. *Am. J. Roentgenol.*, **127**, 393

59   Starling, J. R. and Crummy, A. B. (1979). Hemosuccus pancreaticus secondary to ruptured splenic artery aneurysm. *Dig. Dis. Sci.*, **24**, 726

60   Bivins, B. A., Sachatello, C. R., Chuang, V. P. and Brady, P. (1978). Hemosuccus pancreaticus (hemoductal pancreatitis): gastrointestinal hemorrhage due to rupture of a splenic artery aneurysm into the pancreatic duct. *Arch. Surg.*, **113**, 751

61   Lacey, D. T., Smith, M. J. V. and Koontz, W. W., Jr (1972). Modern trends in the management of urologic trauma. *J. Urol.*, **107**, 641

62   Rizk, G. K., Atallah, N. K. and Bridi, G. I. (1973). Renal arteriovenous fistula treated by catheter embolization. *Br. J. Radiol.*, **46**, 222

63   Chuang, V. P., Reuter, S. R., Walter, J., Foley, W. D. and Bookstein, J. J. (1975). Control of renal hemorrhage by selective arterial embolization. *Am. J. Roentgenol.*, **125**, 300

64   Meng, C. H. and Elkin, M. (1971). Immediate angiographic manifestations of iatrogenic renal injury due to percutaneous needle biopsy. *Radiology*, **100**, 335

65   Bookstein, J. J. and Goldstein, H. M. (1973). Successful management of post biopsy arteriovenous fistula with selective arterial embolization. *Radiology*, **109**, 535

66   Silber, S. J. and Clark, R. E. (1975). Treatment of massive hemorrhage after renal biopsy with angiographic injection of clot. *N. Engl. J. Med.*, **292**, 1387

67   Goldman, M. L., Fellner, S. K. and Parrott, T. S. (1975). Transcatheter embolization of renal arteriovenous fistula. *Urology*, **6**, 386

68   Thomas, T. J., Hodgson, N. B. and Maddison, F. E. (1975). Therapeutic ureteral

obstruction and renal artery embolization. *J. Urol.*, **114**, 518

69 Barbaric, Z. L. and Cutcliff, W. B. (1976). Control of renal arterial bleeding after percutaneous biopsy. *Urology*, **8**, 108

70 Maxwell, D. D. and Frankel, R. S. (1976). Wedged catheter management of a bleeding renal pseudoaneurysm. *J. Urol.*, **116**, 96

71 Chan, J., Katzen, B. T. and Sullivan, K. P. (1978). Transcatheter Gelfoam embolization of post-traumatic bleeding pseudoaneurysms. *Am. J. Roentgenol.*, **131**, 645

72 Kaufman, S. L., Freeman, C., Busky, S. M. and White, R. I. (1976). Management of postoperative renal haemorrhage by transcatheter embolization. *J. Urol.*, **115**, 203

73 Richman, S. D., Green, W. M., Kroll, R. and Casarella, W. J. (1977). Superselective transcatheter embolization of traumatic renal haemorrhage. *Am. J. Roentgenol.*, **128**, 843

74 Kalish, M., Greenbaum, L., Silber, S. and Goldstein, H. (1974). Traumatic renal haemorrhage: treatment by arterial embolization. *J. Urol.*, **112**, 138

75 Blackwell, J. E., Potchen, E. J., Laidlaw, W. W. and Paul, L. H. (1978). Traumatic arteriocaliceal fistula. *Radiology*, **129**, 633

76 Moorhead, J. D., Fritzche, P. and Hadley, H. L. (1977). Management of haemorrhage secondary to renal angiomyolipoma with selective arterial embolization. *J. Urol.*, **117**, 122

77 Schurholz, K. H., Weissbach, L., Thelen, M. and Bueheler, E. (1977). Renal hamartoma – therapeutic aspects. *Eur. Urol.*, **3**, 346

78 Goldstein, H. M., Wallace, S., Anderson, J. H., Bree, R. L. and Gianturco, C. (1976). Transcatheter occlusion of abdominal tumors. *Radiology*, **120**, 539

79 Goldstein, H. M., Medellin, K., Beydoun, M. T., Wallace, S., Ben-Menachem, Y., Bracke, R. B. and Johnson, D. E. (1975). Transcatheter embolization of renal cell carcinoma. *Am. J. Roentgenol.*, **123**, 557

80 Almgärd, L. E. and Slezak, D. (1977). Treatment of renal adenocarcinoma by embolization: a follow-up of 38 cases. *Eur. Urol.*, **3**, 279

81 Mariasoosai, M., Wilson, A. and Gonick, P. (1977). Selective renal artery embolization: treatment for metastatic sarcoma with hematuria. *J. Am. Med. Assoc.*, **237**, 363

82 Hold, T. and Mygind, T. (1974). Control of life-threatening vesical haemorrhage by unilateral hyposgastric artery muscle embolization. *J. Urol.*, **112**, 60

83 Higgins, C. B., Bookstein, J. J., Davis, G. B., Galloway, D. C. and Barr, J. W. (1977). Therapeutic embolization for intractable chronic bleeding. *Radiology*, **122**, 473

84 Bruhl, D. and Thelen, M. (1978). Selective transfemoral embolization of the internal iliac artery in carcinoma of the bladder. *Dtsch. Med. Wochenschr.*, **103**, 737

85 Mitchell, M. E., Waltman, A. C., Athanasoulis, C. A., Kerr, W. S., Jr and Dretler, S. P. (1976). Control of massive prostatic bleeding with angiographic techniques. *J. Urol.*, **115**, 692

86 Bree, R. L., Goldstein, H. M. and Wallace, S. (1976). Transcatheter embolization of the internal iliac artery in the management of neoplasms of the pelvis. *Surg. Gynecol. Obstet.*, **143**, 597

87 Olcott, C., Newton, T. H., Stoney, R. J. and Ehrenfeld, W. K. (1976). Intra-arterial embolization in the management of arteriovenous malformations. *Surgery*, **79**, 3

88 Schwartz, P. E., Goldstein, H. M., Wallace, S. and Rutledge, F. N. (1975). Control of arterial haemorrhage using percutaneous arterial catheter techniques in patients with gynecologic malignancies. *Gynecol. Oncol.*, **3**, 276

89 Athanasoulis, C. A., Waltman, A. C., Barnes, A. B. and Herbst, A. L. (1976). Angiographic control of pelvic bleeding from treated carcinoma of the cervix. *Gynecol. Oncol.*, **4**, 144

90 Miller, F. J., Jr, Martel, R., Mann, W. J. and Jahshaw, A. E. (1976). Selective arterial embolization for control of hemorrhage in pelvic malignancy: femoral and brachial catheter approaches. *Am. J. Roentgenol.*, **126**, 1028

91   Smith, D. C. and Wyatt, J. F. (1977). Embolization of the hypogastric arteries in the control of massive vaginal hemorrhage. *Obstet. Gynecol.*, **49**, 317
92   Patterson, F. P. and Morton, K. S. (1973). The cause of death in fracture of the pelvis. *J. Trauma*, **13**, 849
93   Maull, K. I. and Sachatello, C. R. (1976). Current management of pelvic fractures. *South. Med. J.*, **69**, 1285
94   Margolies, M. N., Ring, E. J., Waltman, A. C., Kerr, W. S. and Baum, S. (1972). Arteriography in the management of hemorrhage from pelvic fractures. *N. Engl. J. Med.*, **287**, 317
95   Ring, E. J., Athanasoulis, C. A., Waltman, A. C., Margolies, M. N. and Baum, S. Arteriographic management of hemorrhage following pelvic fracture. *Radiology*, **109**, 65
96   Ring, E. J., Waltman, A. C., Athanasoulis, C. A., Smith, J. C. and Baum, S. (1974). Angiography in pelvic trauma. *Surg. Gynecol. Obstet.*, **139**, 375
97   Matalon, T. S. A., Athanasoulis, C. A., Margolies, M. N., Waltman, A. C., Novelline, R. A., Greenfield, A. J. and Miller, S. E. (1979). Hemorrhage with pelvic fractures: efficacy of transcatheter embolization. *Am. J. Roentgenol.*, **133**, 859
98   Athanasoulis, C. A., Harris, W. H., Stock, J. R. and Waltman, A. C. (1979). Arterial embolization to control pelvic hemorrhage. Proceedings of the *Hip Society Seventh Open Scientific Meeting*, February. Chapter 12, pp. 247–259. (C. V. Mosby)
99   Goldin, A. R., Walker, W. J. and Goldblatt, M. (1978). Therapeutic embolization for spontaneous retroperitoneal and extravesical haemorrhage. *Australas. Radiol.*, **22**, 158
100 Hood, J. M. and Smyth, B. T. (1974). Nonpenetrating intraabdominal injuries in children. *J. Pediat. Surg.*, **99**, 69
101 Brindle, M. J. (1972). Arteriography and minor splenic injury. *Clin. Radiol.*, **23**, 174
102 Morag, B. and Rubinstein, Z. J. (1978). Conservative management of splenic trauma: Angiographic observations. *ROEFO*, **129**, 517
103 Sherman, R. (1980). Perspectives in management of trauma to the spleen: 1979 Presidential Address, American Association for the Surgery of Trauma. *J. Trauma*, **20**, 1
104 Fischer, K. C., Eraklis, A., Rosello, P. and Treves, S. (1978). Scintigraphy in the follow-up of pediatric splenic trauma treated without surgery. *J. Nucl. Med.*, **19**, 3
105 Goldman, M., Land, W. and Bradley, E. (1976). Transcatheter therapeutic embolization in the management of massive gastro-intestinal bleeding. *Radiology*, **120**, 513
106 Johnsrude, I. S. and Jackson, D. C. (1979). Therapeutic catheterization. In Johnsrude, I. S. and Jackson, D.C. (eds.). *A Practical Approach to Angiography*, pp. 497–520. (Boston: Little Brown & Co.)
107 Probst, P., Castaneda-Zuniga, W. R., Gomes, A. S., Yonebiro, E. G., Delaney, J. P. and Amplatz, K. (1978). Nonsurgical treatment of splenic artery aneurysms. *Radiology*, **128**, 619
108 Thoms, N. W., Wilson, R. F. and Puro, H. E. (1972). Life-threatening hemoptysis in primary lung abscesses. *Ann. Thor. Surg.*, **14**, 347
109 Wagner, R. B., Baeza, O. R. and Stewart, J. E. (1975). Active pulmonary hemorrhage localized by selective pulmonary arteriography. *Chest*, **67**, 121
110 Wholey, M. H., Chamorro, H. W., Rao, G., Ford, W. B. and Miller, W. H. (1976). Bronchial artery embolization for massive hemoptysis. *J. Am. Med. Assoc.*, **236**, 2501
111 Rémy, J., Arnaud, A., Fandou, H., Giraud, R. and Voisin, C. (1977). Treatment of hemoptysis by embolization of bronchial arteries. *Radiology*, **122**, 33
112 Fellows, K. E., Khaw, K. T., Schuster, S. and Shwachman, H. (1979). Bronchial artery embolization in cystic fibrosis. Technique and long term results. *J. Pediatr.*, **95**, 959
113 Sokoloff, J., Wickbom, I., McDonald, D., Brahme, F., Goergen, T. G. and Goldberger, L. E. (1974). Therapeutic percutaneous embolization in intractable epistaxis. *Radiology*, **111**, 285
114 Strother, C. M. and Newton, T. H. (1976). Percutaneous embolization to control epi-

staxis in Render-Osler-Weber disease. *Arch. Otolaryngol.*, **102,** 58

115 Roberson, G. H. and Reardon, E. J. (1979). Angiography and embolization of the internal maxillary artery for posterior epistaxis. *Arch. Otolangngol.*, **105,** 333

116 Higgins, C. B., Siemens, P. T., Bookstein, J. J. and Utley, J. R. (1979). Control of hemorrhage from a common carotid arterial-cutaneous fistula by temporary implantation of a balloon catheter. *Radiology*, **132,** 224

117 Prian, G. W. and Pearlman, N. W. (1978). Permanent control of massive tumor bleeding with intraluminal balloon catheters. *Head Neck Surg.*, **1,** 148

4
Oncofetal antigens in gastrointestinal cancer

E. D. HOLYOKE

Gold identified a glycoprotein antigen associated with fetal gut and colon cancer tissue in 1965[1]. He designated this antigen carcinoembryonic antigen, or CEA for short. Shortly after this Peter Alexander noted that there are a group of substances found in various malignant tumours and in appropriate fetal tissues with either no identifiable, or, as the sensitivity of our techniques has improved, markedly reduced material in the corresponding adult tissue. He called these oncofetal antigens[2]. Since these materials are only quantitatively different in tumour as compared to their tissues of origin and appear in a variety of malignancies, they have also been called 'tumor-associated antigens'. The first clinical studies evaluating CEA as a tumour marker in serum in patients with cancer of the colon and rectum were reported in 1968[3]. Widespread clinical study began shortly thereafter. Under the impetus of the work with CEA, the search for other oncofetal antigens, as well as for more specific antigenic materials, has burgeoned. Because pancreatic, hepatobiliary, gastric, as well as colorectal cancer at different times in their course may be very difficult to diagnose or stage, and because CEA as well as alpha-fetoprotein (AFP) were originally reported in colon and hepatic tumours respectively, it is not surprising that the majority of studies performed in the last decade have sought for and tested tumour markers which might be of potential use in treating patients with gastrointestinal cancer[4,5]. Over the past decade a great deal of information has been accumulated, a number of oncofetal antigens identified, and we are able to make some statements about their use in patients with gastrointestinal malignancy.

PANCREATIC CANCER

Pancreatic cancer is a disease entity which is usually identified at a stage when it is not resectable, or if resectable not curable, with an overall survival rate of 1% at 5 years, so that it is attractive to attempt to improve our treatment success in this disease by developing a means of screening or detection before symptoms occur. A tumour marker with enough sensitivity or specificity to serve as a diagnostic adjunct would also be of assistance in treating such patients. Firstly, a tumour marker for pancreatic cancer might permit earlier diagnosis, at least within the symptomatic population. Secondly, such a marker might be accurate enough to serve as a staging mechanism so that it could reduce the numbers of unnecessary laparatomies for inoperable disease and permit more precise decisions concerning adjuvant and/or combined modality treatment.

Several pancreatic antigens have been identified. Banwo first reported the identification of a pancreatic oncofetal antigen with potential for use as a tumour marker[6]. Although some time has passed, this report has unfortunately not seen further elucidation or follow-up. In Banwo's study antisera were raised in rabbits against homogenates of human fetal pancreas. Using immune electrophoresis techniques, 36 of 37 patients with cancer of the pancreas were found to have demonstrable circulating antigen. This was not identified in a control group of patients, including several with other gastrointestinal tumours with an associated elevation of serum CEA.

A second pancreas-associated oncofetal antigen (POA), a glycoprotein, was reported by Gelder from Chicago[7]. This material has been demonstrated to be distinct from CEA. Wood and Moosa concluded after study that the test had a low accuracy as far as true positivity was concerned, but that a negative test could be considered useful, with a true negativity rate approaching 94%[8]. As seen in Figure 1, except for rare patients with severe pancreatitis, Gelder found an elevated POA to be quite significant for tumour[9]. Unfortunately, patients with other biliary diseases also show a positive POA[10].

It should be apparent to the clinician that initial reports of potentially useful markers for pancreatic cancer must be evaluated with particular care. This was most clearly illustrated for us when we found that by measuring simple light transmittance in serum we could identify 90% of patients with pancreatic cancer compared to a healthy population[11]; however, moderate to severe benign disease caused a similar reduction in light transmittance. It is necessary when evaluating any marker to review adequate information concerning possible elevation of the test substance in the presence of benign disease. In reviewing markers for the detection of pancreatic cancer in particular, it is necessary to examine the stage of the disease reported, as most individuals considered will have moderate to far-advanced disease.

Other glycoprotein antigens have been studied in patients with pancreatic cancer. The Mayo Clinic group studied AFP in patients with pancreatic cancer and found that it offered no real promise, either diagnostically or assisting in treatment[12]. Mihas also immunized rabbits

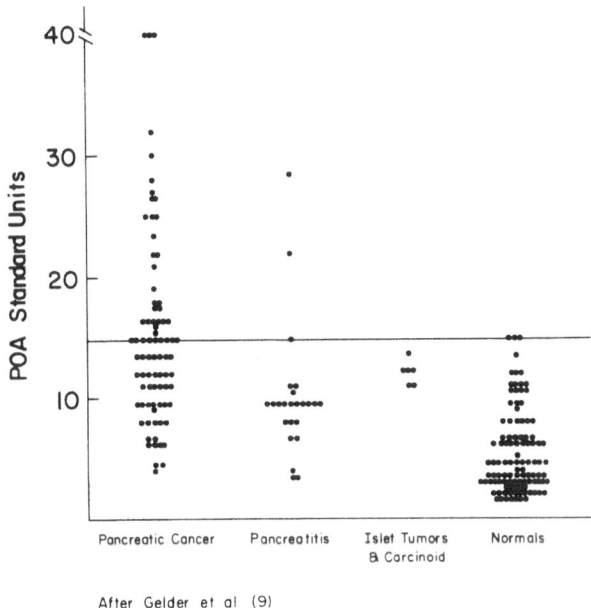

After Gelder et al (9)

Figure 1 Gelder has demonstrated that an elevated pancreatic oncofetal antigen, as seen in this figure, is quite significant in the absence of benign disease

with human fetal pancreas extract and identified an antigen which he called pancreatic oncofetal protein or POP[13]. The material is related to, but distinct from, AFP and is primarily a protein as indicated by enzymatic degradation with trypsin. Clinical data regarding POP are not available. Mesa-Tejada *et al.* prepared an aqueous extract of pancreatic cancer and identified a tumour-associated antigen which was widely cross-reactive, related to lung and colon cancer as well as pancreatic cancer. Indeed, this is more of a gut-associated antigen although it was first identified in the pancreas[14]. Additional markers which have not yet been linked to pancreatic cancer include NCA or non-cross reacting antigen; EDC1, an interesting glycoprotein found in urine; Tennagen; and alpha-2-glycoprotein.

Carcinoembryonic antigen has been tested as a screening marker for pancreatic cancer with banked serum samples from the Framingham Study[15]. CEA, human chorionic gonadotrophin (HCG), and AFP assays were carried out simultaneously using serum samples from nine patients who developed proven pancreatic cancer. CEA appeared elevated up to 10 months before detection of the disease by any other means. HCG levels were only elevated in one patient, and AFP levels demonstrated no significant elevation. However a control test group composed of smokers with diminished vital capacity, but of similar age to our patients with pancreatic cancer, showed a false-positive rate of 20%. This is too high a frequency of spuriously positive values for the assay to be useful in screening an asymptomatic population.

At Roswell Park we reached a similar conclusion after screening an older executive population for possible cancer using the CEA assay for several years[16]. After more than 2000 determinations, only one unknown malignancy which was potentially treatable for cure was identified. This meant a cost of at least $20 000 US spent in order to detect one tumour without considering the problem of false-positive results, which would add a great deal more expense.

The false-positivity problem also severely limits the use of CEA as a diagnostic adjunct for pancreatic cancer. Lurie et al. reported that 52% of their patients with benign disease who were jaundiced demonstrated an elevation in serum CEA[17]. Similarly, Khoo and MacKay reported that CEA is often elevated in biliary cirrhosis[18] and Moore et al. reported that almost 50% of individuals with severe alcoholic cirrhosis showed a rise in CEA[19]. This work agrees with the data of Hansen et al.[20]: 91% of 55 patients with histologically proven pancreatic carcinoma demonstrated a plasma level of CEA greater than 2.5 ng/ml and 60% greater than 5 ng/ml. Ona et al.[21] also reported that 17 of 23 patients with pancreatic cancer demonstrated values greater than 2.5 ng/ml. They found that values greater than 10 ng/ml indicated metastatic disease. Kalser studied 102 patients with proven pancreatic cancer[22] who were divided into three groups. Group I included patients with resectable lesions; group II, patients with locally invasive non-resectable cancer; and group III, patients with distant metastatic disease. Table 1 lists the results of CEA assay in these patients. In group I, as well as in patients with pancreatitis, CEA was highest in patients with jaundice. There was little increase in plasma CEA in the jaundiced patients of group III compared with those who were non-jaundiced. In groups II and III approximately 10% of patients demonstrated a normal CEA.

Using CEA as a parameter, there was some survival discrimination in this series. Patients in group III with elevated CEA values died an

Table 1 Circulating carcinoembryonic antigen in patients with pancreatitis and cancer of the pancreas

Group	Description	Number of patients	CEA in plasma		
			<2.5	2.5–5	>5.0
I	Resectable tumour	11	1	2	8
II	Locally invasive non-resectable tumour	34	5	2	27
III	Metastatic tumour	57	3	8	46
Control	Pancreatitis	26	8	8	10

Details from Ref. 22

average of 2 months earlier than those whose CEA values were not initially elevated. For group II patients this difference was somewhat more significant, 5 months. In this context, possibly only patients with a negative or minimally elevated CEA should be put through regional treatment programmes with one of the various combined modality approaches available; this type of selection might at least insure completion of a reasonable portion of planned treatment. McIntire's Gastrointestinal Tumor Study Group review in 1978 indicated a 25-week longer survival for patients with locally unresectable disease and a normal plasma CEA compared to a similar group of patients with an elevated serum CEA[23]. The Mayo Clinic studies have, on the other hand, indicated that Eastern Cooperative Oncology Group (ECOG) performance staging is as accurate as CEA determination in this regard and that stratification beyond this is probably not helpful, at least in patients with metastatic disease[24]. Nevertheless, we believe that this oncofetal antigen or any other oncofetal antigen of similar or greater sensitivity should be stratified in prospective randomized treatment protocols.

Sharma *et al.* studied CEA levels in pancreatic juice[25] and simultaneously measured CEA serum levels. They reported that 75% of a series of 21 patients who had both levels elevated had known cancer. Other workers have suggested that CEA in pancreatic juice might be diagnostic for pancreatic cancer[26, 27]. The Mayo Clinic group carried out a prospective analysis of CEA, trypsin, lipase and bicarbonate in pancreatic juice[28]. They reported that both enzyme output and bicarbonate following cholecystokinin stimulation were more sensitive as indicators of pancreatic cancer than CEA determinations and they do not feel that the measurement of CEA in pancreatic juice is useful.

Barkin *et al.* studied the course of patients with cancer of the pancreas following treatment[29]; CEA levels fell to normal in three of eight patients following pancreatic resection, and, in general, these workers recorded a decrease in plasma CEA levels even when surgical resection was not curative. Unfortunately, among the eight patients with complete resection, the three with values which fell to normal levels did not survive longer than the others. Radiation alone, or in combination with chemotherapy, did not alter CEA levels in patients with locally unresectable pancreatic cancer. In patients with metastatic disease CEA levels usually progressed as the disease led to death.

At present, aside from possible use in staging, particularly for protocol study, we do not see an established clinical use for any of the oncofetal antigens associated with pancreatic cancer tested to date. We may yet have success in identifying other specific pancreatic cancer antigens which may be demonstrated by *in vitro* tests of active materials, such as the LAI assay (leukocyte adherence inhibition). In a recent report we have described our efforts to identify unique pancreatic tumour antigens[30], and we have marked a promising glycoprotein in the ascitic fluid of pancreatic tumour patients[31]. We have also found a distinct perchloric-acid-soluble glycoprotein preparation in pancreatic tumour tissue[32]. It is hoped that further use of immunological methods of testing, including the LAI assay and the use of hybridomas in the search for pancreatic tissue-specific antigens, will prove fruitful.

GASTRIC CANCER

In spite of extensive endoscopy programmes carried out in Japan and because of a lower incidence of gastric carcinoma in the west, less invasive and more economical screening techniques are needed[33-35]. Because of endoscopic progress and availability, diagnostic serological tests have appeared less necessary for gastric cancer. Because treatment is relatively successful and the natural course of the disease following detection is longer, however, there is more opportunity for using a serological monitor in gastric cancer patients than in those with pancreatic malignancy.

Hakkinen *et al.* described a fetal sulphoglycoprotein antigen (FSA) in gastric juice in 1976[36]. This marker can be identified by histopathological study in malignant gastric cells but this is, once more, a quantitative finding and FSA can be identified in the mucosa of non-cancerous individuals and in fetal gut. FSA is an active secretion product and is always found in higher concentration in gastric secretions than in gastric mucosa.

Unfortunately, in addition to low sensitivity in patients with gastric cancer, FSA screening of a control population aged 40–70 years revealed a 6–9% false-positive rate[37]. Because of this and other vagaries associated with an assay depending on the collection of gastric secretions with a nasogastric tube, FSA determination has proved to be of limited usefulness in screening, diagnosis or monitoring of gastric cancer and is not used.

In 1978 Ishii reported a tumour antigen, serum basic ferroprotein or BFP[38]. This marker is associated with gastric cancer as well as a variety of other malignancies. On the favourable side, over 30% of individuals with gastric cancer are positive on BFP radioimmunoassay but the positive patients are those with more advanced disease. Moreover, up to 40% false-positives are found and are associated with such benign disease as cirrhosis.

Another tumour marker is serum C3DNA-binding protein (C3DP). This fragment of complement has been found elevated in several patients with known gastric cancer[39], but there are apparent problems with stability and consistency with the C3DP assay. Reports involving large and organized series have not appeared. AFP has been studied as a possible marker for gastric cancer[40]. It is clear, however, that from the point of view of clinical utility for gastric cancer, when sera of only 4 of 17 patients with non-hepatic metastases and 8 of 20 patients with hepatic metastases are positive, AFP is neither sensitive nor specific enough.

Björklund et al. have identified a polypeptide in several malignancies which has antigenic properties and which they have designated tissue polypeptide antigen or TPA[41-43]. This polypeptide is identified by haemagglutination assay. Menendez-Botet and Schwartz have surveyed the frequency of TPA elevation for a number of tumour sites[44] and 23 of 31 patients with gastric cancer demonstrated positive assays. In individuals with benign disease, 40 of 112, or 36%, had TPA levels that were elevated and 2 of 67 young and healthy individuals had significantly elevated levels of serum TPA. Holyoke and Chu[45] carried out simultaneous measurements of TPA and CEA in a small group of gastric, pancreatic and colonic cancer patients listed in Table 2. TPA is clearly

Table 2 TPA and CEA determinations in patients with gastrointestinal malignancy

Tumour type	TPA No. elevated/total no.	CEA No. elevated/total no.	Either No. elevated/total no.
Pancreas	6/10	4/10	8/10
Gastric	2/6	2/6	3/6
Colon	21/47	31/47	31/47

not more sensitive in the detection of gastric malignancy than CEA, and there is no evidence for any additive gain. The data with regard to pancreatic cancer may be a little more interesting.

CEA was originally reported as specific for colonic cancer[3]. However, it is now known to be elevated in the plasma of some individuals with a variety of cancers[46, 47]. Early reports of positive radioimmunoassay rates of greater than 70% in patients with metastatic gastric cancer were encouraging[48] but, as seen in our TPA–CEA comparative study at Roswell Park, our figures were considerably lower[45]. Ravry reported that only one of eight patients with regional disease was CEA-positive and in his series of patients with metastatic disease, only 9 of 37 patients demonstrated a plasma CEA greater than 2.5 ng/ml, and for patients with nonhepatic metastases the figure was only 2 of 17[49]. CEA is not useful in the screening, diagnosis, or monitoring of gastric cancer; even in staging it appears of very limited value. For gastric cancer there are no established markers which are presently useful to the clinician in any practical sense.

COLORECTAL CANCER

The use of CEA in patients with colorectal cancer has been extensively studied since 1968. The possible use of CEA screening has been settled in the negative[50]: sensitivity and specificity are simply not good enough. In general, CEA is also of limited use as a diagnostic adjunct in symptomatic patients[51]. It is unfortunate that in those patients in whom it is most difficult to identify malignancy using standard means, either because the disease is early or because of some accompanying benign inflammatory disease, a high percentage of false-negative and false-positive results prevent this assay from being of real assistance. Although comparative diagnostic studies are always difficult to evaluate, most studies would indicate that CEA and barium enema are comparably helpful, so that, in selected instances, CEA determinations could conceivably be of assistance[52, 53]. Good comparison studies with contrast enemas require the use of air contrast studies, however, and colonoscopy appears to be a superior technique in any event[54]. From our studies and a review of the literature we conclude that CEA determinations are of diagnostic help in only a small group of symptomatic individuals.

We reported earlier that an elevated presurgical CEA correlated with a higher incidence of later tumour recurrence[55, 56]. Mach and Zamcheck have recorded similar findings[57, 58]. These observations raise the question as to how CEA levels in plasma relate to stage of disease. Does the CEA level in plasma relate more accurately to outcome than careful clinicopathological staging? We have found in repeated studies that CEA is predictive and that it does correlate with clinicopathological staging[59, 60]. In our hands CEA is a better staging technique than a simple recording of Dukes A, B or C disease. A modified Dukes staging, after Astler Coller, with Stages A, B_1, B_2, C_1, C_2, seems to be about as predictive as CEA assay, but even when compared to this more precise pathological system, the CEA plasma level will identify groups at more or less risk within the C_1 or C_2 categories[61].

Table 3 Roswell Park TNM classification for colorectal cancer

T_0 – No tumour
T_1 – Tumour in mucosa
T_2 – Tumour penetrates muscularis
T_3 – Tumour penetrates through serosa
T_4 – Tumour invades adjacent structures

N_0 – No lymph nodes involved
N_1 – One or two positive nodes close to the primary tumour
N_2 – One to three positive nodes approaching the apex of the resected mesentery
N_3 – Four or more positive nodes, or positive nodes at the apex of the resected specimen

M_0 – No metastases present
M_1 – Metastases present

We have developed an in-house TNM staging programme (Table 3)[62]. In our population the majority of post surgical recurrences have developed in patients originally noted as having T_4 lesions, i.e. those with frank invasion of adjacent structures, or N_2–N_3 patients, those with four or more lymph nodes involved with tumour or with tumour-bearing nodes located near the apex of the surgical specimen. In our study the key group was unfortunately quite small after all the patients were carefully subdivided by stage. There were nine T_2–T_3 patients with disease penetrating or perforating the wall of the colon, and with N_1 nodes, less than four nodes clustered reasonably close to the tumour. None of the patients in this group with a normal presurgical CEA had tumour recurrence but three of four patients with a CEA which was elevated prior to definitive surgery later developed recurrence. Our conclusion has continued to be that overall CEA values are predictive of recurrence and that the level of discrimination approaches that seen with careful and detailed histopathological staging.

The question remains whether or not CEA determinations are additive to careful staging if both techniques are used to attempt to improve stratification. Although CEA does approximate stage, there are some patients who have a very small amount of tumour with rather high plasma CEA, and some patients with a considerable quantity of advanced tumour who show no antigen elevation. CEA evidently measures a parameter other than tumour size or bulk which reflects net amount of material released from the tumour. It is difficult to show that CEA measurement adds to careful staging because of the numbers of patients needed in follow-up to recurrence to reach a definitive answer. Our overall data indicate that there is some addition and that CEA will help define patients at risk within the T_2–T_3 and N_1–N_2 groups[63], but the evidence is less secure than we would like. Perhaps the Gastrointestinal Tumor Study Group data of presurgical CEA levels versus pathological stage and outcome may help, but these data have not yet been fully analysed[64].

At present we recommend that a CEA determination should be done on all patients with colorectal cancer to help the operating surgeon and oncologists in estimating the possible advantage, particularly for rectal cancer, of adjuvant therapy. We believe that CEA staging for stratification in patients undergoing prospective randomized studies is important and should be developed.

We have studied CEA as a monitor of recurrence of colonic cancer, as have many others[65–68]. In a series of 60 patients, we reviewed over 900 post-surgical CEA measurements. About 15% of the patients in our population and assayed in our laboratory demonstrated a spurious elevation of two consecutive values. To assure an 65–70% certainty of finding residual cancer in one of our asymptomatic patients followed after 'curative' resection for colorectal cancer, we required two consecutive CEA values greater than 5 ng/ml. All patients with a single plasma CEA greater than 25 ng/ml demonstrated a recurrence on investigation. Also, on review to date, all patients who have had successively elevated CEA values, with the second value increased by more than 5 ng/ml over the first, have proved to have recurrent cancer[69,70]. In our clinical population, where patients are seen monthly for a physical examination and symptom review with frequent scan and X-ray follow-up, we have found that 30–40% of our patients have a significant elevation of plasma CEA before the disease is detected by other means. As we have pointed out, the usefulness of this finding is limited by the fact that spurious elevations can occur in perhaps 25% of patients as a single event, and two consecutive elevations may still falsely indicate the presence of tumour in 30–35% of our patients. In some of our patients we have found that this type of rise may occur following a course of chemotherapy such as with MeCCNU. Other tumour enzymes may be increased simultaneously and we believe the elevation represents parenchymal damage which is drug induced (Figure 2). If the CEA value is still elevated between 30 and 45 days after surgery, early clinical recurrence is probable.

One outstanding question at present, in the clinical use of tumour markers, is whether or not the CEA assay can assist us in monitoring

patients with colorectal cancer. The basis for any success must be the
timely detection of early clinical recurrence of colorectal cancer using the
CEA assay and the success of second surgery and chemotherapy.
Martin and Minton present the most optimistic findings related to
patient follow-up[71,72]. From their data they believe that CEA levels
should be assayed every month or two for at least the first 2 years following definitive surgery and they do not question that CEA determinations are the most reliable indicators of recurrent colorectal cancer. A
reason for advocating frequent assays for the first 2 years is that in
Morton and Minton's experience two-thirds of recurrences appear in
the first 18 months after removal of the primary tumour. They have
reported two main studies[73,74]. The first was a retrospective series
begun in 1972 which included patients entered through 1975. The
second or prospective study began in 1976. In this work Martin's major
contribution has been the development of a nomogram defining at the
level of two standard deviations the intra- and inter-assay variations
inherent in CEA determinations. This allows us to note small deviations
from normal which occur at low CEA levels. In addition a nadir speci-

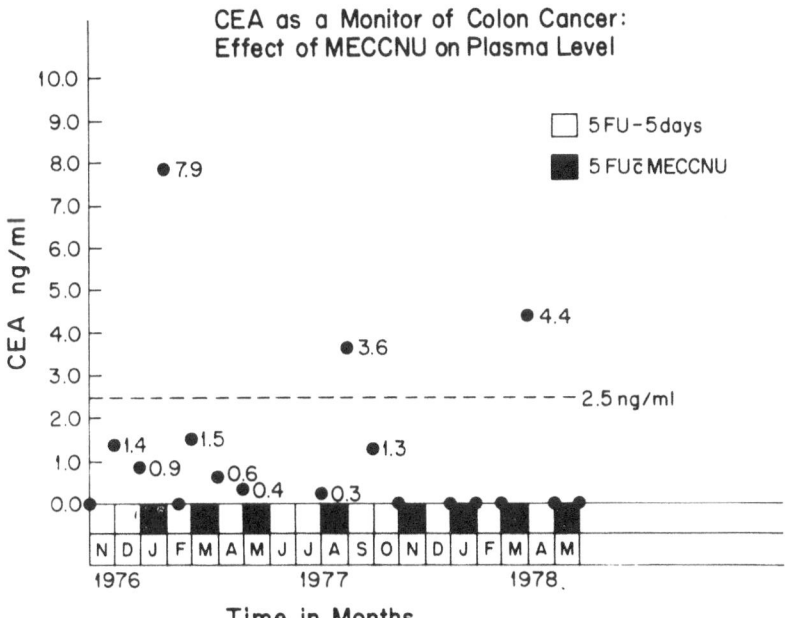

Figure 2 In this patient, sporadic rises in CEA appeared three times over 18 months of
chemotherapy, each time following MeCCNU and 5FU so that a rise was seen following
three of eight courses of both drugs. No rise was seen after nine courses of 5FU alone

men, taken between 1 and 2 months post-reaction, is kept on these patients and if there is evidence of a later elevation, another serum sample is tested against an aliquot of this specimen to further control spurious variation.

In the retrospective study 22 patients underwent a CEA-detected second operation. Recurrent tumour was found in 19 individuals and in six this was resectable so that in slightly more than one in four patients with an elevated CEA, recurrent disease was resectable. The figures reported in 1978 for this prospective study appeared somewhat better. Seventeen of 18 patients demonstrated tumour and it was technically resectable in 13 of these, or 60%. One problem with these reports is that it is not possible to determine whether any of these patients could have been diagnosed as having recurrent tumour by more conventional tests or whether an elevation of CEA was the sole evidence of tumour. However, our experience is not greatly different from these reports overall. If we list those patients operated on for an an elevated CEA, we also found that more than 80% had recurrent tumour but this figure includes patients also found to have other evidence of tumour on endoscopy, X-ray, scan, other enzyme assay or physical examination. We have explored nine patients with two consecutive elevations of CEA who came to laparotomy with no other evidence of tumour aside from an elevated CEA following extensive evalution. Six of these did have tumour and in two the disease was resectable; in one disease was partially resectable and residual tumour was clipped for subsequent radiation therapy and prolonged freedom from disease. It is of interest that in Minton's original series of six patients in whom resection was apparently possible, four were free of disease for more than 3 years.

There are studies which caution against the use of CEA as a monitor for recurrent colorectal cancer. Mach et al. have indicated some of the problems associated with false positivity[75-77]. Moertel report a group of patients with otherwise diagnosable disease recurrence or with clinical evidence of disease progression and a continuing negative CEA assay. The study of Cohen and Wood properly points out that CEA is at its best in reporting liver metastases, a group of patients who may not be much helped by therapy[78]. It is surprising that an organized study of second-look surgery has not been established since only in this way can the CEA assay be convincingly established as a useful means of monitoring colorectal cancer in the initial 2 years following surgery. We recommend that, in addition to the preoperative CEA determination, a CEA level be done following definitive surgery in Dukes B_2, and C_1 and C_2 lesions beginning about 45 days after surgery and continuing for 2 years at 2-month intervals and until 5 years at 3-month intervals thereafter.

The use of CEA to assess and quantitate the effectiveness of chemotherapy or radiotherapy, particularly for advanced disease, has been studied by several clinical groups[79-81]. The results from the Mayo Clinic indicate that there is not a strong correlation between the effects of chemotherapy for metastatic disease and changes in serum CEA[82]. We did find an overall correlation, but it was not as reliable as we would like[83]. One of the problems we found was that near the end of a patient's illness CEA production or release sometimes falls without apparent reduction in tumour bulk.

We also found that chemotherapy did reduce levels of circulating tumour antigen in a percentage of patients who appeared clinically stable. This suggests, in some patients at least, a 5-fluorouracil (5FU) effect which was not apparent by measurement of tumour mass. Even more interesting was the finding that serum CEA following nitrosamine therapy showed a greater and more consistent fall than that seen following 5FU even though clinical response, as measured by other parameters, was not different[84]. While these findings are interesting, we would have to concur with Meyers that with current chemotherapy and variations in CEA assay results this is probably not useful. On the other hand, we believe that monitoring CEA for radiation therapy and for primary disease preoperatively with follow-up for recurrent disease can be useful[85]. Sugarbaker et al. concluded that if CEA titres do not decrease with preoperative radiation, disease should be expected outside the radiation field. These workers also found that tumour escape began after about 8 weeks, so that disease progression began early, at least as measured by the beginning of a rise in CEA titre; optimal surgery should probably be performed within this interval.

Chee et al. reported the presence of a carcinoma-associated antigen in culture media obtained from flasks growing the human colon cancer line HT-29[86]. Using a micro complement fixation (MCF) assay in sera of cancer-bearing and normal individuals, they obtained evidence for carcinoma-associated antigen(s) in media in which HT-29 had grown. They stressed the usefulness of chemically defined media in this study. These antigens were distinct from CEA which was also found in media in which the cell line was grown.

Gold and Miller studied colonic mucoprotein antigen (CMA), a high molecular weight tissue-specific antigen and a normal colonic secretory product[87]. There are distinct chemical composition differences between mucins from normal individuals and those with cancer. It is clear that other colonic cancer-associated antigens which may be oncofetal or may be more specific will probably be identified but there are no data at present. The group at the Sidney Farber Clinic in Boston have pursued simultaneous CEA measurements and immune complex assays with some possible improvement in reliably monitoring colonic cancer[88]. Edginton reported a CEA from colon tissue which he determined was more specific than CEA and which he designated CEA-S[89]. Chu, along with others, performed preliminary analyses with this material, monitoring patients with colon cancer (unpublished data); he felt there were fewer spurious single elevations in CEA as he followed these patients, but the work is incomplete. Furthermore, it has apparently not been possible to reproducibly obtain this material, and this final comparative judgment must be withheld.

SUMMARY

At present as we look over our survey of the current status of oncofetal antigens in gastrointestinal cancer, results are discouraging. There are definite areas of potential usefulness in patients with pancreatic, gastric or colorectal cancer; that is not the main problem. For oncofetal proteins a major problem includes both specificity and sensitivity. The specificity problem is related to the fact that tumour markers are only quantitative departures from normal; thus they are found elevated in the serum in a number of inflammatory and other benign conditions which result in increased cellular turnover. For this reason none of the oncofetal antigen determinations appears useful for screening. In addition, in order for adequate sensitivity in the clinical setting, tumours must release adequate amounts of antigen into the circulation. This usually requires tumours of a certain bulk or stage so that the earliest tumours are not ordinarily detectable by such markers.

For pancreatic cancer CEA or POA may be of some use in diagnosis, used together with other modalities, but such determinations will not help find tumours much earlier than can be done with other techniques; moreover, uncertainty factors are great enough that we cannot rely on assay results alone so that more invasive techniques are not obviated. In a study setting of intense, combined modality therapy POA or CEA are probably useful in looking for shades of sensitivity. In a strict clinical care situation this is probably of no value.

For gastric cancer there is even less evidence for a useful status of any oncofetal antigen marker. The staging problem is not as acute as for pancreatic cancer, and diagnosis is easier.

It is in the area of colorectal cancer that we feel CEA has a useful place. A CEA value should be used preoperatively to help in staging. In our experience a value much above 10 ng/ml, assuming a normal of 2.5 ng/ml, would justify chemotherapy and/or radiation as appropriate adjunct therapy in B_2, C_1 or C_2 patients. Ideally, in follow-up we suggest a CEA value at 45 days, 3 months and then monthly until 2 years after definitive surgery for B_2, C_1 or C_2 patients. CEA levels should then be obtained at perhaps 2-month intervals for the third year, and quarterly during the fourth. If CEA elevation occurs other causes such as liver disease, inflammatory disease or chemotherapy with liver toxicity must be considered. A repeat value should be taken in 2–3 weeks and if it is elevated a second-look procedure should be considered, although it may be reasonable to wait another 3 weeks. At that time, if the CEA level is again elevated with no drop from the two preceding values, or only a minimal drop in level, we suggest laparotomy with, we believe, a better than 60% chance of finding tumour which can be resected with hope of cure in one of three patients. This is the best statement we can make about monitoring and second-look considerations until a proper comparative prospective study has been completed.

On measuring the effects of chemotherapy on residual disease, outside of a study setting, no colon marker would presently be of use. CEA determinations may be helpful, on the other hand, to monitor presurgical radiation or radiation to regional tumour recurrences.

References

1 Gold, P. and Freedman, S. B. O. (1965). Demonstration of tumor specific antigens in human colonic carcinomata by immunologic tolerance and absorption techniques. *J. Exp. Med.*, **121**, 439

2 Alexander, P. (1972). Foetal antigens in cancer. *Nature (Lond.)*, **235**, 137

3 Thompson, D. M. P., Krupeyk, J., Freedman, S. O. and Gold, P. (1969). The radioimmunoassay of circulating carcinoembryonic antigens of the human digestive system. *Proc. Natl. Acad. Sci. (USA)*, **64**, 161.

4 Ruoslahti, E., Seppala, M., Voopio, P., Sakela, F. and Peltokallio, P. (1972). Radioimmunoassay of alphafetoprotein in primary and secondary cancer of the liver. *J. Natl. Cancer Inst.*, **49**, 623

5 Zamcheck, N. and Pusztaszeri, G. (1975). CEA, AFP and other potential tumor markers. *CA – A Journal for Clinicians*, **25**, 204

6 Banwo, O., Versey, J. and Hubbs, J. E. (1974). New oncofetal antigen for human pancreas. *Lancet*, **1**, 643

7 Gelder, F. B., Reese, C. J., Moosa, A. R., Hall, T. and Hunter, R. (1978). Purification, partial characterization and clinical evaluation of a pancreatic oncofetal antigen (POA). *Cancer Res.*, **38**, 313

8 Wood, R. A. B., Hall, A. W., Moosa, A. R. *et al.* (1976). Pancreatic cancer diagnosis: preliminary evaluation of a prospective study. *Surg. Res.*, **21**, 113

9 Gelder, F. B. Reese, C. J. Moosa, A. R. and Hunter, R. (1978). Studies on oncofetal antigen (POA). *Cancer*, **42**, 1635

10 Wood, R. A. B. and Moosa, A. R. (1978). The prospective evaluation of tumor-associated antigens for the early diagnosis of pancreatic cancer. *Br. J. Surg.*, **64**, 718

11 Chu, T. M., Constantine, R. and Holyoke, E. D. Unpublished data.

12 DiMagno, E. P., Malagelado, J. R., Taylor, W. F. *et al.* (1977). A prospective comparison of correct diagnostic tests for pancreatic cancer. *N. Engl. J. Med.*, **14**, 737

13 Mihas, A. A. (1978). Immunologic studies on a pancreatic oncofetal protein. *J. Natl. Cancer Inst.*, **60**, 1439

14 Mesa-Tejada, R., Bhattacharyya, J., Rorat, E., Fenoglio, C. M. and Klavins, J. V. (1977). A widely crossreacting tumor associated antigen in carcinoma of the pancreas. *Fed. Proc.*, **36**, 1075

15 Williams, R. R., McIntire, K. R. and Waldmann, T. A. (1977). Tumor-associated

138 FRONTIERS IN GENERAL SURGERY

antigen levels (carcinoembryonic antigen, human chorionic gonadotrophin and alpha
fetoprotein) antedating the diagnosis of cancer in the Framingham Study. *J. Natl.
Cancer Inst.*, **58**, 1547

16 Chu, T. M. and Holyoke, E. D. (1977). Can CEA assay be used as a screening test for
cancer? *Proc. XI Int. Cancer Congress, Florence, Italy*, **1**, 351

17 Lurie, B. B., Lowenstein, M. S. and Zamcheck, N. (1975). Elevated carcinoembryonic
antigen levels and biliary tract obstruction. *J. Am. Med. Assoc.*, **233**, 326

18 Khoo, S. K. and MacKay, J. R. (1973). Carcinoembryonic antigen in serum in diseases
of the liver and pancreas. *J. Clin. Pathol.* **26**, 470

19 Moore, T., Dhar, P., Zamcheck, N., Keeley, A. Gottlieb, L. and Kupchik, H. Z. (1972).
Carcinoembryonic antigen in liver disease. *Gastroenterology*, **63**, 88

20 Hansen, H. J., Snyder, J. J., Miller, E., Vandervoorde, J. P., Miller, O. N., Hine, L. R.
and Burns, J. J. (1974). Carcinoembryonic (CEA) antigen assay: a laboratory adjunct in
the diagnosis and management of cancer. *Hum. Pathol.*, **5**, 137

21 Ona, F. V., Zamcheck, N., Dhar, P., Moore, T. and Kupchik, N. Z. (1973). Carcinoembryonic antigen in the diagnosis of pancreatic cancer. *Cancer*, **31**, 324

22 Kalser, M. H., Barkin, J. S., Redlhammer, D. and Heal, A. (1978). Circulating carcinoembryonic antigen in pancreatic carcinoma. *Cancer*, **42**, 1468

23 McIntire, J. (1978). Report to Gastrointestinal Tumor Study Group

24 DiMagno, E. P., Malagelado, J. R., Taylor, W. E. *et al.* (1977). A prospective comparison of current diagnostic tests for pancreatic cancer. *N. Engl. J. Med.*, **14**, 737

25 Sharma, M. P., Gregg, J. A., Lowenstein, M. S. *et al.* (1976). Carcinoembryonic
antigen (CEA) activity in pancreatic juice of patients with pancreatic carcinoma and
pancreatitis. *Cancer*, **38**, 2451

26 Zamcheck, N. (1975). Immunology, tumor markers and pancreatic cancer. *J. Surg.
Oncol.*, **7**, 155

27 Molnar, I. G., Vandervoorde, J. P. and Gitnick, G. L. (1976). CEA levels in fluids
bathing gastrointestinal tumors. *Gastroenterology*, **70**, 513

28 DiMagno, E. P., Malagelada, J. R., Moertel, C. G. *et al.* (1977). Prospective evaluation
of the pancreatic secretion of immunoreactive carcinoembryonic antigen enzyme and
bicarbonate in patients suspected of having pancreatic cancer. *Gastroenterology*, **73**, 457

29 Barkin, J. S., Kalser, M. H., Kaplan, R., Redlhammer, D. and Heal, A. (1978). Initial
levels of CEA and their role of change in pancreatic carcinoma following surgery, chemotherapy and radiation therapy. *Cancer*, **42**, 1472

30 Chu, T. M., Holyoke, E. D. and Douglass, H. O. Jr (1980). Tumor antigens as related
to pancreatic cancer. *J. Surg. Oncol.*, **13**, 207

31 Chu, T. M., Holyoke, E. D. and Douglass, H. O., Jr (1977). Isolation of a glycoprotein
antigen from ascites fluid of pancreatic carcinoma. *Cancer Res.*, **37**, 1525

32 Shimano, T., Loor, R. M., Papsidero, L. D. *et. al.* (1981). Isolation characterization and
clinical evaluation of a pancreas cancer associated antigen. *Cancer* (In press)

33 Kasugar, T. (1968). Gastric lavage cytology and biopsy for early gastric cancer under
direct vision by the fiberoscope. *Gastroenterol. Endosc.*, **14**, 205

34 Oscarson, J., Stormby, N. and Sundgren, R. (1972). Selective angiography in fine-
needle aspiration, cytodynamics of gastric and pancreatic tumors. *Acta. Radiol.*, **12**,
737

35 Colcher, H. (1974). Cancer of the gastrointestinal tract. C. Gastric cancer diagnosis.
Diagnostic fiberoptic gastroscopy. *J. Am. Med. Assoc.*, **228**, 891

36 Hakkinen, I., and Wiikari, S. (1969). Occurrence of fetal sulphoglyco-protein antigen
in the gastric juice of patients with gastric diseases. *Ann. Surg.*, **169**, 227

37 Hakkim, I., Jarvi, O. and Giranroos, J. (1968). Sulfoglycoprotein antigens in the
human alimentary canal and gastric cancer. An immunohistochemical study. *Int. J.
Cancer*, **3**, 572

38 Ishii, M. (1978). Basic fetoprotein (embryonic basic protein). *Igaku No Ayami*, **106**, 273

39 Parsons, R. G., Longmire, R. L., Hoch, S. O. and Hoch, J. A. (1977). A clinical evaluation of serum CSDP levels in individuals with malignant disease. *Cancer Res., 37, 692*

40 Waldman, T. A. and McIntire, K. R. (1974). The use of of a radioimmuno-assay for alpha-fetoprotein in the diagnosis of malignancy. *Cancer, 34, 1510*

41 Björklund, B. and Björklund, V. (1957). Antigenicity of pooled human malignant and normal tissues by cyto-immunological technique. Presence of an insoluble heat-labile Antigen. *Int. Arch. Allergy, 10, 153*

42 Björklund, B., Londstrom, R., Eklund, G. *et al.* (1973). A clinically useful antigenic polypeptide in human cancer and placenta. *XVII Scandinavian Congress of Pathology and Microbiology*

43 Björklund, B., Björklund, V., Wilkund, B. *et al.* (1973). III. Clinical Studies of 1483 Individuals with Cancer and Other Conditions. Immunological Techniques for Detection of Cancer. *Proc. Folksam Symposium*, Bonniers, Sweden, p. 164.

44 Menendez-Botet, C. V. and Schwartz, M. K. (1975). A preliminary evaluation of tissue polypeptide antigen (TPA) in serum and/or urine of patients with cancer or benign disease. *Abst. Folksam Symposium*, Bonniers, Stockholm Sweden, 1975. (In press).

45 Holyoke, E. D. and Chu, T. M. (1975). Tissue polypeptide antigen (TPA). *Abst. Folksam Symposium*, Bonniers, Stockholm, Sweden (In press).

46 Reynoso, G., Chu, T. M., Holyoke, E. D., Cohen, E., Nemoto, T., Wang, J. J., Chuang, J., Guinan, P. and Murphy, G. P. (1972). Carcino-embryonic antigen in patients with different cancers. *J. Am. Med. Assoc., 220, 361*

47 Holyoke, E. D., Reynoso, G. and Chu, T. M. (1972). Carcinoembryonic antigen (CEA) in patients with carcinoma of the digestive tract. *Ann. Surg., 176, 559*

48 Laurence, D. J. R., Stevens, V., Bettelheim, R., Darcy, D., Leese, C., Tuberville, C., Alexander, P., Johns, E. W. and Neville, A. M. (1972). Evaluation of the role of plasma carcinoembryonic antigen (CEA) in the diagnosis of gastrointestinal mammary and bronchial carcinoma. *Br. J. Med., 3, 605*

49 Ravry, M., McIntire, K. R., Moertel, C. G., Waldman, T. A. *et al.* (1974). Brief communication: carcinoembryonic antigen and alpha fetoprotein in the diagnosis of gastric and colonic cancer: a comparative clinical evaluation. *J. Natl. Cancer Inst., 52, 1019*

50 Kupchik, H. Z., Zamcheck, N. and Saravis C. A. (1973). Immunological studies of carcinoembryonic antigen, methodological consideration and clinical implications. *J. Natl. Cancer Inst., 51, 1741*

51 Cooper, E. A., Turner, R., Steele, L., Neville, A. M. and MacKay, A. M. (1975). The contribution of serum enzymes and carcinoembryonic antigen to the early diagnosis of metabolic colorectal cancer. *Br. J. Cancer, 31, 111*

52 Costanza, M. E. *et al.* (1974). Carcinoembryonic antigen: report of a screening study. *Cancer, 33, 583*

53 McCartney, W. H. and Hoffer, P. B. (1974). The value of carcinoembryonic antigen (CEA) as an adjunct to the radiological colon examination in the diagnosis of malignancy. *Radiology, 110, 325*

54 Holyoke, E. D., Chu, T. M. and Murphy, G. P. M. (1975). CEA as a monitor of gastrointestinal malignancy. *Cancer, 35, 830*

55 Holyoke, E. D., Reynoso, G. and Chu, T. M. (1976). Carcinoembryonic antigen in patients with carcinoma of the digestive tract. *Ann. Surg., 176, 559*

56 Herrera, M., Chu, T. M. and Holyoke, E. D. (1976). Carcinoembryonic antigen (CEA) as a prognostic and monitoring test in clinically complete resection of coloretal carcinoma. *Ann. Surg., 183, 5*

57 Mach, J. P. (1978). Three years follow-up by repeated CEA assay of 77 patients who had undergone a complete resection of colorectal carcinoma. *Proc. Int. Conf. on Clinical Uses of Carcinoembryonic Antigen*. Lexington, KY, June, 1977. *Cancer, 42, 1439*

58 Zamcheck, N. (1975). The present status of CEA in diagnosis, prognosis, and evaluation of therapy. *Cancer, 36, 2460*

59 Holyoke, E. D., Chu, T. M. and Evans, J. T. (1976). CEA as a prognosticator and monitor in patients with colon cancer. *Proc. 3rd Int. Symp. on the Detection and Prevention of Cancer*, New York, NY, April 1976

60 Evans, J. T., Mittelman, A., Chu, T. M. and Holyoke, E. D. (1978). Pre- and postoperative uses of CEA. *Cancer*, **42**, 1419

61 Holyoke, E. D. and Cooper, E. H. (1976). CEA and tumor markers. *Sem. Oncol.*, **3**, 377

62 Holyoke, E. D., Evans, J. T. and Chu, T. M. (1977). Carcinoembryonic antigen (CEA) in the diagnosis and treatment of colon and rectal cancer. In Enker, W. A. (ed.). *Cancer of the Colon and Rectum*. (Chicago: Year Book Publ. Co.)

63 Holyoke, E. D. and Goldrosen, M. H. (1978). Monitoring of colon cancer through measurement of carcinoembryonic antigen levels, tests of cellular immune competence and tumor specific immunity. *Int. Adv. Surg. Oncol.*, **1**, 85

64 Ramming, K. P., MacIntyre, J., Zamcheck, N. and Holyoke, E. D. (1979). Serum carcinoembryonic antigen (CEA) monitoring of patients at high risk for recurrence following surgery for colorectal carcinoma. *Proc. AACR and ASCO*, May 1979, Vol. 20, ASCO Abst. C-157, 329

65 Joint National Cancer Institute of Canada/American Cancer Society Investigation. (1972). A collaborative study of a test for carcinoembryonic antigen (CEA) in the sera of patients with carcinoma of the colon and rectum. *Can. Med. Assoc. J.*, **107**, 25

66 LoGerfo, P. and Herter, F. P. (1975). Carcinoembryonic antigen in the diagnosis and prognosis in patients with colon cancer. *Ann. Surg.*, **181**, 81

67 Mackay, A. M., Patel, S., Carter, S., Stevens, U., Laurence, D. J. R., Cooper, E. H. and Neville, A. M. (1978). Role of serial plasma CEA assays in detection of recurrent and metastatic colorectal carcinoma. *Br. Med. J.*, **4**, 382

68 Reiger, A. and Wahren, B. (1975). CEA levels at recurrence and metastasis: importance for detecting secondary disease. *Scand. J. Gastroenterol.*, **10**, 869

69 Holyoke, E. D. and Chu, T. M. (1975). Biological markers; our newest weapons against cancer. *Med. Opinion*, **51**

70 Holyoke, E. D., Chu, T. M. and Murphy, G. P. M. (1975). CEA as a Monitor of gastrointestinal malignancy. *Cancer*, **35**, 830

71 Martin, E. W., Jr, Kibbey, W. E., Samson, R., Steward, W., Hardy, T. and Minton, J. P. (1976). Carcinoembryonic antigen in colorectal practice. Report of 3 cases. *Dis. Colon Rectum*, **19**, 99

72 Martin, E. W., Jr, Kibbey, W., DeVecchio, L. *et al.* (1976). Carcinoembryonic antigen, clinical and historical aspects. *Cancer*, **37**, 62

73 Minton, J. P., James, K. K., Hurtubise, P. E., Rinker, L., Joyce, S. and Martin, E. W. (1978). The use of serial carcinoembryonic antigen determinations to predict recurrence of carcinoma of the colon and the time for second-look operations. *Surg. Gynecol. Obstet.*, **147**, 208

74 Minton, J. P. and Jartin, E. W. (1978). The use of serial CEA determinations to predict recurrence of colon cancer and when to do a second-look operation. *Cancer*, **42**, 1422

75 Mach, J. P., Jaeger, P. H., Bertholet, M. M., Ruegsegger, C. H., Loosli, R. M. and Tetlavel, J. (1974). Detection of recurrence of large bowel carcinomas by radioimmunoassay of circulating carcinoembryonic antigen (CEA). *Lancet*, **2**, 2535

76 Sorokim, J. J., Sugarbaker, P. H., Zamcheck, N., Pisick, M., Kupchik, H. Z. and Moore, F. D. (1974). Serial carcinoembryonic antigen assays, use in detection of cancer recurrence. *J. Am. Med. Assoc.*, **228**, 49

77 Sugarbaker, P. H., Zamcheck, N. and Moore, F. D. (1976). Assessment of serial carcinoembryonic antigen (CEA) assays in postoperative detection of recurrent colorectal cancer. *Cancer*, **38**, 2310

78 Cohen, A. M. and Wood, W. C. (1979). Carcinoembryonic antigen level as an indicator for reoperation in patients with carcinoma of the colon and rectum. *Surg. Gynecol. Obstet.*, **149**, 22

79 Wanebo, H. J., Rao, B., Pinsky, C. M. *et al.* (1981). Carcinoembryonic antigen: prognostic and therapeutic guidelines in the management of colorectal cancer. (In press)

80 Mayer, R. T., Harnick, M. B., Steele, G. and Zamcheck, N. (1978). Carcinoembryonic antigen (CEA) as a monitor of chemotherapy in disseminated colorectal cancer. *Cancer*, **42,** 1428

81 Molcare, R. and LoGerfo, P. (1972). Tumor associated antigens in the chemotherapy of solid tumors. *J. Surg. Oncol.*, **4,** 407

82 Skarin, A. T., Delwiche, R., Zamcheck, N., Lokich, J. J. and Frei, E., III (1974). Carcinoembryonic antigen: clinical correlation with chemotherapy for metastatic gastrointestinal cancer. *Cancer*, **33,** 1239

83 Herrera, M. A., Chu, T. M., Holyoke, E. D. and Mittelman, A. (1977). CEA monitoring of palliative treatment for colorectal carcinoma. *Am. Surg.*, **182,** 23

84 Sugarbaker, P. H. *et al.* (1976). Carcinoembryonic antigen (CEA) monitoring of radiation therapy for colorectal cancer. *Am. J. Roentgenol.*, **127,** 641

85 Sugarbaker, P. H., Skarin, A. J. and Zamcheck, N. (1976). Patterns of serial CEA assays and their clinical use in management of colorectal cancer. *J. Surg. Oncol.*, **8,** 523

86 Chee, D. O., Gupta, R. K. and Morton, D. L. (1980). Presence of a carcinoma associated antigen in the spent chemically deformed medium of a human colon carcinoma cell line. *J. Surg. Oncol.*, **13,** 45

87 Gold, D. V. and Miller, F. (1978). Comparison of human colonic mucoprotein antigen from normal and neoplastic mucosa. *Cancer Res.*, **38,** 3204

88 Steele, G., Sonis, S., Stelos, P., Riglgers, R., Zamcheck, N., Finn, D., Maltz, J., Mayer, R., Lokich, J. and Wilson, R. E. (1978). Circulating immune complexes in patients following clinically curative resection of colorectal cancer. *Surgery*, **83,** 648

89 Edgington, T. S., Astarita, R. W., Plow, E. D. and Nakamura, R. (1975). Associates of CEA-s with neoplasia of the GI tract. *N. Engl. J. Med.*, **293,** 103

5
Adjuvant therapy of gastrointestinal carcinoma

F. J. ANSFIELD AND G. RAMIREZ

Due to the fairly dismal prognosis often associated with cancer of the gastrointestinal tract, chemotherapy as an adjuvant to surgery was a logical development for high-risk patients likely to develop recurrence. It was thought merely necessary to await the availability of compounds that showed reasonable effectiveness against such cancers. Regrettably the wait has been a long one and, to a large extent, still prevails.

Adjuvant therapy for the upper gastrointestinal tract or its appendages is chiefly concerned with cancers of the stomach and pancreas. The latter has a median survival of 10.5 months from the onset of symptoms and 3.5 months from proof of incurability, while in gastric cancer the median survival data are 11.5 and 4 months respectively[1]. The National End Results Committee reported that 80% of patients with gastric cancer and 90% of patients with pancreatic cancer are dead within 1 year, emphasizing the grim outlook for victims of such diseases.

Most of the other upper gastrointestinal cancers similarly carry a very dire prognosis and include malignant hepatoma, cancers of the gallbladder, duodenum, bile ducts and ampulla of Vater. The Mayo Clinic Group found the median survival times from proof of incurability to be 9 months for cancer of the small bowel, 30 months for carcinoid (small bowel), and 57 months for islet cell carcinoma, a less rapidly fatal group.

Moertel et al.[2] conducted randomized studies in localized unresectable gastric and pancreatic cancers, treating them with 5-fluorouracil (5FU), $15 \, \mathrm{mg \, kg^{-1} \, d^{-1}} \times 2d$ then $10 \, \mathrm{mg/kg}$ on the third day, plus 4000 r radiotherapy vs. a placebo plus irradiation. Patients with both tumour types showed a significantly increased survival if they were treated with

143

5FU plus radiotherapy.

Since the 5FU, injected intravenously on three successive days, followed by up to 4000 r within an area of 20×20 cm in patients with locally unresected gastric and pancreatic cancers appeared to be useful, it was felt that this combination might be helpful as adjuvant therapy following resection of gastric and pancreatic tumours when the surgeon feels there is a high likelihood of local, remnant cancer.

At the University Hospitals at Madison, WI (University of Wisconsin) we conducted a randomized study[3] of patients with gastric cancer that was incompletely resected or was associated with positive regional lymph nodes. Cards were drawn blindly for treatment with 5FU plus irradiation *vs.* 5FU alone. The 5FU was started on day 1 when radiotherapy was also started, usually 3 weeks following resection providing a fairly good oral protein intake was established. For the combination, the 5FU was given at a schedule of $10 \, \text{mg} \, \text{kg}^{-1} \text{d}^{-1} \times 3 \, \text{d}$, 5 mg/kg on day 4, then 5 mg/kg every Monday, Wednesday and Friday throughout the course of irradiation. Thereafter the patients received 15 mg/kg intravenous 5FU weekly. Patients who were randomized for 5FU alone received a 5FU loading course depending on their intake of protein, then 15 mg/kg intravenous 5FU weekly. No significant difference was found in the small series of patients studied.

In an experimental approach to locally unresectable pancreatic cancer, a catheter was placed percutaneously via a transbrachial approach into the artery supplying the tumour area and patients received intra-arterial 5FU combined with radiotherapy. This pilot study yielded two long survivors of the 18 patients so treated. Patients with a high likelihood of incomplete resection of cancer of the gallbladder and bile ducts were similarly given intra-arterial 5FU ($10 \, \text{mg} \, \text{kg}^{-1} \text{d}^{-1}$) plus concomitant irradiation. With this regimen and with the catheter tip positioned in the common hepatic artery, two patients had complete clearing of their jaundice. After completion of radiotherapy, consisting of 4000 r tumour dose, the arterial catheters were removed and patients were given weekly intravenous doses of 5FU (15 mg/kg).

Possibly due to the increasing prevalence of gastric cancer in Japan, a number of reports from that country have dealt with chemotherapy as an adjuvant to inadequate resection of this tumour. The combination as reported by Hattori *et al.*[4], in gastrectomized patients with a high suspicion of remaining tumour, was given as adjuvant chemotherapy to 180 patients and consisted of Mitomycin-C 20 mg intravenously on the day of gastrectomy and another 10 mg the next day. With suitable randomization of 165 patients the most promising and statistically significant results appeared in the group that received Mitomycin-C, then oral PSK, a protein-bound polysaccharide, and FT-207, a furamyl analogue of 5FU. At 3 year risk 62% or 33 patients survived.

Fujimoto et al.[5] reported a randomized study of 249 patients with resectable stomach cancer. Oral 5FU $3.5\,mg\,kg^{-1}\,d^{-1}$ and FT-207, a furamyl analogue of 5FU, $8\,mg\,kg^{-1}\,d^{-1}$ were given daily to 107 patients as adjuvant therapy following gastrectomy. The 120 patients randomized as controls had gastric resection and no adjuvant therapy. A significantly higher survival was observed in the curatively resected patients who received 5FU and FT-207 as compared to the controls. The two compounds were taken orally on a continuing basis. The results of this study and the previous one of Hattori et al. may be considered mutually supportive.

Gilbert et al.[6] reported encouraging results with the use of Razoxane (ICRF 159), related to the chelating agent EDTA, as an adjuvant to resection of gastric cancer. Five of the first 10 patients survived more than 2 years following purely palliative gastric resections. A large randomized adjuvant study of Razoxane vs. controls (no treatment or 5FU) is currently in progress in patients with cancers of the stomach, pancreas, colon and rectum.

Other than skin cancer the most common malignant tumour afflicting men in the Western hemisphere is colorectal cancer. Despite such technical improvements as early bowel stump ligation to prevent anastomotic tumour cell implantation[7] and the no-touch isolation technique[8], the over-all 5-year survival has remained relatively constant over the past two decades[9].

Surgery alone fails to cure about 80% of patients with Dukes C (spread to serosa or positive regional lymph nodes) and 58% with Dukes B lesions (spread to the muscularis mucosae)[10]. Since Dukes B and C lesions comprise 90% of resectable colorectal cancer[11] the compelling need for effective adjuvant therapy is apparent. Early attempts at adjuvant chemotherapy were aimed at the circulating malignant cells that it was felt were liberated into the blood stream during tumour manipulation at the time of resection[12-16]. Nitrogen mustard was ineffective, as was thio-tepa, except in a subset of women older than 55 years of age who received the larger total course of 0.8 mg/kg. Because of increased morbidity this dose was reduced to 0.6 mg/kg total course. It became apparent that these alkylating agents given on the day of surgery alone, or also for an additional one or two doses over the first two postoperative days were ineffective as adjuvant therapy in colorectal cancer. It was subsequently realized that the major source of spread was not primarily associated with the surgeon's handling of the tumour but that micrometastases had already disseminated in Dukes B and C lesions. Further attempts at cancer chemotherapy against this tumour were desultory for a period, primarily because no effective drug was available.

With the development of 5FU by Heidebergen et al.[17] and Duschinsky *et al.*[18] in 1956, and the demonstration of its clinical utility by Ansfield and Curreri[30] in 1958, there became available for the first time a compound that, given optimally, exhibited significant antitumour activity against colorectal cancer with reasonable consistency. In another 2 years when 5-fluoro-2-deoxyuridine (5FUDR)[19] was developed, we[20] demonstrated that it it had greater antitumour activity against colorectal cancer than 5FU. Our clinical results comparing 5FU to 5FUDR are shown in Table 1.

Table 1   Clinical comparison of 5FU *vs.* 5FUDR in cancer of colon or rectum

	5FU	*5FUDR*	*p*
No. patients improved/No. patients treated	24/141	25/57	<0.001
Percentage improved	17.0	43.8	
Average duration of remission	8.4 months	19.2 months	
Number of complete regressions	3	9	<0.001

The first patient who received a fluoropyrimidine as an adjuvant to resection of a large bowel cancer was a plastic surgeon of Hollywood, CA in 1960. Tumour cells were found in the perineural sheaths and as thrombi in the venules at a resected end of the surgical specimen. Three weeks following surgery he was placed on 5FUDR 30 mg kg^{-1} d^{-1} × 5 d, then a day of rest, then 15 mg/kg every other day for 11 such half doses, all given by intravenous push. The only reactions were occasional nausea and slight anorexia. Two more such courses were given in Hollywood with 30 days between each course. A second-look procedure done 9 months after surgery revealed no recurrence and the patient has remained tumour-free for the past 20 years.

A similar early salutary effect occurred in a 65-year-old female who had a resection for gastric carcinoma with involved lymph nodes. Three weeks following surgery she received the first of three courses of 5FUDR each consisting of 30 mg kg^{-1} d^{-1} × 5 d, a day of rest, then 11 half-doses on alternate days. Subsequent courses were given after a 30-day rest period between courses. She remained free of recurrence for 7 years when she died of a coronary thrombosis. No cases other than the above two received 5FUDR as an adjuvant to resection of gastrointestinal cancer. This compound was to be used in Phase I and later in Phase II studies, but in view of the significantly superior results we observed in advanced cancer with 5FUDR compared to 5FU, it was felt justifiable to administer it to these two high risk patients very likely to develop recurrence.

Higgins[21] reported a series of 1118 patients with colorectal cancer that were entered into two prospective randomized trials to study the utility of 5FU as an adjuvant to surgical resection. The first group consisted of

433 patients of which 308 patients had curative resections and were randomized to receive intravenous 5FU, $12 \, \text{mg} \, \text{kg}^{-1} \, \text{d}^{-1} \times 5 \, \text{d}$, starting 2 weeks postoperatively while the controls received surgery alone. The 5FU-treated group received a second course of five daily infusions of 5FU, 7 weeks later without further adjuvant therapy. Two other subgroups who had palliative resections were also randomized for 5FU or no chemotherapy. Grouping these three subsets showed that the survival was significantly ($p = 0.002$) better for patients who received 5FU compared to those who had surgery alone.

There were also two trials with prolonged intermittent 5FU therapy ($12 \, \text{mg} \, \text{kg}^{-1} \, \text{d}^{-1} \times 5 \, \text{d}$) every 6 weeks for 18 months. Combining all five groups who received 5FU courses *vs.* the controls demonstrates a statistically significant difference in survival favouring 5FU treated patients. Unfortunately the earlier individual studies showed no value for 5FU given as adjuvant therapy and the early negative results still influence physicians to withhold adjuvant chemotherapy today, even for Dukes B and C lesions.

When Moertel and Reitemeirer[22] learned of the superior results we observed with 5FUDR in colorectal cancer they obtained this compound from the National Cancer Institute and conducted a prospective double blind study of 5FU *vs.* 5FUDR given by intravenous push in patients with colorectal cancer. They used 5FUDR at a schedule of $40 \, \text{mg} \, \text{kg}^{-1} \, \text{d}^{-1} \times 5 \, \text{d}$ with plans to then use half-doses every other day to the point of slight toxicity. Unfortunately, with such high doses, toxicity developed very early in most cases, so most patients were not candidates for subsequent half-doses. This randomized study of 5FUDR *vs.* 5FU in colorectal cancer resulted in a 23% response rate for 5FUDR and a 12% response rate for 5FU; the difference approached but did not reach statistical significance.

The Eastern Solid Tumor Group in randomizing 5FU *vs.* 5FUDR *vs.* methotrexate observed early in the study a prohibitive incidence of severe and fatal toxicity. The code in this triple blind study was not broken but instead the five whole doses of each drug were reduced to 3½ doses followed by half-doses on alternate days. When the study was completed and the code broken it was found that 5FU had produced the severe toxicity. By reducing all three drugs the resultant 5FUDR regimen was inadequate: $30 \, \text{mg} \, \text{kg}^{-1} \, \text{d}^{-1} \times 3 \, \text{d}$, half-dose on day 4, and 4 half-doses on alternate days. Since neither of the above studies utilized what we found was an optimal dosage regimen, the incidence of objective regressions did not approach the Wisconsin results and 5FUDR was not approved for subsequent intravenous chemotherapy. We thus lost the most effective compound available and active against disseminated colorectal cancer and the compound most likely to prove beneficial as adjuvant therapy in high-risk patients following surgical removal of gastrointestinal cancers. Unfortunate as this may be, we still have 5FU as a worthy alternative.

It is very disturbing that the majority of physicians believe that adjuvant therapy in colorectal cancer has no merit, and that oncologists too are confused. A brief mention of more of the earlier studies, uncontrolled or randomized, will probably explain the reasons for the diverse opinions that currently exist.

Grage et al.[23] reported the Central Oncology Group's randomized adjuvant study of 5FU vs. untreated controls in 274 patients who had either a curative or palliative resection of colorectal malignancy. Unfortunately the 5FU loading course of $12\,mg\,kg^{-1}\,d^{-1} \times 4\,d$ followed by up to five half-doses on alternate days and weekly doses thereafter at 12 mg/kg is considered inadequate by the authors of this chapter and our recommended schedule will be described. Grage et al's study found no significant benefit from adjuvant chemotherapy except in those treated to toxicity. This could have been predicted in view of the less than optimal dosage schedule. The study summary stated: 'We conclude that a preliminary analysis of the COG data in this trial does not make a convincing case for the use of 5-FU as an adjuvant to the surgical treatment of colorectal carcinoma.' It is readily apparent how the negative results of this and the Veterans Administration studies might adversely influence the decision of physicians and younger oncologists to consider adjuvant 5FU therapy. Unfortunately, it may take several years for the recent reports that show the significant advantage of 5FU adjuvant therapy to reach these personnel.

Rousselot et al.[24] reported on intraluminal instillation of 30 mg/kg of 5FU plus two doses of 10 mg/kg of 5FU intravenously to 77 study patients following resection of colorectal cancers. Seventeen had positive mesenteric nodes and their 8-year survival was 56% which they compared to a 5-year survival rate of 32% for nationwide controls. There appeared to be a favourable trend in long-term survival associated with 5FU use.

Lawrence et al.[25] utilized the same dosage and technique of administration as Rousselot except in a prospective randomized study of 126 patients, and 80 received five monthly courses of oral 5FU after the immediate postoperative adjuvant treatment. They concluded this adjuvant therapy yielded no improvement over the controls.

Only in the last 2 years have reports from the Central Oncology Group and Veterans Administration Adjuvant Studies started to show that 5FU adjuvant therapy, given even suboptimally over an adequate period of time, produces a statistically significant increase in tumour-free survival compared to untreated controls. Unfortunately, for more than half a decade reports claimed no benefit from the 5FU adjuvant therapy. As a result it is our estimate that less than 20% of high-risk

patients (Dukes B and C) are currently being given adjuvant chemotherapy. This stems primarily from the circumstance that earlier randomized studies, which appeared in major medical journals, stated
prematurely that fluoropyrimidine (5FU, 5FUDR) adjuvant therapy had
no significant advantage over no treatment[21, 23, 25–27].

The authors of this chapter have collectively treated well in excess of
6000 patients with 5FU for periods of from 1 to 2 months up to 10 years
with monthly courses of 5FU, each to the point of at least slight reaction,
month after month and year after year if no progression appeared or
with a loading course to slight reaction followed by weekly doses. In a
randomized study that we conducted[28], both regimens were found to be
equally effective so the latter has had preference at the University Hospital at Madison, especially because of greater patient acceptability. Initially in 1957 our monthly courses of 5FU consisted of 15
$mg\,kg^{-1}\,d^{-1} \times 5\,d$. When it appeared the response rate could perhaps
be improved by more aggressive dosage, following the five doses and
then a day of rest, half doses or $7\frac{1}{2}$ mg/kg were added every other day
to the point of slight toxicity or arbitrarily until 11 such half-doses were
given. Each subsequent course was then given after 30-day rest periods
between courses.

Despite added experience and careful daily observation in the hospital by one of us before each dose, the incidence of drug-related deaths
continued at 2.9%, which was considered prohibitive even in patients
with advanced or terminal disease. Therefore, after a phase I study with
200 patients[29], a less toxic 5FU dosage schedule for good-risk patients
was adopted of $12\,mg\,kg^{-1}\,d^{-1} \times 5\,d$, a day of rest, then half-doses or
6 mg/kg every other day to the point of slight reaction or until 11 half-
doses were given. These courses were repeated with 30-day intervals
between the last day of the previous and the first day of the next course.
In retrospect one of us (FJA) has the distinct impression that the earlier
$15\,mg\,kg^{-1}\,d^{-1} \times 5\,d$ plus half-doses produced more remarkable
responses than did the 12 mg/kg schedule but since the lesser schedule
has an incidence of only one toxic death per thousand in the last 3000
patients treated with 5FU and a response rate not significantly different
from that produced by the larger dosage schedule, the 12 mg/kg dose
schedule is the one strongly recommended in good-risk patients.

There are certain definite circumstances when a loading course of 5FU
should not be administered because the incidence of serious fatal toxicity is prohibitive:

(1) Patients on intravenous fluids. Such patients are usually in negative
   nitrogen balance and Wolberg has demonstrated very clearly the
   high toxic mortality 5FU can produce when given to subjects in
   negative nitrogen balance[54]. The VA study regimen, wherein 5FU

adjuvant therapy was begun 2 weeks following resection of a colon cancer, can be hazardous. There is more possibility that such patients will not have recovered nitrogen balance so early following resection of a part of the gastrointestinal tract; hence 3 weeks is recommended post-resection before initiation of therapy.

(2) Patients jaundiced from hepatocellular failure. These patients cannot tolerate an intravenous loading course of 5FU without developing early toxicity which may be severe; on the other hand 5FU given intra-arterially to such patients can be very useful.

(3) Patients with compromised bone marrow caused by either:
  (a) prior prolonged chemotherapy (with alkylating agents, any nitrosourea, mitomycin C, dibramodulcitol, or any compound with alkylating activity);
  (b) extensive pelvic irradiation (regardless of when it was given, even 5 or 10 years ago).

Patients who are likely to develop early and undue toxicity from 5FU are classified as poor-risk patients and cannot safely tolerate the good risk 5FU regimen of $12\,mg\,kg^{-1}\,d^{-1} \times 5\,d$, a day of rest, then $6\,mg/kg$ every other day until slight reaction or until 11 such half-doses are given. They can, however, tolerate $12\,mg\,kg^{-1}\,d^{-1} \times 3\,d$ followed by half-doses as above, but because of the reduced regimen the likelihood of a response may also be decreased[30]. Patients are classified as poor-risk if they have any of the following:

(1) Osseous metastases to bones of the pelvis or lower spine.
(2) Prior pelvic irradiation of 1200–2400 r.
(3) A reduced oral intake, especially of protein, to not less than 50% of the usual food ingestion. This may be caused by anorexia, nausea, vomiting, partial bowel obstruction, moderate to severe stomatitis, pharyngitis, or oesophagitis. If oral intake drops to less than 50% of usual, 5FU should be halted.

It is not unusual for a 'good-risk patient' who is scheduled to receive a 'good-risk regimen' to have his risk status downgraded with the development of any of the above situations and subsequent 5FU doses appropriately curtailed.

Equally important to determining the risk classification of each patient is the decision as to when to halt the course of 5FU. This should be done if any of the following develop:

(1) Diarrhoea, consisting of three or more fluid or semi-fluid stools, any time within the 24 h when a whole or half-dose is due. In a person who normally has two or three soft to semi-fluid stools per 24 h, as

occurs commonly in patients with a portion of the large bowel resected, one could allow up to four or five semi-fluid stools before terminating a course. If the patient has a colostomy, the count of stools is not as useful as is the character of the stools. Ask the patient if they are 'runny' and look at his colostomy bag; if the stools are liquid stop the course.

(2) Stomatitis, in the form of a visible ulceration covered with a whitish pseudomembrane, usually appearing on the inner aspect of the lower lip near the vermilion border. In a small percentage of patients this may develop on the inner aspect of the upper lip.

(3) Leukopenia with a drop in the white blood cell (WBC) count to 3800 if the starting count was 6000 or above. If the starting count was 5000 the cut-off for the course should be 3200 and if the starting count was 4000 the cut-off should be 3000.

(4) A significant decrease in oral intake of protein or failure to retain oral intake.

(5) A moderate pharyngitis or, infrequently, an inflammatory facial dermatitis.

It is essential that the staff-man experienced in administering 5FU to the point of slight reaction give the first course and see the patient every day that a dose is due. A resident who rotates services every month or two should not make the decision for 5FU administration, and of course, neither should an intern. This is equally true in treating patients with disseminated cancer and it is mandatory in patients receiving monthly courses of chemotherapy as an adjuvant to surgical resection. To produce serious or fatal toxicity from 5FU in a patient receiving adjuvant 5FU following resection of a Dukes B colon cancer, in which surgery alone cures 45–55% of patients, would be totally unforgivable. When the staff-man evaluates the patient he inquires carefully regarding the stools for the past 24 h and the oral intake that is being retained; he looks for stomatitis by examining the lower lip and he obtains the result of the WBC count taken earlier that morning before deciding whether the patient is to receive a dose of 5FU.

A WBC count is taken at the start of each course and before the last whole dose (12 mg/kg) and before each half dose (6 mg/kg) of the first course. This is essential because it is often an inadequate WBC count that makes it necessary to terminate a course of therapy. After completion of a course of 5FU, a WBC count every 3 or 4 days for a total of three counts is essential to observe the nadir of the WBC curve, to assist the chemotherapist with subsequent courses. These can be subsequently administered by the patient's physician, guided by a carefully written letter of instructions from the oncologist who sees and evaluates the patient and gives the first dose of each course. Included in the instructions are the dates WBC counts will be required (usually before each of the last three half-doses).

The oncologist who gives the first course of 5FU to the point of slight reaction as described, usually prefers to do it on an in-patient basis so the patient can be carefully observed. If nausea develops the nurse can administer such an anti-emetic as oral compazine without delay, or if vomiting has begun it can be given intramuscularly, probably enabling the patient to maintain an adequate oral intake and thus continue the course of 5FU therapy without premature toxicity. The half-doses of the first course can be given on an out-patient or in-patient basis, but must always be given by an experienced staff-man. If, for example, the patient tolerates five whole doses and eight half-doses on alternate days before he develops some reaction as leukopenia and the course is terminated, in all likelihood, he will be able to tolerate a very similar regimen on subsequent courses. It is such information that the oncologist takes into account when he outlines instructions to the collaborating physician for the next course.

The question is asked not infrequently why we believe 5FU must be administered to the point of slight reaction or slight toxicity. In 1957, we observed a few responses when we used five doses of 5FU then stopped for 30 days. The results improved significantly[31] when we added half-doses on alternate days to the point of some toxicity. Wolberg[30] demonstrated very clearly with tumour slices *in vitro* exposed to different concentrations of 5FU, that the inhibition of thymidilate synthetase activity, which is correlated with antitumour activity, was dependent upon the concentration of FdUMP*. It is recognized that the more 5FU that is present the more FdUMP is formed.

Table 2 Four dosage schedules of 5FU

Regimen no.	Objective response rate	Drug schedule (5FU)
1	33%	$12\,mg\,kg^{-1}d^{-1}\times5$, 1 day of rest, then $6\,mg/kg$ every other day to slight reaction or until 11 half-doses are given; then $15\,mg\,kg^{-1}\,week^{-1}$
2	13%	$15\,mg/kg$ once weekly; if no toxicity increase to $20\,mg\,kg^{-1}\,week^{-1}$; if toxicity occurs, reduce by $5\,mg/kg$
3	14%	$500\,mg/d\times4$ then $500\,mg$ once weekly
4	13%	$15\,mg\,kg^{-1}d^{-1}\times6d$ *orally,* then $15\,mg/kg$ orally weekly

The Central Oncology Group performed a randomized study[32] of four dosage schedules of 5FU in colorectal cancer, as shown in Table 2,

* 5-fluoro-2'-deoxyuridine-5'-monophosphate

where 200 colorectal cancer patients with accurately measurable disease were randomized to one of the four regimens shown in column 1. It is obvious that schedule No. 1, the regimen we have used since 1965, is much more effective than schedules 2, 3 and 4. When one looks at the graphs of the duration of response as well as survival in colorectal cancer with liver metastases, the curve of schedule 1 does not meet the Breslow test for significance, but the median survival and median duration of response (at the 50% point) appear definitely superior to the other three regimens.

The studies of Skipper and Schabel[33, 34] have permitted the observation of a clear dose–response relationship, i.e. higher dose chemotherapy results in higher cure rates. This was seen clinically in our Phase I study of 5FU completed in 1957. In this context, it must be pointed out again that a number of patients, especially with Dukes B lesions, are cured by surgery alone, and severe toxicity or a death from 5FU toxicity is a catastrophe. For these reasons the decision to administer each dose during the first course of 5FU must be made by an oncologist well experienced in giving 5FU to slight toxicity. There are a few occasions when calculated risks with 5FU are justifiable, but not as adjuvant therapy. For example, in a young person who has had a resection of a colorectal cancer and has developed recurrence in the form of lymphogenous spread to the lungs with dyspnoea at rest, I would explain to the patient and family that heroic measures are indicated and would push the first loading course not to slight but to moderately severe toxicity.

This is not to say that an average-risk patient who has had a resection of a Dukes C lesion should be treated lightly and have therapy terminated before any reaction, merely in the interest of preventing toxicity. It is preferable to refer patients to oncologists well experienced in administering optimal courses of 5FU. An oncologist can administer the critical first course and the referring physician can then carry out subsequent courses which are almost always clinically identical to the first course of therapy.

In 1965 we embarked on a programme of 5FU as an adjuvant to resection of Dukes B and C colon cancers[37-40]. Five years had elapsed since the two very high risk patients had been given three courses of 5FUDR as an adjuvant to their surgery and both were alive with no evidence of disease. We hoped that the micrometastases which are presumably present but not discernible could be completely eradicated with 5–8 months of aggressive chemotherapy with 5FU. We felt compelled to begin this study as well because colorectal cancer was the most common malignancy seen in our chemotherapy clinics and the cure rate was not improving. We felt in addition that if adjuvant chemotherapy was to be considered, it would compel the surgeon to inform the patient with

Dukes B or C cancer that although all visible tumour was surgically removed, microscopic examination of the removed tumour showed spread of cancer cells to serosa or regional lymph nodes and a definite probability of recurrence existed. This information is immediately followed with the statement that available treatment (adjuvant to surgery) may eradicate remaining cancer cells.

This frankness is respected by almost all patients and their families, who are happy to learn that adjuvant therapy with demonstrable effectiveness is available. How much more preferable is this honest approach when one realizes that 80% of these high-risk patients are otherwise doomed to develop recurrence[11]? There are very few patients that are more bitter than those who develop recurrence and who were previously told by their surgeon that 'I got it all out'. The patient who develops such a recurrence is convinced that the doctor lied. It is rarely possible to persuade such a patient to return to his doctor for subsequent referral to an oncologist for chemotherapy and follow-up.

To critically dissect the various reasons likely responsible for negative results in other reported adjuvant studies would not prove useful but a few general comments are necessary. To find a short 2- or 3-day course of thio-tepa ineffective as an adjuvant in colorectal cancer is not surprising as this compound was never regarded as useful against this tumour. Similarly, only one or two courses of 5FU would be predictably inadequate, even before the elegant work by Skipper et al.[33] and Schabel et al.[34] demonstrated in animal tumours that total kill of cancer cells was possible with chemotherapeutic compounds when the tumour was small and sufficient quantities of drug were given over repeated courses.

Our plan was to conduct a pilot study and, if it looked promising, to propose this for group study to Central Oncology Group. In this context, each patient with Dukes B cancer received four courses of 5FU starting 3 weeks following resection and all patients with Dukes C cancers received six courses. We also treated for 1–2 years patients with tumour spread to contiguous structures but in whom all gross tumour had been removed and, as well, patients with presumable remaining disease not proven by biopsy. There were over 200 patients in these four groups; there were no operative deaths and no toxicity was sufficiently severe as to require hospitalization. Only those with Dukes B and C lesions will be discussed in this chapter; they had second-look operations 9 months following resection. All patients received each course of 5FU to the point of slight reaction or until they received five whole and 11 half-doses, as described previously, and had 30-day intervals between courses.

A total of 104 patients in these studies received 655 courses of 5FU. Dukes C colonic cancer tumours were present in 53 patients and Dukes

Table 3   Results in 32 patients with Dukes B lesions given 5FU
adjuvant treatment

Results	No. of patients at 6–11 year risk
No tumour or recurrence	29 (91%)
No tumour, later recurrence	3

B in 32. The remaining 19 patients had either tumour attachment to contiguous organs or presumable remaining disease at surgery but not proven by biopsy.

The Dukes B and C lesion patients received careful scrutiny at second-look operations 9 months after initial resection and after all adjuvant chemotherapy was given. Of the 32 Dukes B cancer patients, 29 (91%) had no tumour and no recurrence while three had no tumour at the second-look operation but later developed recurrence. The results are shown in Table 3. There was no serious or fatal toxicity, nor were there any operative deaths. Of the 53 patients with Dukes C lesions 35 (66%) are without evident disease at least 6 years later and an additional three patients had a resectable recurrence at second-look operation and are now free of disease at least 6 years later, yielding a total of 38 patients (71%) alive and without evident disease. The second-look procedure has been discontinued since the CEA determination has become available. CEA levels are quite meaningful if they are elevated prior to surgery, return to a normal level following surgery and then rise again. If a rise is observed a repeat CEA is taken in 7–10 days and if this rises further, it is presumptive evidence of recurrence. Even if studies do not elicit a recurrence, a second look is indicated.

Table 4   Results in 53 patients with Dukes C colon lesions given
5FU adjuvant treatment

Results	No. of patients at 6–11 year risk
No tumour recurrence	35 (66%)
Resectable (and remained tumour free)	3
No tumour, later recurrence	5
Unresectable	6
Resectable, later recurrence	4

Our original plan was to start a Phase I study and, after 12 patients were given 5FU adjuvant therapy, to randomize patients for adjuvant 5FU therapy or no treatment following their original surgery. However, when we observed promising results with adjuvant treatment we simply could not justify denying obviously useful treatment to high-risk patients, so we continued treating all consecutive patients with Dukes B or C cancer. When we presented our results to the Central Oncology

Group they ultimately adopted a prospective randomized trial[23] of adjuvant 5FU for 1 year *vs.* no adjuvant therapy. Unfortunately, despite our protests, they reduced the loading course of 5FU to $12 \, mg \, kg^{-1} \, d^{-1} \times 4$, a day of rest, then $6 \, mg^{-1} \, kg^{-1} \, d$ every other day to toxicity or until five such half-doses were given. Thereafter the patients received $12 \, mg/kg$ once weekly and not the usual $15 \, mg/kg$.

Although the headquarters of the Central Oncology Group was at our institution we did not feel we could participate in a study where half the patients were to receive no adjuvant therapy, especially after we observed superior results in our patients given postoperative 5FU treatment with significantly longer disease-free survivals than in any and all untreated series. Moreover, it would have been difficult to accept the suboptimal dosage regimen of the Central Oncology Group study. Interestingly, of all the Central Oncology Group patients given 5FU adjuvant treatment, there were significantly longer ($p = 0.004$) disease-free intervals for those who became leukopenic compared to those who did not, suggesting that patients treated more aggressively were more likely to respond to therapy.

At this point it is appropriate to discuss the 5FU adjuvant study in colorectal cancer reported by Li and Ross[35]. Significant tumour-free 5-year survival was observed in patients with Dukes B colorectal cancer treated with two courses of 5FU following resection as compared to those treated with surgery alone. All patients with Dukes B and C lesions were given 5FU beginning 4–6 weeks after surgery. Patients under 65 years of age weighing more than 60 kg and in good nutritional status received 1000 mg, 5FU intravenously on day 1 then 500 mg daily on the next 4 days. This course was repeated only once more, after 4 weeks. For patients older than 65, weighing less than 60 kg, and undernourished the regimen consisted of 500 mg 5FU daily for 5 days then repeated after 4 weeks. Leukopenia ($< 3000/mm^3$), thrombocytopenia ($< 120\,000/mm^3$), the appearance of several oral ulcerations, or bouts of diarrhoea prompted suspension of the next dose of 5FU.

This study was not randomized but all 89 consecutive patients with Dukes B and C cancers were resected by the same surgeon in a community hospital from 1965 to 1970 and were then given 5FU. For control purposes they were compared with the results of all patients with Dukes B and C lesions resected by the same surgeon between 1960 and 1965 but untreated with adjuvant 5FU. Patients with Dukes B lesions not treated with 5FU had 58.5% no evidence of disease (NED) status at 5 years compared to 81.6% NED at 5 years for the Dukes B patients who received the two courses of 5FU ($p < 0.02$). Patients with Dukes C lesions not treated with adjuvant 5FU had a 5-year survival of 24.3% compared to 57.5% for those given two courses of 5FU ($p < 0.01$). These results are considerably better than the Veterans Administration Group

Study II as well as the Central Oncology Group Study, with the former group injecting $12 \, mg \, kg^{-1} d^{-1} \times 5 \, d$ every 6 weeks for 18 months and the latter $12 \, mg \, kg^{-1} d^{-1} \times 4 \, d$ then $12 \, mg$/week for 1 year, both delivering considerably more chemotherapy than the Li and Ross study.

It is difficult to reconcile these differences, with only two suboptimal courses of 5FU producing such superior results in patients who received adjuvant 5FU. This minimal, almost homeopathic, dosage violates tenets of pharmacology and the conclusions drawn by Skipper[33] and Schabel[34], indicating that a clear dose–response relationship exists (that is, higher dose chemotherapy results in higher cure rate).

There is no question that the Li 5FU adjuvant regimen will attract many proponents, particularly because of its simplicity and negligible toxicity. We are fearful, however, that these results will not be reproducible and unfortunately will set back the progress implicit in 'multimodal primary treatment', a term coined by Weiss and De Vitta. Since the time Jacobs[36] reported good results with 5FU therapy given only as weekly doses without a loading course, about 90% of physicians (including oncologists) have been happy to adopt this simple, homeopathic dosage regimen and have dropped the loading course like a hot potato. Table 2 clearly demonstrated, in the randomized study of 200 patients with accurately measurable lesions, the significant superiority of the loading *vs.* the other three regimens, one of which constituted weekly therapy without a loading course of 5FU. It would now consume 10 years to compare our 5FU adjuvant treatment *vs.* Li's. We would not propose such study because we cannot withhold what we feel is optimal therapy. To obviate the need for that study we propose to resurrect 5FUDR and test it in a randomized trial *vs.* 5FU in advanced colorectal and stomach cancer with both drugs given intravenously at optimal dosage schedules in monthly courses by a co-operative group. Concomitantly, a randomized study of both compounds would be conducted in Dukes B and C colon cancer and high risk gastric cancer patients with positive lymph nodes.

Combination chemotherapy certainly has the potential of producing greater anti-tumour effect than single drug treatment. However, each of the component drugs of the combination should have proven activity alone against colorectal cancer and it is difficult to find a drug other than 5FU that has this property apart from 5FUDR, which is not available for intravenous administration.

The Southwest Oncology Group performed a randomized experiment[41] on 342 patients with advanced colorectal cancer. In those who received 5FU plus Mitomycin the response rate was 18% and the combination of 5FU plus methylCCNU yielded a 16% response rate: neither regimen showed any advantage over 5FU therapy alone. Still, a number of current randomized studies use MeCCNU + 5FU as one arm of a trial, or combine these two compounds with vincristine administration. Randomizing these three compounds in combination *vs.* 5FU alone showed this combination was more effective in advanced colorectal cancer[42,43]. A search of the literature has failed to reveal any completed randomized studies in man of combinations of drugs used as an adjuvant following resection of colorectal cancer, but some are currently in progress, as are combinations of compounds plus immunotherapy.

Several promising studies of irradiation as an adjuvant in patients with rectal cancer and low sigmoid lesions are currently in progress and some have been completed. Higgins[44] reported on 700 patients randomized to receive either preoperative radiotherapy (2000 r and an additional 500 r for those who were to have an abdominoperineal resection) *vs.* immediate surgery. At 5-year risk the survival of patients who received preoperative radiotherapy was slightly better, particularly for those that had an abdominoperineal resection and received an additional 500 r. In the resected specimens the incidence of metastases to regional lymph nodes was substantially smaller in patients that received preoperative radiotherapy, particularly in those who had abdominoperineal resection; 26% *vs.* 44% in those treated with surgery alone. This observation has been consistent with controlled studies reported in the literature[45-47].

Subsequently the Veterans Administration Surgical Group conducted a trial using 3150 r followed by abdominoperineal resection. Such patients had a smaller percentage of involved lymph nodes than those who did not receive preoperative radiotherapy but survival data are not yet available.

Postoperative radiotherapy has more appeal to the surgeon as he finds it difficult to postpone resection of a resectable cancer while awaiting preoperative radiotherapy. Generally larger doses, 4500–5000 r over an elapsed time of 5–6 weeks, are well tolerated[48] postoperatively in patients with rectal cancer where the surgeon feels the likelihood of recurrence is high. Additionally, the pelvis and abdomen can be thoroughly explored at the time of resection, the surgeon can more accurately determine if irradiation is indicated and can outline with radiopaque clips the precise area requiring irradiation and radiation boosts.

With regard to combined 5FU therapy plus irradiation, it is difficult to administer one without interfering with the other due to the development of leukopenia, diarrhoea or both. After having used this combination in about 25 patients for recurrent or advanced low rectosigmoid or rectal cancer we have abandoned it in favour of using both modalities separately. There has been increasing interest in the use of chemoimmunotherapy as an adjuvant following resection of colorectal cancer and the Mayo Clinic has performed a pilot study with MER BCG, the methanol extraction residue of BCG, in advanced colorectal cancer[49,50]. A preliminary report of adjuvant therapy following resection of colorectal cancer with 5FU MeCCNU plus oral BCG looks promising. An adjuvant study[51] at the M. D. Anderson Hospital found that the results of BCG vs. BCG plus oral 5FU were similar in patients who had Dukes C colonic resected cancer. Combining both groups and comparing them with surgical controls shows a significant advantage ($p = 0.002$) in disease-free interval for the patients who received adjuvant therapy vs. the control group who had surgery alone.

Robinson et al.[53] randomized 53 consecutive patients who had Dukes B_2 and C colorectal cancer. Following surgery the patients were stratified according to stage and location of the tumour and one group received radiotherapy and/or chemotherapy and the second group received the same with the addition of MER, the methanol extraction residue of BCG. The disease-free incidence at 24 months was 84% for the group who received MER and 61% ($p < 0.05$) for the group who did not. The authors recognize that additional patients and longer follow-ups are needed to learn whether such treatment delays recurrence and increases survival.

SUMMARY

In summary it is apparent a great deal of clinical research has been done over the past two decades in an effort to improve our management of gastrointestinal cancer. Many important and promising studies are currently in progress. Some are quite innovative while others search to confirm or even disprove chemotherapeutic results that may appear too glowing. Both approaches are essential.

A word of caution is in order. To make statements such as '5FU is a no treatment' and to term it as the 'breakthrough that never was' confers upon the individual who makes such utterance a mistaken air of omniscient authority. Before one can be critical of claimed or unusual results, it is essential that the exact details of the initial experiment are observed in repeating the study. We do not have 5FUDR available for intravenous use because the Mayo Group would not duplicate the University of Wisconsin dosage schedule, as they would similarly not use our 5FU schedule, selecting instead $13.5 \, \text{mg} \, \text{kg}^{-1} \, \text{d}^{-1} \times 5 \, \text{d}$ with no additional half-doses. In the author's opinion the 5FU dosage implicit in their regimen is too high for a patient in our poor-risk classification and it is inadequate for good-risk patients, over half of the patients that are candidates for 5FU therapy.

A review of the literature shows that 5FU is used either alone or in combination in almost all adjuvant treatment protocols following resection of colorectal cancer. We have gone into considerable detail repeating the dosage regimen we employ and the precautions that we consider mandatory and routine. We are pleased that the Veterans Administration and the Central Oncology studies, both randomized *vs.* no treatment, have eventually shown that 5FU is associated with significant benefit. We hope that the Li and Ross results will be duplicated although we do not hold high hopes, for reasons mentioned. Duplication of the Li and Ross results would be a most important inroad against large bowel cancer since it would be without the hazards associated with our regimen when it is attempted by those with inadequate experience in employing an optimal loading course of 5FU and repeating it at monthly intervals. This therapy has, however, yielded the highest 5-year salvage rate in Dukes B and C colonic cancer and, in our experience it has been eminently safe.

References

1 Moertel, C. G. and Reitemeier, R. J. (eds.) (1969). *Advanced Gastrointestinal Cancer*, p. 6. (New York: Harper & Row)
2 Moertel, C. G., Childs, D. S., Jr, Reitemeier, R. J. *et al.* (1969). Combined chemotherapy and radiation therapy. In Moertel, C. G. and Reitemeier, C. G. (eds.). *Advanced Gastrointestinal Cancer*, pp. 192–204. (New York: Harper & Row).
3 Ansfield, Fred J. (1973) *Chemotherapy of Malignant Neoplasm*, p. 229 (Springfield, Ill: Charles C. Thomas)
4 Hattori, T., Niimoto, M., Koh, T. *et al.* (1979). Post-operative long-term adjuvant immunochemotherapy with miyomycin-C, PSK and FT-207 in gastric cancer patients. *Jpn. J. Surg.*, **9,** 110
5 Fujimoto, S., Akao, T., Itoh, B. *et al.* (1977). Protracted oral chemotherapy with fluorinated pyrimidines as an adjuvant to surgical treatment for stomach cancer. *Ann. Surg.*, April
6 Gilbert, J. M., Ellis, H., Wastell, C. *et al.* (1978). Adjuvant treatment with razoxane (ICRF 159) following resection of cancer of the stomach. *Rec. Results Cancer Res.*, **68,** 217
7 Cole, W. H., Roberts, S. S. and Strehl F. W. (1966). Modern concepts in cancer of the colon and rectum. *Cancer*, **19,** 1347
8 Turnbull, R. B., Kyle, K., Watson, F. R. *et al.* (1967). Cancer of the colon: The influence of the no-touch isolation technique on survival rates. *Ann. Surg.*, **166,** 420
9 National End Results Committee.
10 Falterman, K. W., Hill, C. B., Markey, J. C. *et al.* (1974). Cancer of the colon, rectum, anus: a review of 2313 cases. *Cancer*, **34,** 951
11 Weiss, R. B. and De Vitta, V. T., Jr (1979). Multimodal primary cancer treatment (adjuvant chemotherapy): current results and future prospects. *Ann. Intern. Med.*, **91,** 251
12 Mrazek, R., Economou, S., McDonald, G. O. *et al.* (1959). Prophylactic and adjuvant use of nitrogen mustard in the surgical treatment of cancer. *Ann. Surg.*, **150,** 74
13 Dwight, R. W., Higgins, G. A. and Keehan, R. J. (1969). Factors influencing survival after resection in cancer of the colon and rectum. *Am. J. Surg.*, **117,** 512
14 Higgins, G. A., Serlin, O., Hughes, F. *et al.* (1962). The Veterans Administration Surgical Adjuvant Group-Interim report. *Cancer Chemother. Rep.*, **16,** 141
15 Holden, W. D., Dixon, W. J. and Kuzma, J. W. (1967). The use of triethylenethiophosphoramide-adjuvant to the surgical treatment of colorectal carcinoma. *Ann. Surg.*, **165,** 481

16 Dixon, W. J., Longmire, W. P. and Holden, W. (1971). Use of triethylenethiophospha-
    mide as an adjuvant to the surgical treatment of gastric and colorectal carcinoma – Ten
    year followup. *Ann. Surg.*, **173**, 26
17 Heidelberger, C., Chaudhuri, N. K., Danneberg, P. *et al.* (1957). Fluroinated pyrimi-
    dines; a class of tumor-inhibitory compounds. *Nature (Lond.)*, **179**, 663
18 Duschinsky, R., Pleven, E. and Heidelberger, C. (1957). The synthesis of 5-fluoro-
    pyrimidines. *J. Am. Chem. Soc.*, **79**, 4559
19 Heidelberger, C., Griesbach, L., Cruz, O. *et al.* (1958). Studies on fluorinated pyrimi-
    dines. VI. Effects of 5-fluorouridine and 5-fluoro-2'-deoxyuridine on transplanted
    tumors. *Proc. Soc. Exp. Biol. Med.*, **97**, 470
20 Ansfield, F. J. and Curreri, A. R. (Division of Clinical Oncology, University of Wiscon-
    sin, Madison) (1963). Further clinical comparison between 5-fluorouracil (5-FU)[1] and
    5-fluoro-2'-doxyuridine (5-FUDR). *Cancer Chemother. Rep.*, No. 32
21 Higgins, G. A., Dwight, R. W., Smith, J. V. *et al.* (1971). Fluorouracil as an adjuvant to
    surgery in carcinoma of the colon. *Arch. Surg.*, **102**, 339
22 Moertel, C. G., Reitemeier, R. J. and Hahn, R. G. (1969). Therapy with the fluorinated
    pyrimidines. In Moertel, C. G. and Reitemeier, R. J. (eds.). *Advanced Gastrointestinal
    Cancer*, pp. 86–107. (New York: Harper & Row)
23 Grage, T. B., Metter, G. E., Cornell, G. N. *et al.* (1977). Adjuvant chemotherapy with
    5-fluorouracil after surgical resection of colorectal carcinoma (COG Protocol 7041). A
    preliminary report. *Am. J. Surg.*, **133**, 59
24 Rousselot, I. M., Cole, D. R., Grossi, C. E. *et al.* (1968). A five year progress report on
    the effectiveness of intraluminal chemotherapy (5-fluorouracil) adjuvant to surgery
    for colorectal cancer. *Am. J. Surg.*, **115**, 140
25 Lawrence, W., Terz, J. J., Horsley, S. *et al.* (1975). Chemotherapy as an adjuvant to
    surgery for colorectal cancer. *Ann. Surg.*, **181**, 616
26 Higgins, G. A., Jr, Humphrey, E., Juler, G. L. *et al.* (1976). Adjuvant chemotherapy in
    the surgical treatment of large bowel cancer. *Cancer*, **38**, 1461
27 Dwight, R. W., Humphrey, E. W., Higgins, G. A. *et al.* (1973). FUDR as an adjuvant
    to surgery in cancer of the large bowel. *J. Surg. Oncol.*, **5**, 243
28 Ramirez, G., Korbitz, B. C., Davis, H. L., Jr *et al.* (1969). A comparative study of
    monthly courses *vs.* weekly maintenance dose of 5-fluorouracil (NSC 19893). *Cancer
    Chemother. Rep.*, **53**, 243
29 Ansfield, F. J. (1964). A less toxic fluorouracil dosage schedule. *J. Am. Med. Assoc.*,
    190, 686
30 Wolberg, W. H. and Morin, J. (1981). Thymidylate synthetase activity and fluorouracil
    sensitivity of human colonic cancer and normal mucosal tissue preparations. *Cancer*
    (In press)
31 Ansfield, F. J. and Curreri, A. R. (1958), Clinical studies with 5-fluorouarcil. *Proc.
    Am. Assoc. Cancer Res.*, **2**, 276
32 Ansfield, F. J., Klotz, J., Nealon, T. *et al.* (1977). A Phase III study comparing the clini-
    cal utility of four regimens of 5-fluorouracil – a preliminary report. *Cancer*, **39**, 34
33 Skipper, H. E. (1978). Adjuvant chemotherapy. *Cancer*, **41**, 936
34 Schabel, F. M., Jr (1975). Concepts for systemic treatment of micrometastases. *Cancer*,
    35, 15
35 Li, M. C. and Ross, S. T. (1976). Chemoprophylaxis for patients with colorectal cancer:
    prospective study with five-year follow-up. *J. Am. Med. Assoc.*, **235**, 2825
36 Jacobs, E. M., Reeves, W. J., Wood, D. A. *et al.* (1971). Treatment of cancer with
    weekly intraveous 5-fluorouracil. *Cancer*, **27**, 1302
37 Curreri, A. R. and Mackman, S. (1966). Reoperation in carcinoma of the colon follow-
    ing resection and adjuvant chemotherapy. *Surg. Gynecol. Obstet.*, **123**, 724
38 Mackman, S. and Curreri, A. R. (1968). The second look operation for carcinoma of
    the colon after administration of 5 FU. *Am. J. Surg.*, **115**, 227

39 Mackman, S., Curreri, A. R. and Ansfield, F. J. (1970). Second-look operation for colon carcinoma after 5-FU therapy. *Arch. Surg.*, **100**, 527

40 Mackman, S., Ansfield, F. J., Ramirez, G. *et al.* (1974). A second look at the second-look operation in colonic cancer after the administration of fluorouracil. *Am. J. Surg.*, **128**, 763

41 Buroker, T., Kim, P. N., Groppe, C. *et al.* (1978). 5-FU infusion with mitomycin-C versus 5-FU infusion with methyl-CCNU in the treatment of advanced colon cancer: a Southwest Oncology Group Study. *Cancer*, **42**, 1228

42 Falkson, G. and Falkson, H. C. (1976) Fluorouracil, methyl CCNU, and vincristine in cancer of the colon. *Cancer*, **38**, 1468

43 Moertl, C. G., Schutt, A. J., Hahn, R. J. *et al.* (1975). Therapy of advanced colorectal cancer with a combination of 5-FU, methyl 1,3 cis (chloroethyl)-1-cyclohexyl nitro-sourea and vincristine. *J. Natl. Cancer Inst.*, **54**, 69

44 Higgins, G. A., Jr, Humphrey, E. W., Amadeo, J. H. *et al.* (1977). Preoperative radiotherapy for colorectal cancer. In Gerard, A. (ed.). *Gastrointestinal Tumors: a Clinical and Experimental Approach* (Proceedings of an International Symposium sponsored by the European Organization for Research and Treatment of Cancer, Brussels, 14–15 April)

45 Buroker, T., Nigro, N., Correa, J. *et al.* (1976). Combination preoperative radiation and chemotherapy in adenocarcinoma and the rectum. *Dis. Colon Rectum*, **19**, 660

46 Kligerman, M. M., Urdaneta, N., Knowlton, A. *et al.* (1972), Preoperative irradiation of rectosigmoid carcinoma including its regional lymph nodes. *Am. J. Roentgenol.*, **114**, 498

47 Quan, S. H., Deddish, M. R. and Stearns, M. W. Jr (1960). The effect of preoperative roentgen therapy upon the 10 and 5 yr results of the surgical treatment of cancer of the rectum. *Surg. Gynecol. Obstet.*, **111**, 507

48 Turner, S. S., Vieira, E. F., Ager, P. J. *et al.* (1977). Elective postoperative radiotherapy for locally advanced colorectal cancer. *Cancer*, **40**, 105

49 Moertel, C. G., Ritts, R. E., Schutt, A. J. *et al.* (1975). Clinical studies of methanol extraction residue fraction of Bacillus Calmette-Guerin as an immunostimulant in patients with advanced cancer. *Cancer Res.*, **35**, 3075

50 Moertel, C. G., O'Connell, M. J., Ritts, R. E., Jr *et al.* (1978). A controlled evaluation of combined immunotherapy (MER-BCG) and chemotherapy for advanced colorectal cancer. In Terry, W. D. and Windhurst, D. (eds.). *Immunotherapy of Cancer: Present Status of Trials in Man.* (New York; Raven Press)

51 Valdivieso, M. and Mavligit, G. M. (1978), Chemotherapy and chemoimmunotherapy of colorectal cancer – role of the carcinoembryonic antigen. Symposium on Colon and Anorectal Surgery. *Surg. Clin. N. Am.*, **58**, 619

52 Pannettiere, F. J. and Jones, S. E. (eds.) (1977). Adjuvant chemotherapy and che-moimmunotherapy for locally advanced large bowl adenocarcinoma. Preliminary report of a continuing Southwest Oncology Group Study. *Adjuvant Therapy of Cancer* (Amsterdam: Elsevier/North-Holland Biomedical Press)

53 Robinson, E., Batal, A., Cohen, Y. *et al.* (1979). Adjuvant therapy in colorectal cancer (a randomized trial comparing radio-chemotherapy and radio-chemotherapy combined with the Methanol Extraction Residue of BCG, MER). *Biomedicine*, **31**, 8

54 Wolberg, W. H., Johnson, R. O. and Curreri, A. R. (1960). Toxicity studies of 5-flurouracil used as an adjuvant to surgery. *Am. Med. Assoc. Arch. Surg.*, **81**, 244

6
Combined modality (adjuvant) therapy in breast cancer

K. COWAN AND M. LIPPMAN

Breast cancer remains the leading cause of death due to cancer in women. A woman living in the USA currently has a lifetime risk of developing breast cancer of one chance in eleven. In 1980 alone there will be over 100 000 new cases in the USA. Despite the fact that the majority of patients present with 'operable' lesions, nearly half will relapse. Although therapy of advanced disease is successful in prolonging survival, virtually all of these women will eventually die of their disease. Over the past several years basic research has provided new insights into the biology of breast cancer which have resulted in new therapeutic approaches to this disease. In addition, the development of effective and relatively safe combination chemotherapy for metastatic disease has encouraged the earlier use of cytotoxic drugs in breast cancer treatment.

New hope for patients with breast cancer has been recently provided by the demonstration that early systemic chemotherapy (adjuvant chemotherapy) is effective in at least delaying the appearance of recurrent disease in certain patients. The rationale for the use of adjuvant therapy is quite simple. If a tumour is detected before metastases occur, local therapy, either surgery or radiation therapy, will be curative. If, however, tumour metastases have already developed, obviously local procedures will no longer be sufficient. Under these conditions effective systemic therapy must be employed to treat the metastatic lesions.

The fact that undetectable micrometaststic lesions already exist in most patients with breast cancer at the time of initial diagnosis is all too apparent from an examination both of recurrence rates and sites of recurrence in patients following 'curative' resection of the primary tumour. Thus, despite extensive local therapy (radical mastectomy ± radiation therapy), almost 50% of all breast cancer patients with apparently localized disease will subsequently die from distant metastases[1]. While many factors influence the rate of tumour recurrence including tumour size, menopausal status, oestrogen receptor concentration, and histological type and grade, one of the most significant factors is the histological status of the axillary nodes at the time of diagnosis. Seventy-five per cent of all patients with positive axillary nodes and 90% of all patients with more than four positive axillary nodes will relapse within 10 years following initial 'curative' surgery. Even more disappointing is the fact that at least one-quarter of patients with negative axillary nodes will also subsequently relapse. Since the ability to cure patients who develop tumour recurrence is limited, the figures for relapse-free survival are virtually equivalent to overall survival data.

These data for disease-free survival in the breast cancer patient have remained relatively constant over the past several decades despite increasingly aggressive approaches to local control. It is beyond the scope of this chapter to review the various primary therapies employed over the years in the treatment of breast cancer and the reader is instead referred to several recent reviews[2-4]. Suffice it to say that the various local surgical and radiotherapeutic approaches employed, in spite of their ever-expansive nature, while reducing the incidence of local recurrences, have failed to significantly alter overall patient survival. This failure on the part of aggressive local primary therapy implies that breast cancer is truly a systemic disease, even at the time of initial diagnosis. In light of the dismal results with primary local therapy in breast cancer, several adjuvant chemotherapy trials were initiated in the hope that early intervention with effective systemic therapy would prevent tumour recurrence. Before discussing the results of recent clinical trials, several basic principles regarding early multimodality (adjuvant) therapy will be reviewed.

TUMOUR CELL KINETICS AND ANIMAL STUDIES

It has been estimated from animal studies that the minimal detectable tumour contains approximately 10^9 cells. Thus a cancer arising from a single neoplastic cell would take at least 30 cell doublings before it became clinically apparent by routine physical or radiographic examination. The growth rate of human breast cancers is quite variable and the mean doubling time has been estimated to average between 90 and 166 days[5]. Thus, even when a breast cancer is barely palpable it has probably already existed for several years. These findings are consistent with the long period (>10 years) of risk of recurrence following mastectomy for primary breast cancer. The variability in tumour doubling time is a reflection of the fact that the growth rate of breast cancers is no doubt a complex function of various factors, dependent not only on tumour growth fraction and cell doubling time, but also on various host factors including hormonal influences (in endocrine-dependent tumours) and immune defence mechanisms.

It has been shown that the growth of most malignant tumours is not logarithmic but rather can be described by a Gompertzian equation. That is, as the size of the tumour increases the growth fraction of the tumour decreases and the tumour doubling time increases[6,7]. Since most cytotoxic drugs are more effective against actively dividing cells, chemotherapy should be more effective on tumours with higher growth fractions. If it is assumed that the kinetics of minimal microscopic disease parallel the equations derived from studies of macroscopic disease, it follows that cytotoxic chemotherapy should be even more successful at this stage of disease, when a greater fraction of cells should be actively dividing. This concept has been tested in several transplantable animal tumour sytems. For example, B16 melanoma subcutaneously inoculated into mice responds to therapy with methyl-CCNU. Griswold has shown that the number of mice cured after a single dose of methyl-CCNU is directly proportional to the size of the initial tumour cell inoculum[8]. If the tumour initially contains 10^9 cells, only 13% of the tumours respond to a single dose of this drug and all the mice die from disease. However with smaller tumour inocula there is a progressive increase in the percentage of long-term survivors. Thus when there are only 10^3 tumour cells there are 70% cures following a single dose of chemotherapy. When the tumour cell number is intermediate, between 10^3 and 10^9 cells, the chemotherapy cure rate is directly proportional to the tumour burden.

Additional animal studies have explored the effectiveness of 'adjuvant' chemotherapy given after surgical resection of transplanted tumours. As noted previously, the risk of recurrence in human breast cancer following mastectomy is directly proportional to the size of the primary lesion at the time of surgery. A similar relationship is observed in several animal tumour models, i.e. the rate of recurrence following surgical resection of the transplanted tumour is directly related to the primary tumour cell burden. At the Southern Research Institute primary multimodality (adjuvant) therapy was investigated using four different animal tumour models: C3H mammary carcinoma, B16 melanoma, Lewis lung carcinoma, and line 26 colon carcinoma[9]. Effective single-agent chemotherapy was given in each case after surgical reduction of the primary tumour. Several important observations were made in these studies. First, combined modality therapy (surgery plus chemotherapy) was more effective in increasing survival than either therapy alone. Second, delaying surgery following tumour implantation (increasing primary tumour cell burden) reduces the effectiveness of multimodality therapy. Third, delaying chemotherapy following surgery (presumably allowing growth of micrometastatic tumour burden) also decreased the therapeutic advantage of adjuvant chemotherapy. Finally, the effect of adjuvant therapy was dose-related: more aggressive chemotherapy resulted in higher disease-free survival rates. Similar results demonstrating the effectiveness of post-surgical adjuvant chemotherapy have been obtained in several other animal tumour systems using both single agent[10-13] and combination chemotherapy[13,14]. These experimental data on cell kinetics and adjuvant therapy have been useful in generating the following principles with which adjuvant trials in human breast cancer have been designed:

(1) Effective chemotherapy should be employed at maximum doses with acceptable toxicity.
(2) Chemotherapy should be given intermittently in order to reduce toxicity.
(3) Adjuvant therapy should be initiated as soon as possible after local therapy, when micrometastatic tumour burden is least.
(4) Treatment should be given over a prolonged period of time (to encompass several tumour cell doubling periods).

CLINICAL TRIALS

The first large study of adjuvant chemotherapy in the treatment of breast cancer patients was begun in 1957 by the National Surgical Adjuvant Breast Project (NSABP)[1]. The concept of micrometastatic tumour burden was not considered at that time. Instead it was believed that the failure of local therapy resulted from dislodging tumour cells during the initial surgery. In order to test this hypothesis, patients with localized disease were first treated by radical mastectomy and then were randomized to receive a single course of thio-tepa given over a 72 h period following surgery. The overall results from 826 patients were analysed according to both axillary lymph node status and menopausal status, and indicated that there was no therapeutic advantage in the patients who received postoperative chemotherapy. However subsequent analyses of the individual patient subgroups revealed that one group did benefit from chemotherapy. Premenopausal patients with four or more positive axillary nodes who received a single course of postoperative chemotherapy had a 40% lower rate of recurrence between 18 and 36 months following surgery than the control group. This difference decreased with time, but there were still 21% fewer recurrences in this treatment subgroup at 10 years and a 21% increase in survival.

Another trial using one course of adjuvant chemotherapy was initiated in Scandinavia in 1967[15]. In this multicentre trial 1136 patients with operable breast cancer were randomized following surgery (plus radiation therapy) to receive cyclophosphamide 30 mg/kg intravenously over a 6-day period. With a median follow-up of 12 years there was a statistically significant decrease in recurrences. Overall, there was an increase of 11% in patient survival in the chemotherapy group ($p < 0.02$). Given current concepts regarding adjuvant chemotherapy, it is indeed quite remarkable that any beneficial effects were found in both of these studies in which such limited adjuvant chemotherapy was given. Other clinical studies of adjuvant chemotherapy were initiated at this time using both short-course[16] and more prolonged chemotherapy[17,18]. These series were either uncontrolled or too small and the results are at best ambiguous.

Since those initial studies much has been learned regarding the most effective way to administer chemotherapy in the treatment of metastatic breast cancer. Several cytotoxic agents are now known to be active in this disease and various combination chemotherapy regimens have been shown to be safe and effective in the treatment of patients with advanced breast cancer. Following the suggestion derived from the preceding studies that limited adjuvant chemotherapy was beneficial in some patients with breast cancer, several trials were initiated to examine the efficacy of more prolonged and more aggressive administration of cytotoxic agents in the post-surgical adjuvant setting[19-21]. The two largest studies with the longest follow-up data are those by the NSABP[20] and the National Cancer Institute in Milan, Italy[21]. The trials were essentially identical with respect to patient selection and basically consisted of women with operable breast cancer and histologically positive axillary nodes. The two groups differed primarily in their choice of adjuvant chemotherapy. The NSABP selected single-agent therapy with l-phenylalanine mustard (L-PAM), $0.15\,\mathrm{mg\,kg^{-1}\,d^{-1}}$ day given orally for 5 consecutive days every 6 weeks for 2 years. The Milan group used a combination chemotherapy regimen (CMF) previously shown to be effective in advanced disease. It consisted of cyclophosphamide $100\,\mathrm{mg/m^2}$ by mouth on days 1–14, methotrexate $40\,\mathrm{mg/m^2}$ intravenously on days 1 and 8; 5-fluorouracil (5FU) $600\,\mathrm{mg/m^2}$ intravenously on days 1 and 8. This regimen was given every 28 days for a total of 12 cycles. Both groups adjusted their chemotherapy for myelotoxicity.

The results of both studies have been reported with a median follow-up of 5 years[20,21]. In both studies there was a statistically significant increase in disease-free interval for premenopausal patients who received adjuvant chemotherapy. In the NSABP trial, 55% of patients less than 50 years old treated with L-PAM were free of disease 4 years following surgery, as compared to 45% of placebo-treated women ($p = 0.005$). The greatest benefit of adjuvant therapy in this study was observed in premenopausal patients with one to three positive axillary nodes. In this group 87% of the L-PAM-treated patients remain free of disease as opposed to 57% of the control group of patients ($p = 0.005$). While there was a trend towards apparent benefit in postmenopausal patients and the other subgroup of premenopausal patients (four or more positive axillary nodes) the results were not statistically significant.

Table 1   Milan trial – 4-year disease-free survival and overall survival[25]

	Control	CMF	p-value*
Premenopausal patients	43.4	70.0	0.00002
One node	52.2	80.9	0.01
Two or three nodes	49.3	84.2	0.0005
More than three nodes	26.7	45.4	0.005
Overall survival	70.6	89.6	0.02
Postmenopausal patients	51.7	56.5	0.22
One node	63.2	72.0	0.24
Two or three nodes	45.4	53.0	0.10
More than three nodes	43.6	46.2	0.23
Overall survival	75.4	76.5	0.60

*On time distribution
Data from Ref. 25, with permission

In contrast, the Milan data demonstrate that there was a statistically significant benefit in disease-free survival in all groups of premenopausal patients treated with adjuvant CMF, regardless of the number of axillary nodes involved (see Table 1). Thus, 4 years following initiation of therapy, 70% of premenopausal patients treated with adjuvant CMF have not yet developed recurrence of tumour, as compared to only 43% of the premenopausal control group ($p = 0.00002$). This therapeutic advantage observed in the premenopausal patients has already resulted in a statistically significant improvement of overall survival in the treated group (90% *vs.* 71%; $p = 0.02$). Although early analysis of the Milan data had indicated a significant decrease in relapse rate for post-menopausal patients treated with chemotherapy, subsequent follow-up reveals that the difference between treatment and control groups of postmenopausal patients is now statistically insignificant. Thus 4 years following initiation of therapy 52% of all untreated postmenopausal patients remain free of disease as opposed to 57% of patients treated with CMF ($p = 0.22$).

These two important trials have clearly demonstrated that in certain subgroups of patients with breast cancer early systemic therapy is effective in at least delaying tumour recurrence and prolonging survival. The major question emerging from these two studies is why the benefits from adjuvant chemotherapy were seen only in premenopausal patients. Since alkylating agents such as cyclophosphamide and phenylalanine mustard are known to affect ovarian function, it has been suggested that the beneficial effect of adjuvant chemotherapy in premenopausal women actually reflects the indirect result of medical castration. There are several arguments against this hypothesis. First, several prospective studies have failed to demonstrate any increase in overall survival for patients treated with prophylactic oophorectomy at the time of mastectomy when compared to a control group[22-24]. Second, in the Milan Study there was no correlation between the incidence of drug-induced amenorrhoea and the rate of relapse[25].

Furthermore, a recent report of endocrine studies done by the NSABP on patients receiving L-PAM provides additional evidence against the hypothesis that chemically induced ovarian failure resulted in improved disease-free survival[26]. In this study premenopausal patients were further subdivided into two separate age groups, i.e. ≤39 years and 40 to ≤49 years. Examination of relapse rates reveals that while the benefit from L-PAM adjuvant therapy was most pronounced in the younger age group (≤39 years), it was the older premenopausal patients (40–49 years) who reported a higher incidence of drug-induced alteration in menses following treatment with L-PAM. In addition, serial FSH, LH, and oestradiol levels were obtained from 37 premenopausal patients treated with chemotherapy (L-PAM or L-PAM plus 5FU). Consistent with previous observations on the effect of cytotoxic drugs on ovarian function, serum values of both FSH and LH rose during therapy while oestradiol values remained essentially unchanged. In particular, the greatest changes in these endocrine studies were seen in the older group of patients (39–49 years), in whom the benefit of adjuvant chemotherapy was less. These studies thus confirm previous observations that chemotherapy, particularly alkylating agents, may alter menses and even result in irreversible amenorrhoea. Most significantly, even though chemotherapy-induced endocrine changes occurred more frequently in older premenopausal patients, the major clinical benefit from adjuvant L-PAM therapy was observed primarily in younger patients. As will be discussed below, a final argument against the hypothesis that the benefit of adjuvant chemotherapy in breast cancer patients occurs primarily via indirect hormonal mechanisms is provided by several more recent trials, in which a significant decrease in relapse rate was observed in both postmenopausal as well as premenopausal patients given adjuvant chemotherapy.

Alternatively, it has been suggested that the difference in patient benefit resulting from adjuvant chemotherapy observed in both the NSABP and Milan trials, may actually reflect a true difference in the biology of the tumours in premenopausal and postmenopausal patients. Several diverse observations have suggested an association between the absence of oestrogen receptor and response to cytotoxic chemotherapy in metastatic breast cancer. These include the following facts:

(1) less well differentiated tumours recur earlier;
(2) patients with oestrogen receptor-negative tumours have a shorter disease-free survival[27-29];
(3) thymidine labelling indices are higher in oestrogen receptor-negative tumours[30]; and
(4) cytotoxic chemotherapy is in general more effective against actively dividing cells.

In a recent retrospective analysis in which receptor-positive and receptor-negative patients appeared well balanced with respect to important prognostic and treatment variables, receptor-negative patients had highly significant increased response rates to cytotoxic chemotherapy[31]. Since publication of these results several independent investigations of this issue have yielded markedly divergent results[32-34]. At the present time it is not possible to explain the different results in these studies. However these findings may in part explain why the major benefit of adjuvant chemotherapy was seen in premenopausal patients since their tumours more often lack oestrogen receptors.

Since both trials adjusted the chemotherapy doses for myelotoxicity it has also been suggested that the difference seen between premenopausal and postmenopausal breast cancer patients given adjuvant chemotherapy in both the NSABP and the Milan trials may simply reflect differences in the total amount of chemotherapy given to older and younger patients. Indeed in the Milan trial of adjuvant CMF, patients over the age of 60 were automatically begun at reduced doses of methotrexate (75%) and 5FU (70%) in anticipation of possible increased toxicity in older patients. Furthermore, retrospective analysis of the Milan trial revealed that the postmenopausal patients actually required more frequent dose modifications and overall received less total chemotherapy than the premenopausal patients[25].

The influence of the amount of chemotherapy given on the 5-year relapse-free survival and overall patient survival in the Milan trial have recently been reported[35]. Patients who received less than 65% of the expected total dose of CMF had no difference compared to the control untreated group in either 5-year relapse-free survival (46% treated *vs.* 48% control) or overall patient survival (67% *vs.* 66%). In contrast, patients who received greater than 85% of the total expected dose of adjuvant chemotherapy had both a greater incidence of relapse-free survival (76% *vs.* 48%) and overall survival (82% *vs.* 66%) at 5 years. This correlation between total amount of adjuvant chemotherapy and subsequent patient benefit was seen regardless of axillary lymph node status (one to three nodes or more than three nodes) or menopausal status. In the patients who received ≤ 85% of the predicted total dose of CMF there was an increase in 5-year relapse-free survival compared to the control group in both premenopausal (76% treated *vs.* 44% control) and postmenopausal patients (74% treated *vs.* 52% control). Thus, it appears that the difference in benefit between premenopausal and postmenopausal patients given adjuvant chemotherapy in the Milan trial, and perhaps also the NSABP trial, may reflect overall differences in total amounts of drugs given to each group. This clinical observation is consistent with animal studies of adjuvant chemotherapy in which increases in the dose of effective chemotherapy have resulted in increased long-term survival[9].

Several recent trials lend additional support for the hypothesis that adjuvant chemotherapy may be of value in postmenopausal as well as premenopausal patients. In one historically controlled trial, breast cancer patients with positive axillary nodes were treated after postoperative radiation therapy with adjuvant chemotherapy consisting of cyclophosphamide, adriamycin, and 5FU (FAC) and adjuvant immunotherapy with BCG, repeated at monthly intervals for 2 years[36]. Analysis at a median follow-up of 30 months revealed a statistically significant decrease in the rate of recurrence and an increase in overall patient survival in both premenopausal and postmenopausal patients. In another historically controlled trial, 100 breast cancer patients with four or more positive axillary nodes were given adjuvant chemotherapy consisting of cyclophosphamide, methotrexate, 5FU, vincristine, and prednisone (CMFVP) for 9 months[37]. Approximately half of the patients treated were postmenopausal. The results from this trial were recently published at a median follow-up of 5½ years and again both premenopausal and postmenopausal patients treated with adjuvant chemotherapy had significantly increased overall survival compared to historical controls. Although neither of these trials have contemporaneous control groups, a large review of end-results obtained from several sources, examined both prospectively and retrospectively, has demonstrated no change in the relapse rate or survival in breast cancer patients with positive axillary nodes over the past two decades. The importance of these two trials is the suggestion that postmenopausal as well as premenopausal patients with breast cancer may benefit from adjuvant chemotherapy.

Results from several ongoing adjuvant trials have also been encouraging. The Southwest Oncology Group is currently comparing the effectiveness of single-agent chemotherapy (L-PAM) vs. combination (CMFVP) in a prospective randomized trial of adjuvant therapy in women with stage II disease[38]. A preliminary report was recently published of the results in 334 patients followed for a median duration of 26 months. Overall, the patients treated with the five-drug regimen had a markedly decreased rate of recurrence (15.4%) as compared to the single-agent treatment group (33.1%). This increased benefit from combination chemotherapy was statistically significant in both premenopausal (12.5% vs. 32%) and postmenopausal (17.3% vs. 34%) patients and was observed throughout all subgroups of axillary node involvement.

The NSABP is also investigating the efficacy of combination chemotherapy in the adjuvant setting. Treatment with single-agent chemotherapy (L-PAM) is being compared to two-drug therapy (L-PAM plus 5FU), while another trial is comparing this two-drug regimen to a three-drug combination (L-PAM, 5FU, and methotrexate)[20]. While the time of follow-up is quite limited, in each of these trials preliminary results indicate that the combination chemotherapy regimens appear to be more effective than single-agent therapy. Furthermore, the benefit of multiple-drug therapy is being observed in both premenopausal and postmenopausal patients. It must be reiterated that the results from these controlled trials, while encouraging, are quite preliminary and must be interpreted with caution. However, there is increasing evidence that adjuvant chemotherapy may prove to be beneficial for postmenopausal as well as premenopausal patients with breast cancer.

RISKS OF ADJUVANT CHEMOTHERAPY

While the use of early multimodalitity therapy appears to be effective, at least in delaying recurrence of tumour in certain patients with breast cancer, enthusiasm must be tempered by the realization that longer follow-up of patients in present clinical trials is necessary not only to ascertain if early survival benefits persist, but also to generate information regarding long-term toxicity of adjuvant therapy. Since many of the cytotoxic drugs employed are in themselves carcinogenic, the long-term risk of future development of second malignancies following treatment with adjuvant chemotherapy is an important consideration.

Indeed, there have been increasing reports of second malignancies arising in cancer patients treated with chemotherapy. Alkylating agents in particular have been implicated as a strong risk factor in patients treated for multiple myeloma, ovarian cancer, and lymphomas[39]. Furthermore, it appears that the combination of radiation therapy and chemotherapy increases the risk of developing a second malignancy. At present a small amount of data appears in the literature regarding the risk of development of second malignancies in breast cancer patients treated with adjuvant chemotherapy. In one retrospective analysis of breast cancer patients treated with thio-tepa as adjuvant chemotherapy, no statistical increase in development of second malignancies (either breast or non-breast) was found compared to historical control[40]. However it was noted that the overall incidence of second malignancy did increase with more prolonged administration of chemotherapy. In a small series reported by Lerner, there were three cases of acute leukemia among 13 patients with breast cancer treated for more than 1 year with chlorambucil[41]. At present neither the NSABP nor Milan trials have noted any increase in development of second malignancy, but the duration of follow-up is limited and there may be a relatively long latency period before detection of such a trend.

Other toxicities of chemotherapy must be considered before recommending their universal use in an adjuvant setting. Infertility, for example, is a common occurrence in patients treated with alkylating agents. As discussed previously, alteration in menses is a frequent finding in breast cancer patients treated with chemotherapy and the possibility of infertility may be a special concern in individual cases. Finally, individual drug toxicities must also be carefully analysed prospectively. For example, the long-term risk of cardiotoxicity observed following therapy with doxorubicin may limit the usefulness of this drug in the adjuvant setting. In a recent adjuvant breast cancer trial there were three cases of congestive heart failure possibly related to the use of this drug[36]. Studies at the National Cancer Institute (Surgery Branch) indicate that the risk of cardiac toxicity from adjuvant therapy with doxorubicin may be substantial (Barr, L. and Rosenberg, S., personal communication). In their trial, patients with localized soft tissue sarcoma were treated following surgical resection ± radiation therapy with adjuvant chemotherapy consisting of cyclophosphamide, doxorubicin (total dose $\leq 510 \, mg/m^2$) and methotrexate. Following completion of adjuvant chemotherapy, cardiac ejection fractions were subsequently measured both at rest and during exercise. Preliminary results indicate that 17 of the 40 patients studied following doxorubicin therapy have detectable abnormalities in cardiac function compared to normal controls. Although only five of these patients are presently symptomatic, longer follow-up will be necessary to determine the precise risk of this complication and to determine whether the cardiac abnormalities which occur will improve or worsen with time following cytotoxic therapy. Since it is expected that a significant proportion of the original patient population will live for a prolonged period, the long-term risk of cardiac toxicity must be given serious attention before routine use of doxorubicin is recommended in this setting.

RECOMMENDATIONS AND FUTURE GOALS

The use of early systemic therapy in the treatment of primary breast cancer has proved beneficial in at least some patients. Our recommendations for the management of early stage breast cancer according to histological status of the axillary lymph nodes and the receptor status of the primary lesion are shown in Table 2. At present it has certainly been

Table 2 Management of early stage breast cancer

Histological status of axillary lymph nodes	Oestrogen receptor status	Recommended adjuvant therapy
Premenopausal Patients		
Axilla positive	Positive	Combination chemotherapy – combined endocrine therapy plus chemotherapy encouraging but requires further evaluation
Axilla positive	Negative	Combination chemotherapy
Axilla negative	Positive	No therapy indicated
Axilla negative	Negative	?Combination chemotherapy
Postmenopausal patients		
Axilla positive or negative	Positive or negative	Preliminary results with combination chemotherapy now encouraging
All patients		
1. *Adequate therapy for local control of disease*		
2. *Evaluation of axillary lymph nodes status*		
3. *Oestrogen receptor and progestetone receptor analyses of primary tumour*		

demonstrated that the use of adjuvant chemotherapy is successful in delaying recurrence and prolonging survival in premenopausal patients with positive axillary nodes. The recent encouraging results observed in postmenopausal patients are still quite preliminary and must be viewed with caution. However the outlook for this group of patients also appears promising and only longer follow-up data from present trials will determine whether the current benefit from adjuvant therapy in postmenopausal patients will remain obvious.

Only 25% of patients with negative axillary nodes will relapse following mastectomy and at present no additional therapy is indicated. A preliminary report from a Swiss co-operative group suggests, however, that breast cancer patients with negative axillary nodes may also benefit from adjuvant chemotherapy[42]. In this study all patients, regardless of nodal involvement, were randomized following surgery to receive adjuvant chemotherapy with chlorambucil, methotrexate, 5FU, and prednisone (LMF-P) for 6 months. With a median follow-up duration of 34 months only 7% of the treated patients with negative axillary nodes have relapsed, as compared to 37% in the control group ($p = 0.007$). Although the relapse rate in the control group is higher in this study than in other reported series, these results indicate that further study of adjuvant chemotherapy in this subgroup of breast cancer patients is warranted. Since 75% of patients with negative axillary nodes will be cured by surgery alone the risk of adjuvant chemotherapy must be carefully considered. However, it has been shown that patients whose primary tumours are oestrogen receptor-negative have been observed to have substantially increased rate of recurrences[27-29] and decreased overall survival[43]. This association is independent of other variables known to affect tumour recurrence including menopausal status, tumour size, histological grade, and axillary lymph node status. Therefore patients with stage I breast cancer whose tumours lack receptor should be considered for an appropriate clinical trial of adjuvant chemotherapy.

Another area of particular interest is the role of adjuvant hormonal therapy in the treatment of primary breast cancer. Two studies involving prophylactic ovarian irradiation indicated a prolongation of disease-free interval in patients with stage I and II breast cancer[22,23]. In contrast, a controlled study by the NSABP failed to find any benefit in rates of recurrence in patients treated by adjuvant surgical oophorectomy[24], and all three trials failed to demonstrate any benefit in overall patient survival in the endocrine treatment group. However, these studies were completed before the availability of oestrogen receptor analysis and the appreciation of its role in the prediction of endocrine dependence. A small, uncontrolled but provocative study reported by Dao et al. indicates that perhaps there is a role for endocrine manipulation in adjuvant therapy[44]. They treated 17 postmenopausal patients with four or more axillary nodes with radical mastectomy and bilateral adrenalectomy. In this series there was a decrease in recurrences and prolongation of survival in the treated patients compared to historical controls. Furthermore, there has been one prospective randomized trial in which adjuvant hormonal therapy was successful in prolonging overall patient survival[45]; in this study patients were randomized following mastectomy to receive either no further therapy or ovarian irradiation. For patients 45 years old or over, there was randomization to a third treatment group which consisted of ovarian irradiation plus oral prednisone 7.5 mg daily for up to 5 years. This latter therapy presumably combined ovarian ablation with at least partial suppression of adrenal androgen production, particularly androstenedione, which could be peripherally converted to oestrogens. After 10 years of follow-up, premenopausal patients more than 45 years old treated with both ovarian irradiation and prednisone had a significant improvement in both disease-free survival and overall patient survival compared to the control group. Thus the role of adjuvant hormonal therapy needs further careful evaluation, particularly in conjunction with oestrogen receptor analysis.

The use of combination chemotherapy and hormonal therapy in the adjuvant setting must also be investigated. Preliminary results of a trial using adjuvant chemotherapy and tamoxifen appear quite encouraging[46]. In this prospective randomized trial, 296 patients with stage II breast cancer were treated following mastectomy with one of three treatment regimens: (1) CMF; (2) CMF plus tamoxifen (CMFT); or (3) CMFT plus BCG vaccination. Patients were stratified according to oestrogen receptor status and axillary node status (one to three, and four or more). After a median follow-up of 33 months it was noted that oestrogen receptor-negative patients had more recurrences and a higher mortality than the receptor-positive group. As expected, there was no benefit from the addition of anti-oestrogen to adjuvant chemotherapy in the oestrogen receptor-negative patients. However, patients with oestrogen receptor-positive tumours treated with combination chemotherapy and anti-oestrogen therapy (CMFT) had a significantly decreased rate of recurrence compared to the CMF treatment group ($p = 0.0176$). The benefit from addition of tamoxifen therapy to CMF is apparently seen in both premenopausal and postmenopausal patients with receptor-positive tumours. However the number of patients in each subgroup is quite small and the differences at present remain statistically insignificant. These data are still preliminary and it is too early to detect any overall survival benefit from the combined therapy.

Another area for further clinical evaluation involves the use of different drug schedules in adjuvant therapy. It has been suggested, in particular, that the intensity of chemotherapy should be adapted to the expected sensitivity of the tumour. It has always been assumed that small tumours, because of their large proportion of actively dividing cells, must be more sensitive to chemotherapy. A recent mathematical model proposed by Norton and Simon has raised serious questions regarding this hypothesis[47]. In the previous section on tumour cell kinetics it was noted that the growth of most malignant tumours follows a Gompertzian equation. Norton and Simon emphasize that the growth rate of a tumour described by this equation is slowest for both very large and very small tumours and is maximal at the tumour inflection point, i.e. a size approximately 37% of its maximum size. These workers propose a mathematical model, relating tumour size and sensitivity to therapy, which appears consistent with clinical and experimental data. In their model both the growth rate and the sensitivity to chemotherapy decrease with decreasing size of small tumours. This model does not mean to imply that a smaller tumour is less 'curable', but rather that a given dose schedule of chemotherapy, sufficient to cause significant regression in a tumour of intermediate size, may be insufficient to cause regression in small tumours. Norton and Simon suggest that the most efficient therapy for advanced tumours would be to apply therapy of moderate intensity initially and then to use increasingly more intense therapy as the tumour regresses. Clinical trials designed to test this hypothesis are currently under way[48,49].

On the other hand the Milan group, in an effort to try to reduce the toxicity of therapy, has initiated a trial in premenopausal patients comparing 6 months of therapy with CMF to 12 months of the same regimen[25]. The results are still preliminary and thus far no difference exists between the two therapy schedules. However, it should be noted that although there is no statistical difference, the results in the 12 month schedule were slightly better for each subgroup of axillary node stratification. At present there is thus no evidence to support the routine use of only 6 months of adjuvant CMF chemotherapy.

In conclusion, the value of postsurgical adjuvant chemotherapy has been proven to be successful in prolonging survival in at least some patients with breast cancer. The aim of future clinical trials should be directed toward answering some of the following questions:

(1) what types and numbers of drugs should be used (including combination with endocrine therapy);
(2) what are optimal drug schedules;
(3) what should be the duration of such therapy; and
(4) what should be the role, if any, of radiation therapy and of immunotherapy in combination with adjuvant chemotherapy?

In addition, attention should be directed towards identification of other prognostic factors which may help select certain high-risk subgroups who might benefit from adjuvant therapy.

Acknowledgment

The authors wish to thank Mrs Vikki Wells for her assistance in preparation of this manuscript.

References

1   Fisher, B., Slack, N., Katrych, D. and Wolmark, N. (1975). Ten year follow-up results of patients with carcinoma of the breast in a co-operative clinical trial evaluating surgical adjuvant chemotherapy. *Surg. Gynecol. Obstet.*, **140**, 528

2   Fisher, B. (1977). Surgery of primary breast cancer. In McGuire, W. L. (ed.). *Breast Cancer: Advances in Research and Treatment. Current Approaches to Therapy*, pp. 1–42. (New York: Plenum Medical Book Company)

3   Harris, J. R., Levene, M. B. and Hellman, S. (1978). The role of radiation therapy in the primary treatment of carcinoma of the breast. *Sem. Oncol.*, **5**, 403

4   Stjernsward, J. E. (1977). Adjuvant radiotherapy trials in breast cancer. *Cancer*, **39**, 2846

5   Schiffer, L. M. (1978). The cell kinetics of mammary cancers. In McGuire, W. L. (ed.). *Breast Cancer: Advances in Research and Treatment. Experimental Biology*, pp. 259–282. (New York: Plenum Medical Book Company)

6   Skipper, H. E. (1971). Kinetics of mammary tumor cell growth and implications for therapy. *Cancer*, **28**, 1479

7   Schabel, F. M. (1969). The use of tumor growth kinetics in planning curative chemotherapy of advanced solid tumors. *Cancer Res.*, **29**, 2384

8   Griswold, D. S. (1975). The potential for murine tumor models in surgical adjuvant chemotherapy. *Cancer Chemother. Rep.*, **5**, 187

9   Schabel, F. M. (1977). Surgical adjuvant chemotherapy of metastatic murine tumors. *Cancer*, **40**, 558

10 Shapiro, D. M. and Fugman, R. A. (1957). A role for chemotherapy as an adjunct to surgery. *Cancer Res.*, **17**, 1098

11 Chirigos, M. A., Colsky, J., Humphreys, S. R. *et al.* (1962). Evaluation of surgery and chemotherapy in the treatment of mouse mammary 755. *Cancer Chemother.*, **22**, 49

12 Humphreys, S. R. and Karrer, K. (1970). Relationship of dose schedules to the effectiveness of adjuvant chemotherapy. *Cancer Chemother. Rep.*, **54**, 379

13 Strauss, M. J., Sege, V. and Choi, S. C. (1975). The effect of surgery and pretreatment or posttreatment adjuvant chemotherapy on primary tumor growth in an animal model. *J. Surg. Oncol.*, **7**, 497

14 Martin, D. S., Hayworth, P. W. and Fugman, R. A. (1970). Enhanced cures of spontaneous murine mammary tumors with surgery, combination chemotherapy, and immunotherapy. *Cancer Res.*, **30**, 709

15 Nissen–Meyer, R., Kjellgren, K., Malmio, K. *et al.* (1978). Surgical adjuvant chemotherapy results with one short course with cyclophosphamide after mastectomy. *Cancer*, **41**, 2088

16 Finney, R. (1971). Adjuvant chemotherapy in radical treatment of carcinoma of the breast – a clinical trial. *Am. J. Roentgenol.*, **111**, 137

17 Donegan, W. L. (1974). Extended surgical adjuvant thio-TEPA for mammary carcinoma. *Arch. Surg.*, **109**, 187

18 Kholdin, S. A., Deemarsky, L. Y. and Bavly, J. L. (1974). Adjuvant long term chemotherapy in complex treatment of operable breast cancer. *Cancer*, **33**, 903

19 Multicentre Breast Cancer Chemotherapy Group (1977). Multimodal therapy for histological stage-II breast cancer. *Lancet*, **2**, 396

20 Fisher, B. and Redmond, C. (1979). Breast cancer studies on the national surgical adjuvant breast and colon project (NSABP). In Jones, S. E. and Salmon, S. E. (eds.). *Adjuvant Therapy of Cancer*, Vol. II, pp. 215–226. (New York: Grune & Stratton)

21 Bonadonna, G., Rossi, A., Valagussa, P. *et al.* (1977). Combination chemotherapy as an adjuvant treatment in operable breast cancer. *N. Engl. J. Med.*, **294**, 405

22 Cole, M. P. (1968). Suppression of ovarian function in primary breast cancers. In Forrest, A. P. M. and Kunkle, P. B. (eds.). *Prognostic Factors in Breast Cancer*, pp. 146–156. (Edinburgh: Livingstone)

23 Nissen-Meyer, R. (1968). Suppression of ovarian function in primary breast cancer. In Forrest, A. P. M. and Kunkle, P. B. (eds.). *Prognostic Factors in Breast Cancer*, pp. 135–145. (Edinburgh: Livingstone)

24 Ravdin, R. G., Lewison, E. F., Slack, N. H. *et al.* (1970). Results of a clinical trial concerning the worth of prophylactic oophorectomy of breast cancer. *Surg. Gynecol. Obstet.*, **131**, 1055

25 Bonadonna, G., Valagussa, P., Rossi, A. *et al.* (1979). CMF adjuvant chemotherapy in operable breast cancer. In Jones, S. E. and Salmon, S. E. (eds.). *Adjuvant Therapy of Cancer*. Vol. II, pp. 227–237. (New York: Grune & Stratton)

26 Fisher, B., Sherman, B., Rockette, H. *et al.* (1979). l-Phenylalanine mustard (L-PAM) in the management of premenopausal patients with primary breast cancer: lack of association of disease-free survival with depression of ovarian function. *Cancer*, **44**, 947

27 Knight, W. A., Livingston, R. B., Gregory, R. J. *et al.* (1977). Estrogen receptor as an independent prognostic factor for early recurrence in breast cancer. *Cancer Res.*, **37**, 4669

28 Walt, A. J., Singhawinta, A., Brooks, S. C. *et al.* (1976). The surgical implications of estrophile protein estimations in carcinoma of the breast. *Surgery*, **80**, 506

29 Allegra, J., Simon, R. and Lippman, M. (1979). The association between steroid hormone receptor status and the disease free interval in breast cancer. In Jones, S. E. and Salmon, S. E. (eds.). *Adjuvant Therapy of Cancer*. Vol. II, pp. 47–54. (New York: Grune & Stratton)

30 Meyer, J. S., Rao, B. R., Stevens, S. C. *et al.* (1977). Low incidence of estrogen receptor in breast carcinomas with rapid rates of cellular proliferation. *Cancer*, **40**, 2290

31 Lippman, M. E., Allegra, J. C., Thompson, E. B. *et al.* (1978). The relation between estrogen receptors and response rate to cytotoxic chemotherapy in metastatic breast cancer. *N. Engl. J. Med.*, **298**, 1223

32 Jonat, W. and Mass, H. (1978). Some comments on the necessity of receptor determination in human breast cancer. *Cancer Res.*, **38**, 4305

33 Kiang, D. T., Frenning, D. H., Goldman, A. I. *et al.* (1978). Estrogen receptor and responses to chemotherapy and hormonal therapy in advanced breast cancer. *N. Engl. J. Med.*, **299**, 1330

34 Samal, B., Singhakowinta, A., Brooks, S. C. *et al.* (1978). Estrogen receptors and response of breast cancer to chemotherapy. *N. Engl. J. Med.*, **299**, 604

35 Bonadonna, G. and Valagussa, P. (1980). Dose response effect of cyclophosphamide, methotrexate, and 5-fluorouracil (CMF) in breast cancer. *Proc. Am. Soc. Clin. Oncol.*, **21**, 413

36 Buzdar, A. U., Blumenschein, G. R., Gutterman, J. U. *et al.* (1979). Post-operative adjuvant chemotherapy with fluorouracil, doxorubicin, cyclophosphamide, and BCG vaccine. *J. Am. Med. Assoc.*, **242**, 1509

37 Cooper, R. G., Holland, J. F. and Glidewell, D. (1979). Adjuvant chemotherapy of breast cancer. *Cancer*, **44**, 793

38 Glucksberg, H., Rivkin, S. E. and Rasmussen, S. (1979). Adjuvant chemotherapy for stage II breast cancer: a comparison of CMFVP versus L-PAM. In Jones, S. E. and Salmon, S. E. (eds.). *Adjuvant Therapy of Cancer*. Vol. II, pp. 261–268. (New York: Grune & Stratton)

39 Donehower, R., Erlichman, C., Schilsky, R. *et al.* (1979). Pharmacologic considerations in adjuvant chemotherapy. In Jones, S. E. and Salmon, S. E. (eds.). *Adjuvant Therapy of Cancer*. Vol. II, pp. 37–46. (New York: Grune & Stratton)

40 Chan, P. Y. M., Sadoff, L. and Winkley, J. H. (1973). Second malignancy following first breast cancer in prolonged thiotepa adjuvant chemotherapy. In Jones, S. E. and Salmon, S. E. (eds.). *Adjuvant Therapy of Cancer*, pp. 597–607. (Amsterdam: Biomedical Press)

41 Lerner, H. J. (1978). Acute myelogenous leukemia in patients receiving chlorambucil

as long term adjuvant chemotherapy for stage II breast cancer. *Cancer Treat. Rep.*, **62**, 1135

42 Senn, H. J., Jungi, W. F. and Amgwerd, R. (1979). Divergent results in node-negative and node-positive breast cancer. In Jones, S. E. and Salmon, S. E. (eds.). *Adjuvant Therapy of Cancer*. Vol. II, pp. 245–252. (New York: Grune & Stratton)

43 Knight, W. A., Livingston, R. B., Gregory, E. J. *et al.* (1978). Absent estrogen receptor and decreased survival in human breast cancer. *Proc. Am. Soc. Clin. Oncol.*, Abstr. No. C–342

44 Dao, T. L., Nemoto, T., Chamberlain, A. and Bross, I. (1975). Adrenalectomy with radical mastectomy in the treatment of high-risk breast cancer. *Cancer*, **35**, 478

45 Meakins, J. W., Allt, W. E. C., Beale, F. A. *et al.* (1977). Ovarian irradiation and prednisone following surgery and radiotherapy for carcinoma of the breast. In Jones, S. E. and Salmon, S. E. (eds.). *Adjuvant Therapy of Cancer*, pp. 95–99. (Amsterdam: Biomedical Press)

46 Hubay, C. A., Pearson, O. H., Marshall, J. S. *et al.* (1980). Antiestrogen, cytotoxic chemotherapy, and bacillus Calmette Guerin vaccination in stage II breast cancer: a preliminary report. *Surgery*, **87**, 494

47 Norton, L. and Simon, R. (1977). Tumor size, sensitivity to therapy, and design of treatment schedules. *Cancer Treat. Rep.*, **61**, 1307

48 Fisher, R. I., DeVita, V. T., Hubbard, S. M. *et al.* (1980). ProMACE-MOPP Combination chemotherapy: treatment of diffuse lymphoma. *Proc. Am. Soc. Clin. Onc.*, **21**, 468

49 Brambilla, C., Valagussa, P., Bonnadonna, G. *et al.* (1980). Sequential adjuvant chemotherapy in postmenopausal (≤ 65 yrs) breast cancer. *Proc. Am. Soc. Clin. Oncol.*, **21**, 189

7
Principles of intravenous hyperalimentation

M. DEITEL AND I. SANDERSON

INTRODUCTION AND HISTORICAL ASPECTS

While the concept of providing sufficient nutrition parenterally to patients who are either unable or unwilling to eat adequately has been developing for some time, it has been relatively recent changes that have established the techniques for safe intravenous administration of total nutrients.

This concept was impossible before 1616, when William Harvey in London described the circulation of blood[1]. Shortly thereafter investigators began to look into the possibilities and consequences of intravenous infusion of a variety of substances. The first intravenous infusion was attributed to Sir Christopher Wren in Oxford, who in 1656 used a goose quill attached to a pig's bladder to infuse ale, wine and opium into the veins of dogs[2,3]. His attempts to infuse venum emeticum into the vein of a man failed when his subject apparently swooned. Wren's studies were soon expanded, including experiments into the possibilities of blood transfusion. An excellent review of these early experiments was published in 1904 by Fortescue-Brickdale[3].

After these experiments some technical improvements were made, but the only therapeutically satisfying results were obtained in the 1830s with infusion of salt solutions into the veins of cholera victims[4]. However, it was not until the discovery of microbial infection by Pasteur[5] in Paris (1877) and the pioneering of aseptic technique by Lister[6] in Edinburgh and Glasgow (1870) that serious complications of intravenous injections could be overcome. By the end of the nineteenth century infusion of sugar and saline solutions into humans was routine. With the intravenous route still considered unsafe, physicians generally used subcutaneous injections of sugar, salt, and protein solutions plus olive oil in an attempt to provide nutritional support, and some successes were reported[7].

In the early 1900s, protein hydrolysate solutions were further developed and refined, and fat emulsions for intravenous use began to be developed[4]. Febrile reactions to the infusions were still common, and this final barrier to safe parenteral fluid administration was removed in 1923 when Florence Siebert[8] in Philadelphia discovered pyrogens as the cause. However, it was not until 10 years later that sterile pyrogen-free water was generally available.

In the 1930s Rose[9] in Urbana, USA defined mammalian protein and essential amino acid requirements. In 1939 Robert Elman in St Louis successfully infused protein hydrolysates into humans, and investigators began experimenting with a wide variety of nutrient solutions in an attempt to provide long-term infusion by vein[10]. However, the hyperosmolarity of these solutions resulted in thrombosis and phlebitis in peripheral veins. Investigators tried to overcome this by infusing large volumes of less hypertonic nutrient fluids together with diuretics, and by attempting to use fat as a major source of energy, or by infusing hypertonic solutions into a central vein via peripherally inserted catheters. Problems arose in each case; in particular, the early fat emulsions were associated with coagulopathy, jaundice and chills, due to a non-extractable toxin in the emulsifying agent, and were finally withdrawn from the United States market in 1964[4].

Meanwhile, investigators such as Francis Moore[11] in Boston and David Cuthbertson[12] in Glasgow were doing much to unravel the complex metabolic effects of trauma and sepsis, and the need for safe parenteral nutrition became increasingly evident. In 1961, Arvid Wretlind[13] in Stockholm introduced a safe parenteral fat emulsion, and while European investigators went the lipid route, it was Stanley Dudrick who with Jonathon Rhoads in Philadelphia decided to investigate the possibilities of providing total nutrition via central vein, using hypertonic glucose as the energy source. This was the inception of what was termed *intravenous hyperalimentation* (IVH). In 1967, Dudrick and his colleagues reported an effective method of long-term intravenous nutrition using glucose, protein hydrolysate, vitamins, and minerals into the superior vena cava as the sole diet in beagle puppies[14]. Normal growth and development occurred in these animals for more than 8 months, when compared to their litter-mates who had been fed kennel diets of similar nutritional value. IVH was then successfully adapted for use in humans[15]. Infusion of the markedly hypertonic solutions into the large-bore, valveless central veins allows immediate dilution, which avoids the intimal damage seen with peripheral infusion.

During the last decade intravenous hyperosmolar alimentation (or *hyperalimentation*) has been the lifeline for numerous critically ill and/or malnourished patients. It has permitted positive nitrogen balance with anabolism where prior forms of nutritional treatment could not. Further refinements proved the method to be both practical and safe. As the period during which patients were maintained on IVH became more prolonged, the need for the addition to the regime of sufficient lipid to provide essential fatty acid requirements and trace elements such as zinc, copper, iodine, manganese and chromium became realized. As a result of these advances it appears that humans can be sustained solely on an intravenous diet for indefinite periods of time[4]. The growing number of patients currently receiving IVH at home attests to this fact[16].

NUTRITIONAL METABOLISM

Body fuels

Man has three energy sources, namely carbohydrate, protein, and fat. Carbohydrate supplies 16.7 kJ (4 kcal)/g, and is stored as glycogen, in limited amounts (200 g in liver – available for systemic use, and 300 g in muscle – not available to provide glucose to the rest of the body). The hepatic glycogen stores are generally conserved for emergencies, such as anoxia or severe exercise. There is no storage form of protein as such; each molecule of protein has some useful function, such as structure, contractile potential, enzymes, antibodies, etc. Although 1 g of protein can supply 16.7 kJ (4 kcal) of energy, it is normally spared for its important non-fuel functions. Any excess dietary intake of protein is metabolized, and the nitrogen is excreted as urea, with the consequent energy either utilized or stored as fat. Fat is the body's major and most efficient energy source. It is present in large (about 15 kg), often excessive, amounts, and supplies 38.0 kJ (9 kcal)/g. Any excess or deficit of energy is met by increasing or decreasing the fat reserves.

In adult man the daily food intake should supply his energy needs and sufficient protein to replace that lost to the body due to normal protein turnover (mucosa, skin, nails, etc.). During periods of starvation the body must call upon its own energy reserves to meet the deficit produced by inadequate intake. Blood glucose levels are maintained by breaking down skeletal muscle to amino acids (mainly alanine), which are converted in the liver to glucose (gluconeogenesis).

Brief starvation

During *brief* starvation (less than 72 h) 10–15 g of nitrogen per day are lost in the urine, reflecting protein catabolism for gluconeogenesis, and this figure includes the basal, obligatory nitrogen losses of 1.5 g/day. If

100 g of carbohydrate per day is provided, this spares protein catabolism, and urinary nitrogen loss is reduced to 2–5 g/day, and ketosis from products of fat metabolism is prevented. Body fat is broken down to glycerol and fatty acids, and the latter are metabolized by tissues which are not obliged to use glucose for energy (heart, muscle, kidney, etc.). Fatty acids may be metabolized directly from the circulation or after they have been oxidized to keto acids by the liver. Protein catabolism, however, is a significant source of energy needs during brief starvation.

Prolonged starvation

If the period of starvation is *prolonged* (more than 72 h), the body adapts to the use of more energy from fat breakdown, thus conserving protein. Total body protein is approximately 13 kg, and it has been estimated that if more than 25% of body protein is lost, survival is threatened. At a rate of protein breakdown losing 10–15 g of nitrogen per day (multiply by 6.25 to convert to corresponding protein mass), this will not take very long. The majority of tissues switch from glucose to fatty acids as their energy source, and the brain adapts to keto acids (beta-hydroxybutyrate, acetoacetate) for energy. Thus the body's need for glucose is decreased, and protein breakdown is reduced[17]. Nitrogen losses in the urine drop to 3–4 g/day, which is still above basal, obligatory losses, since some glucose continues to be required by the healing wound (fibroblasts), adrenal cortex, and haemopoietic tissue (red and white cells); also, some of the amino acids derived from protein breakdown are used for visceral protein anabolism, namely as building blocks for formation of plasma proteins, antibodies, and cells necessary for survival (red and white blood cells). The shift therefore in prolonged starvation is to provide energy needs from fat stores.

Trauma and/or sepsis

The body's response to stress such as trauma (injury, operation) and sepsis is almost the opposite to that observed during prolonged starvation. There is both a hypermetabolic and catabolic response in proportion to the severity of injury. The basal energy expenditure (BEE)* can be calculated reasonably from the Harris–Benedict equation[18]:

* BEE is the metabolic rate after a total night (12 h) fast and after lying at complete rest for at least 30 min. The Harris–Benedict equation is a formula originally derived from multiple regression analysis based on the BEE using indirect calorimetry (computed from gaseous exchange and respiratory CO_2/O_2 quotient) on more than 200 normal men and women, correlating the contribution of each of weight, height, age and sex to the BEE. The formula is different for males and females.

Male: BEE (kcal) = 66 + {13.7 × wt (kg)} + {5 × ht (cm)} − {6.8 × age (years)}

Female: BEE (kcal) = 655 + {9.6 × wt (kg)} + {1.7 × ht (cm)} − {4.7 × age (years)}

The BEE is increased by about 13% for every degree centigrade rise in body temperature, 20–35% after surgery, 40–60% with sepsis and even greater than 100% with major burns[18, 19].

The catabolism observed is not due to lack of energy stores, since even with infusion of carbohydrate tissue breakdown continues. Visceral protein metabolism is affected, and there is increased synthesis of plasma proteins, antibodies and cellular components, such as red and white blood cells and reparative tissues. During trauma and sepsis there is a decreased ability to handle a glucose load, as insulin response is insufficient and peripheral tissues are insulin-resistant. It is theorized that the alterations in central nervous system hypothalamic function and increased adrenergic activity are related to the hypermetabolic, catabolic and hyperglycaemic responses observed in these conditions[20].

For some time it was thought that the nitrogen losses associated with trauma or sepsis were obligatory. However, if sufficient energy and protein are administered, in excess of that required to meet the increased BEE and nitrogen excretion, these losses can be drastically reduced. IVH can accomplish this[21]. IVH will not avoid or reverse the catabolic response to trauma, but it does lessen the effect during the critical period by promoting a favourable nitrogen balance[22]. Continued use of IVH in the post-traumatic phase will achieve positive nitrogen balance with anabolism.

NUTRITIONAL ASSESSMENT

The body's responses are well designed to accommodate short periods of trauma, infection and nutritional deprivation. However, there comes a time during prolonged periods of stress and/or starvation when signs of malnutrition begin to appear, and specialized nutritional support may be considered. Assessment of nutritional status plays an important role in any IVH programme. It detects nutritional deficiencies, and, with serial follow-up, allows measurement of the effects of nutritional therapy (Table 1).

A nutritional assessment begins with a history and physical examination. The patient's present weight, usual weight and ideal weight based on height and habitus are recorded, and the percentage loss of body weight determined. A greater than 10% loss in the previous 3 months is an indication for nutritional support. Such clinical features as

Table 1 *Nutritional assessment* (initial; may be repeated serially to assess needs and response)

Clinical
  Weight for height: actual   usual   ideal (sex)   % loss
  Disease
  Dietary history
  Oedema, skin scaling, decubiti, etc.

Visceral protein status
  Albumin (half-life 20 days)
  Transferrin (half-life 8 days)
  Thyroxine-binding prealbumin (half-life 2 days)
  Retinol-binding protein (half-life 12 h)
  Total lymphocyte count in peripheral blood

  Cell-mediated immunity
    Delayed hypersensitivity skin-testing to recall antigens: candidin, mumps, SK/SD, PPD (repeated at 7–10 day intervals)
    Primary sensitization to topical application of dinitrochlorobenzene (DNCB) with challenge after 14 days may be used in long-term situations.

Fat reserves
  Triceps skinfold (TSF) in mm

Somatic (skeletal) protein status
Mid-arm muscle circumference in cm =
  mid-arm circumference cm − 0.314 × TSF mm
        (*or* − 3.14 × TSF cm)
        where 3.14 = π (pi)
  Creatinine/height index

Nitrogen (N) balance may be indirectly determined from:
N Intake (protein/6.25) − N Output (urinary urea N + 3.5).
(The factor 3.5 allows for N losses in urine (uric acid, NH_3, etc.) plus skin and faecal losses.)

decubitus ulcers, dependent oedema, scaling skin, breaking nails, recent hair loss on the comb and anaemia are recorded.

Visceral protein status is evaluated from measurement of serum albumin, serum transferrin and total lymphocyte count. The more sensitive indicator is the serum transferrin level due to its shorter half-life, but due to their even shorter half-lives, prealbumin and retinol-binding protein are very sensitive indicators of dietary protein restriction and repletion (Table 1)[23].

In the kwashiorkor type of malnutrition (protein deficiency with some energy intake), the visceral protein compartment is deficient.

Response of the cell-mediated immune system to delayed hypersensitivity skin-testing with a battery of common recall antigens (purified protein derivative of tuberculin, mumps, candida, streptokinase–streptodornase) reflects visceral protein status. If there is less than 5 mm of induration after 48 h to all the recall antigens, the patient is said to be anergic. Primary sensitization to topical application of dinitrochlorobenzene (DNCB) with challenge 14 days later may also be used to measure immunocompetence. Anergy almost always develops in the critically ill patient and is closely correlated with susceptibility to infection and mortality; it can be reversed with IVH[24].

To assess the patient's skeletal muscle (somatic) protein status, a variety of tests may be performed. Creatinine, the anhydride of creatine, is formed in muscle as a preliminary step for excretion of creatine. Creatinine is liberated from muscle at a constant rate and excreted in the urine. The 24 h urinary creatinine expressed in terms of body weight is fairly constant among different individuals of the same sex and age. Creatinine/height index (actual urinary creatinine over ideal urinary creatinine × 100) is a sensitive indicator of muscle protein depletion. Another indicator of skeletal muscle metabolism is measurement of urinary 3-methylhistidine, which is released upon breakdown of actin and myosin[25].

Anthropometric measurements such as triceps skinfold (TSF) thickness and mid-arm circumference (MAC) are measured at the midpoint between acromion and olecranon in the non-dominant arm. The TSF thickness is an indicator of fat reserves[26]. The mid-arm muscle circumference (MAMC) is calculated as follows: MAMC = MAC − 3.14 × TSF (in cm). A comparison of the MAMC with standard tables gives a measure of somatic protein status. Marasmus is a protein-energy malnutrition characterized by depressed anthropometric measurements, i.e. loss of fat and skeletal muscle. Malnourished patients may present with kwashiorkor, marasmus, or a combination of both.

As a measure of protein intake minus protein output, nitrogen balance has classically been measured biochemically using the Kjeldahl method. However, clinically it can be determined by noting the nitrogen intake of the IVH solution and subtracting the nitrogen output as calculated by adding 3.5 to the 24 h urinary urea nitrogen excretion. The constant of 3.5 is added to account for skin and faecal loss of nitrogen and non-urea urinary nitrogen (ammonia, uric acid and creatinine)[26]. It is invalid in the presence of diarrhoea and high-output fistula losses.

A routine nutritional assessment will indicate the degree of malnutrition, establish guidelines for nutritional support, and dictate when a patient should start or stop nutritional therapy.

188 FRONTIERS IN GENERAL SURGERY

INDICATIONS FOR NUTRITIONAL THERAPY

Generally speaking, any patient who has not been receiving adequate nutrition for a period of 7 days or more, and who will possibly be unable to begin adequate nutritional intake in the near future, is a candidate for nutritional support.

Delivery of nutrients through a functioning gastrointestinal tract is best; if the gut is working, it should be used. Assuming that normal food cannot be tolerated, *enteral hyperalimentation* using specialized liquid diets should be used. Compared to IVH, enteral feeding is less expensive, has less potential complications and maintains efficient gut function.

The elemental or chemically defined diets are non-residue, predigested, balanced liquid diets of basic constituents – L-amino acids or hydrolysates, oligosaccharides, minerals, vitamins and essential fat. They usually supply 4.184 kJ (1 kcal)/ml in full-strength solution. When taken orally, flavouring is required to mask the organic amino acid taste. This taste cannot be masked, however, in the preparations which contain increased amino acid content to meet the proper energy: nitrogen ratio of 630 kJ (150 kcal)/g of nitrogen, and these have to be given by tube-feeding. A very fine tube is passed into the stomach and its location is confirmed by X-ray (Figure 1). These hyperosmolar diets are delivered by continuous infusion, with the head of the bed elevated to avoid regurgitation and aspiration. Fine tubes have also been inserted directly into the stomach[27] or jejunum[28] safely at the time of surgery for postoperative feeding.

Because these diets are hyperosmolar, they are started slowly as half-strength solutions to avoid diarrhoea. First the rate and then the concentration is gradually increased. Enough water must be added to avoid hypertonic dehydration. These elemental diets are absorbed in the proximal intestine after minimal or no digestion; they stimulate no significant digestive enzyme secretion[29]. Hence, they may be used for low small-bowel or colonic fistulas or pancreatitis, where secretory and mechanical rest for the gut is advantageous. As the nutrients are presented in a form ready for absorption, they may also be used in the short bowel syndrome, where exposure of the remaining small bowel mucosa to nutrients is important for adaptive hyperplasia[30].

Semi-elemental diets contain albumin as the protein source as well as simple sugars. Since some proteolytic enzyme secretion is stimulated by the undigested albumin, they are generally not used in fistulas or pancreatitis. They are, however, useful when an ultra-low-residue diet is desirable, such as in active inflammatory bowel disease. These diets are more palatable than the elemental diets, and while tube-feeding may be necessary, they are often tolerated when given orally. They are also less

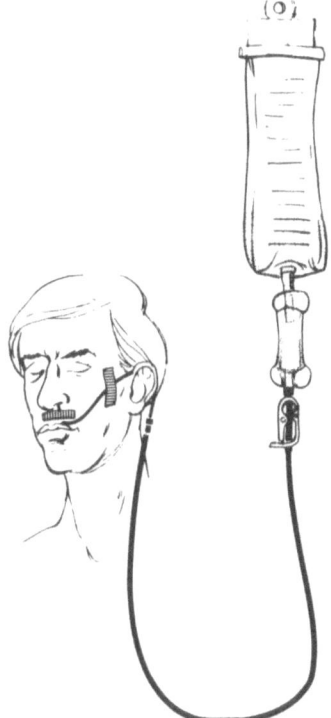

Figure 1   Enteral hyperalimentation via fine nasogastric tube

hyperosmolar and less expensive than elemental diets.

A variety of other ultra-low-residue liquid complete diets have been developed for oral feeding (including between-meal supplements) and for feeding down very fine tubes, whose formulas vary in osmolality, lactose content, and digestive requirements[31].

INDICATIONS FOR IVH

Apart from obvious situations in which the gastrointestinal tract is mechanically obstructed, severely malnourished patients often have compromised absorption secondary to mucosal oedema and atrophy, so that rapid nutritional repletion by enteral feeding cannot be achieved. Thus all patients with an abnormal nutritional assessment who cannot be rehabilitated enterally are considered for IVH. The indications for IVH are summarized in Table 2. Basically these are patients who either

Table 2   Indications for IVH

1. Oral intake impossible
   (a) Unable to swallow
   (b) Oesophageal obstruction
   (c) Pyloric obstruction
   (d) Bowel obstruction

2. Oral intake inadvisable
   (a) Enteric fistula
   (b) Crohn's disease
   (c) Ulcerative colitis
   (d) Short bowel syndrome
   (e) Acute pancreatitis
   (f) Complicated gastrointestinal operations

3. Oral intake inadequate
   (a) Chronic sepsis/malaise
   (b) Chronic obstructive lung disease
   (c) Short gut syndrome/malabsorption syndrome
   (d) Burns
   (e) Malignant disease (adjunctive therapy)
   (f) Anorexia nervosa

4. Special situations
   (a) Renal failure
   (b) Hepatic failure

cannot eat (e.g. oesophageal obstruction), should not eat (e.g. entero-cutaneous fistula, fulminant pancreatitis) or will not eat (e.g. anorexia nervosa, cancer chemotherapy). IVH is also used preoperatively in malnourished patients for nutritional repletion, so that they can better tolerate surgery with less risk of postoperative complications. IVH is also used where elimination of oral intake, providing mechanical and secretory rest for the gut, plus anabolism are required. A postoperative high-output enterocutaneous fistula, where losses of fluid, electrolytes and nutrients occur, is an ideal case for IVH. Even the hospital full-fluid diet stimulates digestive enzyme secretion, which would attack surrounding tissues as the corrosive enzymes spill out through the fistula, and with elemental diets, there would be significant volume and nutritional loss. However, IVH, by providing total gut rest, allows fistulas to close spontaneously, while adequate nutrition is maintained. Fistulas with distal obstruction or major anastomotic disruption require surgical intervention, and fistulas due to inflammatory bowel disease, prior irradiation or foreign bodies in the fistulous tract are difficult to heal. However, the mortality associated with alimentary fistulas has fallen from 40% prior to 1968 to less than 10% with the use of IVH[32].

Other postoperative complications, such as prolonged ileus or bowel obstruction, wound disruption or evisceration and sepsis are indications for IVH. IVH affords pancreatic rest, which is useful when confronted with necrotizing pancreatitis, and it provides the nutrients needed to combat the catabolism associated with this disease.

Active inflammatory bowel disease (Crohn's disease and ulcerative colitis) may result in severely malnourished patients. IVH can both replenish these patients and provide bowel rest, and may result in remissions in Crohn's disease, although IVH does not generally lead to a permanent cure with ulcerative colitis[33]. If surgery is required, these patients are in a better nutritional state to withstand it. Patients who have had massive intestinal resections develop malabsorption due to rapid transit through the short gut. Though gradual adaptive improvement in absorptive function can be expected, it is often 2 years before the patient can be adequately nourished by oral intake alone. During this period, IVH is essential to maintain adequate nutrition while adaptations are proceeding. If the adaptive period is to be a long one, programmes have been established to allow the patient to carry on IVH at home[16]. Patients have been on ambulatory home IVH, leading an active life for more than 8 years now. Some patients with very short bowel may require IVH permanently.

IVH as an adjunct to cancer therapy has minimized catabolism and improved the immune response[34]. Immunocompetent patients with good nutritional status respond significantly better to chemotherapy[35]; they also tolerate increased doses of chemotherapy or radiation. However, in patients who are both depleted and inoperable, IVH is best reserved only for those patients in whom significant palliation with improvement in quality of life is anticipated, and who are expected to live for longer than 3 months after IVH[36].

The use of IVH in infants has been invaluable[37]. Premature infants who cannot be adequately nourished orally or by tube, infants with severe gastrointestinal anomalies such as atresia of the small bowel or omphalocele with postoperative ileus, and infants with prolonged diarrhoea are candidates for IVH.

INFUSION CONSTITUENTS

General additives

Before the patient can begin IVH, the clinician and the pharmacist have to develop a nutrient formula. One plans to provide approximately the following:

water, 40 ml (kg body weight)$^{-1}$ day^{-1} (2500–3500 ml)
energy, 167 kJ [40 kcal] (kg body weight)$^{-1}$ day^{-1}
protein, 1 g (kg body weight)$^{-1}$ day^{-1}
sodium, 100–120 mmol/day
potassium, 80–100 mmol/day
calcium, 20 mmol/day
magnesium, 30 mmol/day
phosphorus, 45 mmol/day
chloride, 110 mmol/day.

The recommended daily oral requirements of vitamins for patients over 6 years of age and excluding pregnant or nursing women are as follows:

vitamin A, 2500–5000 IU/day (500–1000 µg of retinol equivalents/ day)
vitamin D, 200–400 IU/day (5–10 µg/day)
vitamin E, 6–10 mg/day
vitamin K, 70–140 µg/day
thiamine (vitamin B$_1$), 0.9–1.5 mg/day
riboflavin (vitamin B$_2$), 1.0–1.7 mg/day
niacin, 11–19 mg/day
pantothenate, 4–7 mg/day
pyridoxine (vitamin B$_6$), 1.3–2.2 mg/day
ascorbic acid (vitamin C), 45–60 mg/day
folic acid, 200–400 µg/day
vitamin B$_{12}$, 2.5–3 µg/day

Trace element requirements are approximately as follows:

zinc, 3 mg/day
copper, 1.6 mg/day
manganese, 2 mg/day
selenium, 30 µg/day
chromium, 15 µg/day
fluoride, 1–2 mg/day
iodine, 120 µg/day
iron, 1–1.5 mg/day.

Essential fatty acid requirements are supplied as linoleic acid equivalent to about 0.2 g (kg body weight)$^{-1}$ day^{-1}

Water

Water comprises 60% of body weight in adults and 75% of body weight in the newborn. It serves as a major transport medium throughout the body. In the adult, daily water intake is about 2500 ml[38] (1200 ml is imbibed as fluids, 1000 ml is derived from water in foods, and 300 ml results from oxidation of body fuels). This input is balanced by the output from the kidneys, lung, skin and in stool. Water requirements are greater in the neonate (125 ml (kg body weight)$^{-1}$ day^{-1}). Water needs are increased by fever, burns, diarrhoea, vomiting and fistula losses. Some diseases (renal failure, congestive heart failure) result in water retention, and requirements will be decreased in these. Reasonable estimates of fluid needs can be made by recording daily fluid balance and body weight.

Energy

Energy requirements depend on age, size, nutritional status, physical activity and degree of hypermetabolism caused by injury or sepsis. The normal adult requirement is about 150 kJ [36 kcal] (kg body weight)$^{-1}$ day^{-1}. In injury and sepsis, an increase to 200–250 kJ [40–60 kcal] (kg body weight)$^{-1}$ day^{-1} may be required depending on severity[19], and in major burns an extra 170 kJ [40 kcal]/percentage of body burned is required per day[39]. Infants have higher energy demands, mainly due to increased growth rate, and infusion of 400 kJ [96 kcal] (kg body weight)$^{-1}$ day^{-1} is often required. Premature and low-birth-weight infants may even require more. The glucose concentration of IVH solution for infants, however, should not exceed 25%, as osmotic diuresis could ensue.

Carbohydrate

Energy is usually provided as carbohydrate in IVH (glucose or occasionally fructose). Advantages for the use of fructose which does not require endogenous insulin have been put forward, but are more theoretical than real in the ill patient: a major portion of infused fructose will be converted to glucose before utilization[40], and fructose in the critically ill can lead to lactic acidosis[41].

Lipid

Fat is added to the IVH regime either to provide essential fatty acids or, in larger amounts, to provide a portion of the energy requirements. The effects of fat administration on nitrogen balance in the catabolic patient at first appear confusing. When lipid is given for the first 3 days following trauma, it does not exert the protein-sparing effect seen when carbohydrate alone is given[42]. When a combination of fat and carbohydrate is given for a few days after trauma, they are less effective in promoting nitrogen utilization than is carbohydrate alone[43]. After several days, however, isocaloric regimens of carbohydrate alone, and carbohydrate and lipid in approximately equal amounts, show no significant difference, in their effect on protein-sparing and anabolism[43, 44]. Improvement in protein-sparing with time parallels the body's adaptation to starvation, since in prolonged starvation the body adapts to using fatty acids and ketones for energy. It is not surprising, therefore, that nitrogen balance improves with either fat or carbohydrate administration. The ideal combination during periods of extreme stress has yet to be ascertained.

MacFadyen et al.[45] showed that when large amounts of lipid were infused, anabolism improved as the relative carbohydrate portion of the infusion was increased. On the other hand, Askanazi and co-workers[46] found that in septic, injured, hypermetabolic patients, excess glucose appears to be converted to glycogen while endogenous fat is used preferentially as an energy source. They suggest that fat emulsions could replace glucose as a source of energy in these patients.*

The lipid preparations available are obtained from vegetable oils (soyabean or safflower) emulsified with 1.2% egg-yolk phospholipids in 2.5% glycerol to attain isotonicity with plasma. The 10% emulsions contain lipid particles with average size $0.13 \mu m$, which is within the range of natural chylomicrons, which have a particle diameter of 0.10–$0.21 \mu m$. The delicate emulsion will destabilize if anything such as electrolytes is mixed with it, and must be infused into a separate intravenous line, which may be unerminally by a Y-connector to the amino acid–dextrose line. Heparin, however, is compatible with the lipid emulsion, and 1 unit/ml of lipid may be added to the bottle. Since heparin activates plasma lipoprotein lipase, it helps clear the lipid from the plasma.

The fat emulsions contain the essential fatty acid (EFA) linoleic. To meet basal EFA requirement, linoleic acid should supply about 4% of energy requirements per day[47]. In the adult this is achieved by giving 500 ml of 10% fat emulsion two or three times a week. Biochemical EFA deficiency may occur with fat-free IVH within 1 week in the infant[48] and within 4 weeks in the adult[49]. The diene linoleic acid ($18 : 2\omega 6$) and tetraene arachidonic acid ($20 : 4\omega 6$) are the EFA; arachidonic is formed from linoleic acid. In deficiency states, the mono-ene oleic ($18 : 1\omega 9$)

---

* Infusion of lipid for protein-sparing or, with nitrogen, as an energy source in the starved or injured/septic patient (as well as the optimal proportions of carbohydrate and fat) is presently a controversial area in clinical nutrition, which hopefully will be resolved in the next decade.

forms the triene $\Delta^{5,8,11}$-eicosatrienoic acid (20:3ω9) which is normally absent from body lipids*. Blood fatty acid levels are measured by gas–liquid chromatography. A triene : tetraene ratio of greater than 0.4 (i.e. $\Delta^{5,8,11}$-eicosatrienoic acid divided by arachidonic acid) indicates biochemical EFA deficiency. The time it takes for this biochemical abnormality to become clinically manifest varies widely among individuals, and appears to be partially dependent upon the state of fat stores present[50]. Clinical EFA deficiency manifests as scaling skin, sparse hair growth, retarded wound healing, increased susceptibility to infection and thrombocytopenia secondary to decreased prostaglandin synthesis from EFA precursors[51]. The intravenous fat emulsions presently available are 10% soybean oil containing 55% linoleic acid, and 10% safflower oil containing 77% linoleic acid. Fat administered as an energy source in large amounts (> 3–4 g (kg body weight)$^{-1}$ day^{-1}) results in hyperlipidaemia.

Protein

Protein is required to replenish losses and promote healing. In healthy adults the daily protein intake is 0.73–0.80 g/kg body weight. For infants and children (1–3 years) the recommended daily intake is 1.67 g/kg, and for children 10–12 years[38] it is 1.3 g/kg. These figures include a considerable margin for safety and assume that the individual is in good health and is consuming adequate amounts of other nutrients. In depleted adults amounts are similar to those required by an actively growing child[52].

In order for protein synthesis to take place, the body requires an amino acid source and a supply of energy. The amount of energy required for optimal nitrogen utilization is about 630 kJ [150 kcal]/g of nitrogen infused. If less energy is infused, the amino acids will be deaminated and metabolized for energy instead of being used as building blocks for protein, and the nitrogen will be excreted in the urine. However, since Elman's work in 1947[53], it has been known that if only amino acids are given, in sufficient quantity, they will exert a protein-sparing effect. This has recently been confirmed and used postoperatively in short-term clinical situations[54].

It is important that any intravenous amino acid mix contain all of the

---

* In fatty acids, the first number indicates the number of carbon atoms and the second the number of double bonds; ω indicates the position of the first double bond, counting from the methyl (left) end of the molecule. The Δ nomenclature indicates the position of all double bonds, counting from the carboxyl (right) end of the molecule. Mammals do not have the ability to place a double bond by desaturation at the ω6 position, and if ω6 is not supplied in the diet, the same elongating enzyme which ordinarily changes linoleic to arachidonic will now elongate oleic (18 : 1ω9) which is desaturated to eicosatrienoic (20 : 3ω9).

eight essential amino acids in adequate quantities. Essential amino acids are those which cannot be synthesized in the human and are as follows: leucine, isoleucine, valine, phenylalanine, lysine, methionine, threonine and tryptophan. In addition, histidine is required by infants. The percentage of essential amino acids to the total amino acids given (the E/T ratio) is approximately 19% in the adult, 36% in the adolescent and 40% in the infant [52, 55].

IVH solutions contain amino acids either as protein hydrolysates or crystalline amino acids. Complete (acid) hydrolysates of fibrin or partial (enzymatic) hydrolysates of casein were originally used, but now crystalline amino acid solutions are used almost exclusively. With the hydrolysates more than twice as much is needed to maintain positive nitrogen balance compared to the properly proportioned crystalline amino acid solutions[56]. With acid hydrolysis of fibrin there is destruction of tryptophan, and this expensive amino acid has to be supplemented. The enzymatic hydrolysis of casein cannot be carried to completion, which results in about 45% of the solution being di- and tri-peptides, with 36–53% of these peptides being excreted in the urine[57]. The relative proportions of the essential amino acids in protein hydrolysates do not correspond to the requirements in man as determined by Rose[58], nor do they conform to the pattern of the World Health Organization ideal protein (egg albumin for adults, human breast milk for infants)[59]. The proportionately most deficient essential amino acid limits the rate at which protein synthesis may proceed. Some protein hydrolysates were deficient in valine and phenylalanine, so that these were added by the manufacturers to meet the minimal daily requirements and improve utilization for protein synthesis[60]. Furthermore, hyperammonaemia occurred in some infants receiving the protein hydrolysates, because of the high ammonia content of the hydrolysates and the inefficient conversion of ammonia to urea in the infant liver[61].

There are now a variety of crystalline amino acid preparations available on the market for use in IVH solutions. Products containing all the essential amino acids plus 10 to 12 non-essential amino acids, with the pattern of egg albumin, promote the best nitrogen utilization[62]. Although non-essential amino acids can be synthesized by the body, utilization of infused amino acids is greater if some non-essential ones such as alanine, proline and glutamic acid are provided. Moreover, the body has limited capacity to synthesize arginine, and this too should be provided[55].

In early crystalline amino acid preparations, there was a cation gap which resulted in a hyperchloraemic metabolic acidosis[63]. These solutions contained an excess of cationic amino acids (histidine, arginine, lysine) as hydrochloride salts, which, when metabolized, generated sufficient hydrogen ion to cause the acidosis. This was corrected by replacing hydrochloride with acetate. Another problem was an excess of glycine and a deficit in arginine, which resulted in hyperammonaemia in infants, and this has been corrected by addition of arginine[64]. The crystalline amino acids support virtually no microbial or fungal growth, whereas hydrolysates support microbial growth, with fungi predominating over bacteria[65]. The amino acid solutions have different electrolyte contents, and electrolyte additions to the IVH solution will have to be adjusted according to the total daily requirements.

Electrolytes

Generally, 100–120 mmol/day of sodium, usually added as sodium chloride, is required. In those patients with large sodium losses, such as from fistulas, more may be required, while in patients with cardiac failure or certain forms of high- or low-output renal failure, little or no sodium may be required. Potassium requirements can be quite labile, depending on the patient's nutritional status prior to infusion. Initially large daily amounts may be required to correct reduced total potassium stores. Administration of insulin to control the hyperglycaemia, often seen in the critically ill and septic patient, tends to drive potassium into the cells, and additional potassium may be needed at first. However, once equilibrium has been obtained, about 80 mmol/day of potassium is usually adequate. In renal failure, very little potassium may be required. Chloride usually accompanies the sodium and potassium additives. However, it should not be present in amounts greatly exceeding the daily sodium requirements, as acidosis may result.

Requirements for calcium (20 mmol/day), magnesium (30 mmol/day) and phosphate (45 mmol/day) are less variable. However, frequent checks on serum levels of these macro-minerals are advisable. Magnesium deficiency is characterized by neurological disturbances, with tetany, irritability and convulsions. Hypophosphataemia is associated with greater affinity of haemoglobin for oxygen due to decreased levels of 2,3-diphosphoglycerate and ATP[66]. The resulting cellular hypoxia may lead to hyperventilation and respiratory alkalosis. Craddock et al. attributed impaired chemotactic, phagocytic and bactericidal activity to depressed leukocyte ATP levels secondary to hypophosphatemia[67]. Phosphate supplementation of the solution must be coupled with addition of calcium to prevent hypocalcaemia.

Vitamins

Vitamins are needed in the amounts previously indicated[68]. It is reasonable to assume, just as requirements for energy and nitrogen are elevated in sepsis and trauma, so too are vitamin requirements (especially water-soluble vitamins which are not stored)[69]. Vitamin C requirements are particularly increased, and are necessary for wound collagen formation. Vitamins A and D are probably required in amounts somewhat less than the daily oral recommended allowance. Daily parenteral amounts of 2500 IU of vitamin A and 250 IU of vitamin D are sufficient to maintain normal plasma vitamin levels[70]. Vitamin E is present in parenteral fat emulsions as well as parenteral vitamin preparations, but its importance is not clear. However, low serum levels of tocopherol have been associated with red blood cell haemolysis in infants and possibly with creatinuria, ceroid pigment deposition and muscular lesions in children[68]. Vitamin K in the normal adult is present in the diet (300–500 µg) and is synthesized by bacteria in the colon. Lack of oral intake, and particularly the ingestion of wide-spectrum antibiotics, greatly reduce the numbers of colonic organisms. Hence, vitamin K must be provided parenterally. The amount needed parenterally is unknown, with reports varying from 10 mg two times per week to 10 mg once every 3 weeks. The new RDA advises 70–140 µg/day in total[68]. The water-soluble vitamins (B complex – except B_{12}, C and folic acid) are not stored in the body, and become deficient before the fat-soluble vitamins (A, D, E, and K) which are stored. Vitamin B_{12} is stored in liver (2 mg) and elsewhere in the body (2 mg) and is not depleted until after 3–6 years. While deficiency states are more commonly seen, overdoses of fat-soluble vitamins[69] and on rare occasions trace elements have occurred.

Trace elements

The trace elements, iron, copper, zinc, manganese, iodine and chromium are essential solution components for sustained IVH. Deficient iron stores or blood losses increase the patient's requirements for iron. Deficiency leads to anaemia and fatigue in the adult and retarded growth in the child. It may be given daily into the solutions, e.g. 0.5 mg/1000 ml.

Copper is required for formation of several enzymes, and is important in iron metabolism. Copper deficiency in experimental animals is associated with anaemia, neutropenia, defective collagen and elastin synthesis and degeneration of the nervous, skeletal and cardiac system[71]. When IVH is given without added trace elements, a fall in copper and zinc levels may be noted. Zinc is also a component of enzymes such as carbonic anhydrase, alkaline phosphatase, and alcohol dehydrogenase. Zinc deficiency with a fall in serum zinc levels to below 20 µg/ml will result in a severe dermatitis about orifices resembling acrodermatitis enteropathica, hair loss, poor wound healing, growth retardation and CNS disturbances[72]. Zinc deficiency in mice has been associated with an inadequate immune response[73]. Zinc, copper and chromium deficiencies have been reported on long-term IVH[74-76]. Zinc deficiency can be encountered early in zinc-free IVH therapy. Since zinc is excreted in large amounts in pancreatic juice, and is then absorbed as it passes down the gastrointestinal tract, zinc losses will be greater in patients with pancreatic or duodenal fistulas or short gut syndrome; in these patients, 15–20 mg/day of zinc may be needed to replace these losses[77]. In fistulas more distally in the bowel or in Crohn's disease of the terminal ileum, 5–10 mg/day may be required to maintain zinc balance. Chromium deficiency produces glucose intolerance and peripheral neuropathy, and is required for long-term IVH patients[76].

Iodine is an essential component of thyroid hormones. It is stored in the thyroid gland and deficiencies are unlikely to develop for many months or even years in the previously normal patient. It is, however, important to provide iodine for long-term IVH patients.

Manganese is a component or activator of several enzymes (alkaline phosphatase, arginase, pyruvate dehydrogenase) and is considered an essential trace element. Deficiencies in animals result in impaired growth, skeletal deformities, defects in carbohydrate and lipid metabolism and ataxia[71].

A host of other trace elements such as selenium, molybdenum, arsenic, cadmium and silicone are necessary for normal growth and prevention of disease in some animals. Their requirements for man, if any, have yet to be established. In the usual patient requiring short-term IVH where no trace elements are provided, only zinc and perhaps copper deficiencies are likely to occur.

PREPARATION OF SOLUTIONS

Amino acid solutions are mixed with the appropriate hypertonic glucose solution under strict aseptic conditions[78]. Solutions are prepared in the hospital pharmacy by an essentially closed transfer system with additions under a laminar airflow hood. Electrolytes, vitamins and trace elements are added in the required amounts. Sometimes heparin (0.5–1.0 IU/ml) and insulin are also added. The pharmacist should provide the clinician with a sterile, accurately labelled solution.

These solutions cannot be heat-sterilized, since the Maillard reaction (browning) which occurs between reducing sugars (glucose or fructose) and amino acids is enhanced by heat. The laminar airflow hood controls the risk of contamination from airborne particles. The hood takes in room air and directs it through a high efficiency particle arresting (HEPA) filter, which removes 99.9% of particles 0.3 μm or larger[78, 79].

Use of the hood *complements* proper aseptic technique, by providing a clean working environment. A direct, open path between the air filter and the working area is a necessary precaution against contamination. If a break in technique occurs, the solution is discarded. The prepared solutions are stored at 4 °C until used, to prevent microbial growth.

The next time the solutions are exposed to possible contaminations is during their attachment to the patient's intravenous line. Making up solutions in 2000 ml quantities means less frequent changing of bottles or bags, with less chance of contamination.

CATHETER INSERTION

Central venous catheterization

The high osmolality and acid pH of the solutions make central venous catheterization imperative. The tip of the catheter should be located in the superior vena cava, where high blood-flow assures immediate dilution of the nutrient solutions with avoidance of phlebitis and thrombosis[80].

While peripheral venous introduction of a long catheter can be used, various problems can arise. There is often a lack of available peripheral veins, forearm movement is restricted, catheter malpositioning is common, and there is a greater incidence of thrombosis and sepsis. The use of a Silastic catheter can reduce the latter. The direct method, percutaneous catheterization of the subclavian vein or internal jugular vein, is advantageous in terms of patient comfort and mobility, easier catheter care and low incidence of complications.

The infraclavicular, subclavian puncture used by Dudrick *et al.* is the technique of choice[15]. It is performed at the bedside using strict aseptic technique. With the patient in Trendelenburg position to distend the subclavian vein, the skin is prepared with povidone–iodine (fungicidal and bactericidal) solution. The skin and tissue through which the needle will be passed are infiltrated with local anaesthetic, and a percutaneous subclavian puncture is performed using a 5 cm needle and a 3 ml plastic syringe (Figure 2a). A 20 cm polyvinyl catheter is threaded into the vein through the needle and the needle withdrawn over the catheter. The intravenous line is then attached (Figure 2b) and the bottle transiently lowered to confirm free flow of blood back up the catheter. The catheter is sutured to the skin with 3–O silk and a needle-guard is applied to prevent catheter shearing. A sterile occlusive dressing is then applied (Figure 2c). A chest X-ray is taken to confirm the catheter-tip location[81]. If the catheter has been misdirected, e.g. up into the jugular vein, it has to be either manipulated fluoroscopically down into the superior vena cava, or withdrawn and the puncture repeated. Once the tip is confirmed in the superior vena cava, IVH administration may begin.

Infants

In infants under 5 kg the subclavian vein is too narrow to allow safe cannulation, so the catheter has to be introduced surgically into the external or internal jugular vein, and threaded into the superior vena cava. The catheter is then tunnelled under the skin to exit out of the parietal scalp (Figure 3a and 3b)[82]. This location eliminates the risk of dislodgement with movement and of contamination of the exit site by the infant's oral and nasal secretions.

Home IVH

In patients on long-term or permanent IVH, silastic rubber catheters are used, as they are inert, soft and flexible[83]. They are inserted in the operating room, and threaded into the right atrium (beyond the superior vena cava) where the tip lies free, preventing damage that could occur to the caval intima with long-term infusion[84]. Polyvinyl and Teflon catheters are relatively stiff and could erode the wall of the atrium with prolonged use, and fibrin sheaths tend to form along these catheters, predisposing them to clotting and infection[85].

To permit full ambulation without risk of dislodging the home IVH catheter, the extravascular portion is tunnelled subcutaneously down the anterior chest wall; its entrance site is below the nipple level, beyond the focal length of the eye, so that the patient can maintain catheter care (Figure 4a). The tunnelled portion of the catheter has a Dacron cuff which becomes fixed by ingrowth of fibrous tissue, and serves as an anchor and also as a barrier against outside organisms (Figure 4b). These patients are trained in aseptic techniques of catheter care, setting up the system, solution addition, etc. Solutions are obtained monthly or weekly from the hospital pharmacy and kept refrigerated. Multiple vitamins are added prior to infusion, and the solutions are usually infused overnight wih an infusion pump which includes an electronic eye alarm system to wake the patient and shut off the pump if the container is empty. Some lipid will be required (e.g. two to three 500 ml units per week) and this is infused through the same catheter. At the end of the infusion, the catheter is filled aseptically with 1–1.5 ml of heparin (1000 units/ml) to prevent clotting in the catheter between infusions, and capped. Dudrick *et al.* have reported the use of a lightweight vest with pockets which hold all the components of the IVH system, which allows free movement and ambulation at work while the infusion continues[84].

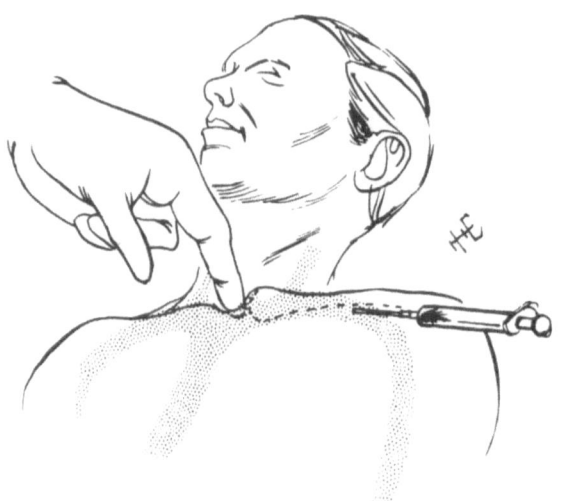

(a)

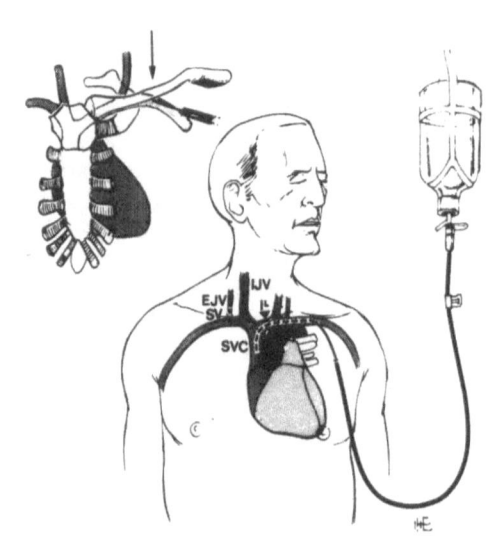

(b)

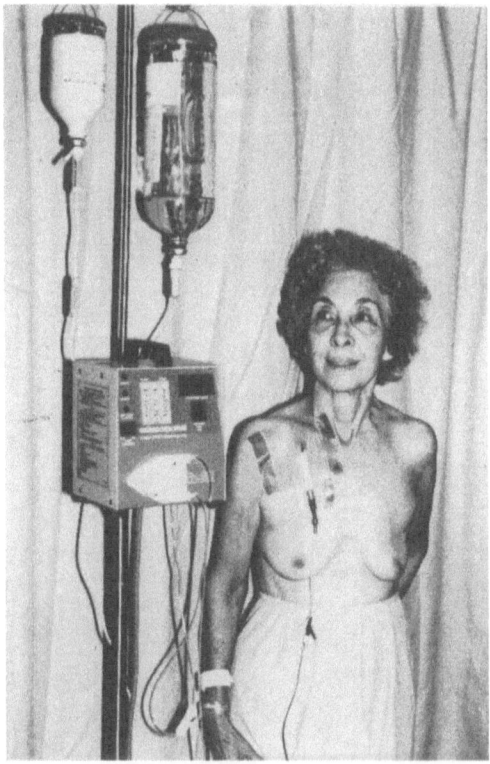

(c)

Figure 2 (a) Percutaneous subclavian puncture below midpoint of clavicle, with needle directed towards finger in sternal notch. Aspiration of blood indicates needle in subclavian vein, and catheter will now be inserted through the 14-gauge needle (a 16-needle is used in smaller patients) (b) The system for IVH. SVC = superior vena cava; SV = subclavian vein; I^L = left innominate vein; IJV = internal jugular vein; EJV = external jugular vein. (c) Catheter sutured, needle-guard in place, and sterile occlusive dressing applied. The 2 litre bottle, pump and tubing system are shown. Lipid is being piggy-backed centrally, under sterile precautions

MANAGEMENT OF THE INFUSION

Once the catheter-tip has been confirmed radiologically to be in the correct position, the infusions may proceed either by gravity drip or by using an infusion pump. It is advisable to begin the infusion slowly, either infusing supplemental isotonic intravenous fluids peripherally together with the full concentration of IVH solution or infusing lower

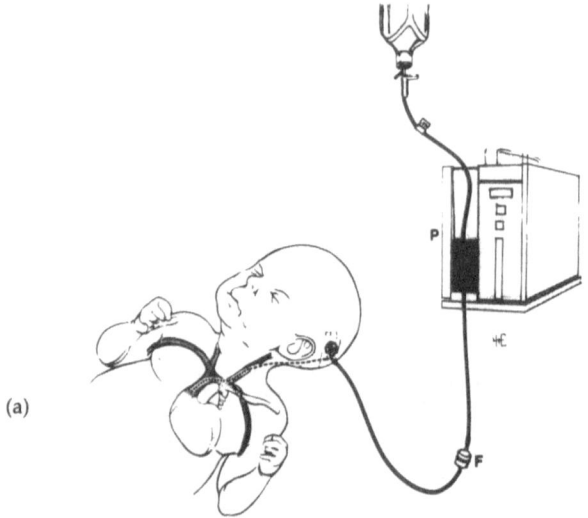

(a)

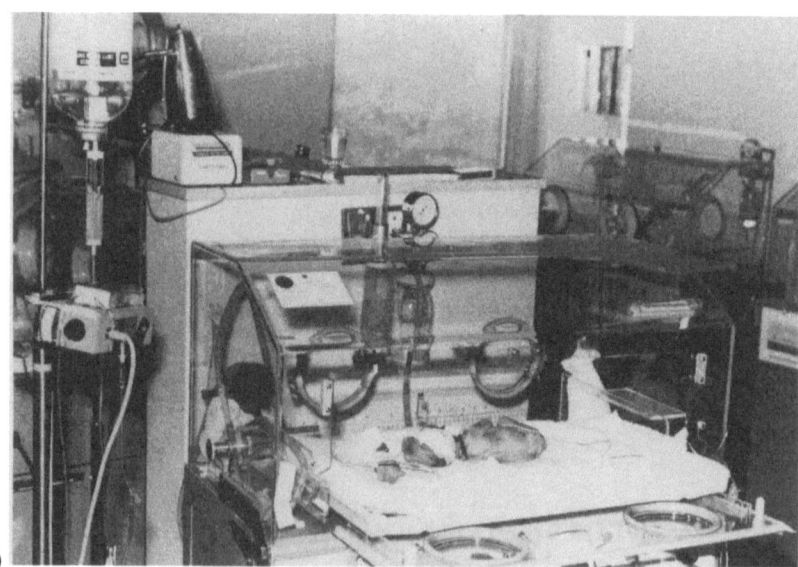

(b)

Figure 3 (a) System for IVH in the infant. P = pump; F = filter. (b) 900 g immature infant who had attacks of cyanosis on tube-feeding and was deteriorating on intravenous fluids. In the operating room, through a transverse supraclavicular incision, the superior vena cava was cannulated via the jugular vein and the proximal part of the silastic catheter was tunnelled out the retroauricular scalp for aseptic care. The patient is now 6 years old and a normal child

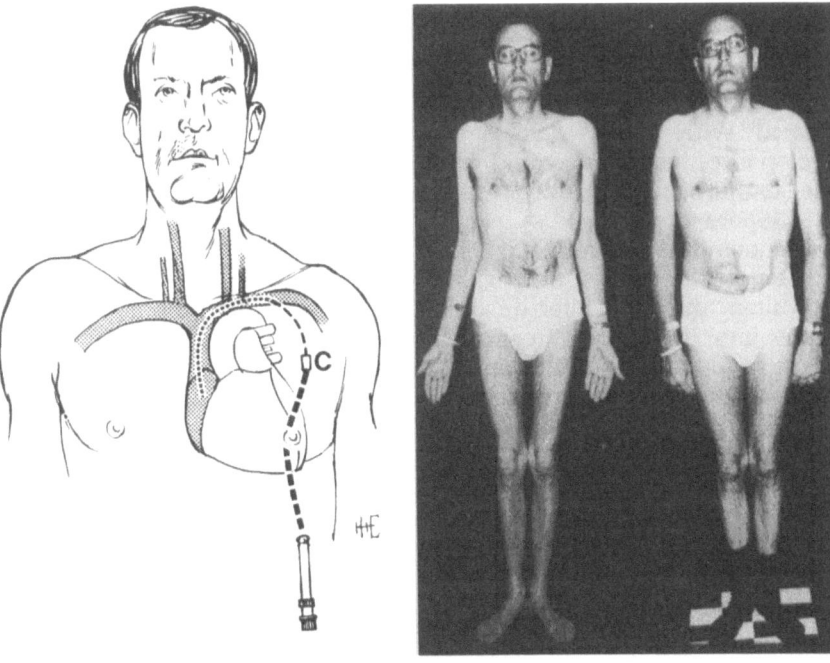

(a)   (b)

Figure 4 (a) Arrangement of silastic catheter for home IVH. C = cuff. Patient is fully trained, and usually administers infusions overnight. During the day, 1 ml of heparin is instilled, and line capped (shown). (b) Patient with antithrombin III deficiency, who had massive bowel resection for gangrene leaving 29 cm of small bowel, equally divided between jejunum and ileum. During postoperative intestinal adaptation, he was supported with IVH, which was stopped as medications appeared to control his diarrhoea and malabsorption. However, he returned in a depleted state (shown on left) and home IVH was instituted, while he carried on an active life during the day. Note appearance on right, after being on home IVH for 2 months. (We would now use the Op-Site dressing.) Adequate intestinal adaptation occurred over 10 months so that he could thrive on oral intake and medication, and home IVH was stopped

glucose concentrations in the IVH solution with a gradual increase to full concentrations, depending on the patient's tolerance. Sudden marked increase or decrease in the rate causes hyper- or hypo-glycaemia. Though expensive, pumps will maintain control of the infusion rate. The current models have an electronic eye which detects air in the tubing and automatically shuts off the pump and sounds an alarm. In infants, the use of a pump is mandatory to ensure constancy of the very slow infusion rate.

Millipore (0.45 or 0.22 µm) filters are sometimes inserted into the intravenous line between the infusion bottle and the patient's catheter to serve as a barrier against organisms, particulate matter and air. The larger filter prevents the passage of all bacteria except pleomorphic pseudomonas[86]. The 0.22 μm filter blocks passage of all bacteria and fungi, but will not permit a gravity drip and requires the use of a pump[87]. With the slow, almost stagnant infusion rates used in infants, bacterial contamination could result in a significant proliferation within the solution, and here a 0.22 μm filter is mandatory.

Millipore filters must be changed daily, which adds interruptions and thus potential contaminations of the infusion lines[88]. If organisms are present in the bottles, they will be concentrated on the 'bottle side' of the filter, and with filter breakdown these would be discharged as a bolus into the blood stream. Most workers therefore stress proper aseptic precautions in all areas of preparation and infusion, rather than using filters in adults, and have excellent results[89].

IVH PROTOCOLS

Once IVH has begun, careful monitoring plays a key role in prevention of complications and assessment of patient progress. Before the infusion commences, one obtains baseline laboratory values for haemoglobin, white cell count, total lymphocyte count, electrolytes, BUN, blood sugar, liver function tests, proteins and A/G ratio, serum transferrin, calcium, phosphate and magnesium. After starting IVH, electrolytes, BUN and blood sugar are obtained regularly, often daily at first, then three times a week. These values provide a basis for the alteration of formulation and nutrient concentration of the solution. The other blood indices are checked periodically (e.g. weekly). The patient's urine is checked by a nurse for glucose every 6 h. The nurse also checks the infusion rate, the patient's general well-being, and the catheter and intravenous tubings regularly.

Meticulous care is required in the management of the indwelling catheters to avoid infection. The occlusive dressing is changed three times a week (more often if soiled) under sterile precautions. The intravenous tubing is usually changed at the same time and is used solely for IVH solutions.* In recent years, Op-Site dressing has been used widely, and is changed every 7 days; this transparent, hypoallergenic, adhesive membrane is permeable to air and water vapour but is impervious to bacteria and liquids.

The central line should not be used for blood transfusions, administration of medications, measurement of central venous pressure, or drawing blood samples. These manipulations increase the opportunity

* A short intravenous extension set can be used between the intravenous line and the subclavian catheter, and can be clamped when changing the intravenous tubing; this extension set is changed once weekly.

for entry of organisms and infection. The catheter may be changed to the opposite side every 30 days, depending on the clinician's routine. The site is changed if catheter sepsis is suspected. A fever which persists with no obvious cause after the bottle and tubings have been changed is indicative of possible catheter sepsis. Blood cultures are withdrawn through the catheter; the catheter is then removed and the tip sent for culture. IVH infusion is resumed through a new catheter on the opposite side, usually 24 h later. If IVH protocols are carefully drawn up and maintained by an organized team, complications can be kept to a minimum.

COMPLICATIONS OF IVH

Technical complications

Due to the proximity of several important anatomical structures, problems may arise during subclavian vein catheterization. These are summarized in Table 3. Pneumothorax may arise from puncture of the apex of the lung. The experienced clinician avoids this by keeping the needle-tip as close to the clavicle as possible. The chest radiograph taken to confirm catheter-tip position will also check for pneumothorax. Haemothorax can occur if the patient's clotting mechanism is impaired, and deficient clotting is a contraindication to this technique. Hydrothorax and hydromediastinum occur if the solutions are infused outside the vein. Injury to the brachial plexus, phrenic nerve and thoracic duct is more potential than real. Puncture of the subclavian artery is unlikely in skilled hands, but if this happens, removal of the needle from the artery is generally all that is necessary to stop the bleeding. Air embolism can occur if the patient is hypovolaemic or not in the Trendelenburg position when the catheter is inserted. Some clinicians ask the patient to perform a Valsalva manoeuvre during catheter insertion. Air embolism is more likely to occur if the intravenous tubing becomes disconnected from the catheter, especially when the patient is upright.

The large diameter and large flow of the central veins minimize the occurrence of venous thrombosis. However, if the catheter is malpositioned, e.g. coiled up and distending the vein, administration of the hypertonic solution may cause thrombosis. The brittle polyvinyl catheter may work its way through the atrial wall into the pericardial sac, so that positioning it in the superior vena cava or innominate vein is necessary to avoid this possibility. A skilled approach and in-hospital education will avoid such complications.

Table 3 Complications of subclavian venepuncture

(A) Complications of catheter insertion
     Pneumothorax   Air embolism
     Haematoma   Hydrothorax
     Hydromediastinum   Brachial plexus injury
     Arterial puncture (injury)   Subclavian haematoma
     Subclavian vein thrombosis   Superior vena caval thrombosis
     Catheter embolism   Thromboembolism
     Catheter misplacement   Innominate or subclavian vein laceration
     Thoracic duct laceration   Phrenic nerve paralysis
     Horner's syndrome

(B) Complications of catheter maintenance
     1. Septic (bacterial or fungal)
          contaminated insertion site
          catheter contamination, e.g. used to draw blood
          intravenous tubing contamination
          solution contamination
             ward
             pharmacy
     May result in septicaemia, septic shock, septic emboli and endocarditis.

     2. Mechanical
          catheter pulled out
          catheter cracked and leaking
          intravenous line disconnection, with air embolism
          catheter thrombosis
          catheter kinking
          blood in intravenous line (poor venting of vacuum bottle)
          intravenous tubing breaks
          catheter-tip perforation through caval or right atrial wall
          venous thrombosis

Septic complications

The incidence of septicaemia varies among institutions and is usually
the result of inadequate surveillance and techniques. Infection rates
from 1 to 27% have been reported, with some deaths, especially from
infections with Candida organisms[89, 90]. The source of contamination
may occur anywhere in the IVH system – in the solutions, the tubings,
and around the catheter tract itself. Ingrowth of skin organisms along
the catheter, and contamination of the infusion apparatus due to interruptions in the closed system, have been frequent sources of infection[91].
With meticulous technique, catheter sepsis in less than 2% of patients is
attainable; this possibly represents haematogenous spread of bacteria
from abscesses elsewhere in the body with seeding on the catheter or

fibrin sleeve. Patients who receive IVH are often severely ill and/or mal-nourished, have impaired immune response, and are often being treated with broad-spectrum antibiotics, steroids, radiation or chemo-therapy. These factors, plus the occasional presence of diabetes mellitus, further interfere with defence mechanisms and predispose the patient to antibiotic-resistant or fungal infections[89].

The most common septicaemia reported with the use of protein hydrolysates was fungal (usually Candida strains)[92]. Candida multiply in hydrolysates at 20–37 °C but not at 4 °C, and protein hydrolysates select for growth of Candida over bacteria[93]. However, the incidence of solution-related infection has decreased since the change from hydroly-sates to crystalline amino acid solutions, and indeed there is no growth of bacteria or fungi in crystalline amino acid solutions at 37 °C for 24 h[65]. However, lipid emulsions can support both bacterial and fungal growth at 20 and 37 °C, and care must be exerted in their administration to prevent contamination[94].

Metabolic complications

Many of the earlier metabolic complications were caused by omission or excessive administration of various substances. Omission or inadequate administration of a key patient requirement will eventually lead to a de-ficiency state. Reported deficiency and excess states are listed in Table 4. More commonly, however, metabolic upsets are related to infusion rate. It is important to begin the infusion of the hypertonic solution slowly and gradually increase to the desired rate based on the patient's toler-ance. Too rapid administration causes hyperglycaemia, and if the renal threshold for absorption is exceeded glycosuria occurs. Glycosuria in excess of 2 mg/dl can cause osmotic diuresis, which will progress to cellular dehydration, lethargy and ultimately coma[95, 96]. This hyperos-molar, hyperglycaemic, non-ketotic coma can be prevented by careful monitoring of urine and blood glucose levels, and this should be done routinely. Blood glucose levels above 180 mg/dl are treated with the ad-dition of insulin to the regime. Occasionally the glucose concentration in the solutions may have to be reduced and supplemental isotonic fluids may be necessary. Patients who originally required exogenous insulin when IVH was started may gradually tolerate the high glucose load without added insulin. Diabetic patients may require insulin in the IVH bottles, and must be closely monitored.

Abruptly stopping IVH has resulted in severe hypoglycaemia in low-birth-weight infants[97]. In adults, however, this has only occurred after inadvertent acceleration of the infusion was followed by abrupt ces-sation; this could happen if the nurse, finding that the patient has

Table 4 Possible metabolic complications

Hyperglycaemia
Hyperosmolar non-ketotic dehydration and coma
Ketoacidosis in diabetes mellitus
Hypoglycaemia

Hyperchloraemic metabolic acidosis
Serum amino acid imbalance
Hyperammonaemia
Prerenal azotaemia

Essential fatty acid deficiency
Hypercholesterolaemia
Hypertriglyceridaemia

Hypokalaemia
Hyperkalaemia
Hyponatraemia
Hypernatraemia

Hypophosphataemia
Hyperphosphataemia
Hypocalcaemia
Hypercalcaemia
Hypervitaminosis D
Hypovitaminosis D
Hypomagnesaemia
Hypermagnesaemia

Anaemia

Hypervitaminosis A
Biotin deficiency
Trace element deficiency
   Zinc
   Chromium
   Iodine, etc.

Hypertransaminaemia
   SGOT
   SGPT
   Alkaline phosphatase

received too much solution over a short period, suddenly stops the infusion[95]. In such circumstances the nurse should be instructed to resume the infusion at the prescribed hourly rate.

Electrolyte imbalances may occur with IVH. The commonest is perhaps hypokalaemia. During IVH with an anabolic patient, requirements for intracellular electrolytes (potassium, magnesium and phosphate) are increased, as these are incorporated in cell synthesis. The insulin response to a glucose load causes potassium to move into cells with glucose, and adequate potassium must be provided. However, as the body's potassium stores are repleted, it is important to decrease the

the body's potassium stores are repleted, it is important to decrease the daily potassium addition so that hyperkalaemia will not result. Hypokalaemia is associated with cardiac arrhythmias, muscular weakness and mental confusion, and hyperkalaemia may result in cardiac arrest.

Sodium requirements may also vary, with hyponatraemia resulting from excessive fistula losses or renal losses and inadequate intake. Hypernatraemia may occur in hyperosmolar coma, or if renal excretion of sodium is impaired. An excessive sodium load may result in cardiac failure. With properly formulated solutions, metabolic complications are usually minimal and easily correctable.

NEW HORIZONS IN INTRAVENOUS FEEDING

As knowledge of biochemical processes and nutrient requirements accumulates, special IVH solutions for the treatment of specific diseases are being investigated.

Amino acid mixtures have been formulated which decrease or avoid encephalopathy in hepatic failure. The cerebral effects seen with severe liver damage were previously thought to be caused by toxic accumulation of ammonia from amino acid breakdown, due to inability of the liver to convert this to urea. However, it has now been shown that there is an abnormal pattern of amino acids in these patients' blood, which can alter neurotransmitter synthesis in the brain and contribute to the aetiology of hepatic coma[98]. Patients in hepatic failure have increased blood levels of aromatic amino acids (phenylalanine, tyrosine, tryptophan) plus methionine and a decrease in the branched-chain amino acids (leucine, isoleucine, valine). An IVH solution containing decreased aromatic amino acids and increased branched-chain amino acids, when given to animals with liver damage along with large amounts of glucose, has produced dramatic improvement in cerebral function and normalization of plasma aromatic : branched-chain amino acid ratios[99].

In renal failure, amino acid catabolites normally excreted by the kidney (urea, creatinine, ammonia) accumulate in the blood. A specialized amino acid solution containing only the minimum daily requirements of the eight essential amino acids has been formulated to be infused with a high concentration of glucose for energy. The theory is to use the nitrogen from endogenous urea for synthesis of non-essential amino acids, which together with the infused essential amino acids and energy will result in anabolism[100]. Benefit from this therapy remains to be proven.

Innovative amino acid mixtures have potential use in curtailing the body's catabolic response to trauma. When muscle protein is metabolized for gluconeogenesis, the branched-chain amino acids are metabolized directly by the muscles for energy. If branched-chain amino acids are infused, they go directly to muscle or kidney to be metabolized and are not changed into glucose by the liver. In the traumatized or septic patient, where there is glucose intolerance due to insulin resistance in the peripheral tissues, muscle is still able to utilize branched-chain amino acids to meet energy requirements[101]. However, their value as therapy during trauma has yet to be confirmed.

At present, IVH is used in cancer patients to replenish them or sustain them nutritionally in order to tolerate therapies. In the future it may be possible to create specialized amino acid mixtures for IVH which will actually deprive the cancer cells of specific needs but still maintain the patient.

SUMMARY

The 1970s will go down in medical history as the decade in which safe, total nutrition by vein became a reality. Since the inception of IVH in the 1960s, remarkable advances have been made. Catheter insertion techniques, materials for delivery, care of the system, and infusion constituents have improved to the point where the benefits of this treatment strongly outweigh the risks. With improved balanced amino acid solutions, safe lipid emulsions to supply essential fatty acids, and better understanding of vitamin, mineral and trace element requirements, the clinician can confidently proceed in the knowledge that he is providing a total diet intravenously. The multitude of clinical conditions for which IVH is indicated continues to grow as the importance of attaining normal nutritional indices in disease is realized. As specifically formulated solutions are developed, the potential for IVH as a curative therapy will probably increase. Intellectual contemporaries of Harvey and Wren in the seventeenth century would probably have rejected a prediction that in the 1980s it would be possible to nourish a human completely by vein from cradle to grave.

Acknowledgments

We acknowledge the assistance of Dr Kevin H. Wong, Research Associate, the St Joseph's Hospital (Toronto) Research Foundation; the Nelson Arthur Hyland Foundation; and the Department of Photography of St Joseph's Health Centre.

References

1 Annan, G. L. (1939). An exhibition of books on the growth of our knowledge of blood transfusion. *Bull. N.Y. Acad. Med.*, **15**, 622

2 James, R. (1745). Transfusion. *In a medical dictionary*, **3** (London)

3 Fortescue-Brickdale, J. M. (1904). A contribution to the history of the intravenous injection of drugs. *Guys Hosp. Rep.*, **58**, 15

4 Sanderson, I. (1980). History of nutrition in surgery, in M. Deitel (ed.). *Nutrition in Clinical Surgery*, Chapter 1. (Baltimore: Williams & Wilkins)

5 Pasteur, L. and Joubert J. V. (1877). Charbon et seticémie. *Compt. V, Hebd Séave. Acad. Sci. Paris*, **85**, 101

6 Lister, J. (1870). On the effects of the antiseptic system of treatment upon the salubrity of a surgical hospital. *Lancet*, **1**, 4, 40

7 Friedrich, P. L. (1904). Die kunstliche subcutane Ernahrung in der praktischen Chirurgie. *Arch. Klin. Chir.*, **73**, 507

8 Siebert, F. D. (1923). Fever producing substance found in some distilled waters. *Am. J. Physiol.*, **67**, 90

9 Rose, W. C. (1938). Nutritional significance of amino acids. *Physiol. Rev.*, **18**, 109

10 Elman, R. and Weiner D. O. (1939). Intravenous alimentation with specific reference to protein (amino-acid) metabolism. *J. Am. Med. Assoc.*, **112**, 796

11 Moore, F. (1959). *Metabolic Care of the Surgical Patient*. (Philadelphia: W. B. Saunders)

12 Cuthbertson, D. P. (1932). Observations on the disturbance of metabolism produced by injury of the limbs. *Q. J. Med.*, **25**, 233

13 Schuberth, O. and Wretlind, A. (1961). Intravenous infusion of fat emulsions, phosphatides and emulsifying agents. *Acta. Chir. Scand.*, **278**, (Suppl.), 1

14 Dudrick, S. J., Rhoads, J. E. and Vars, H. M. (1967). Growth of puppies receiving all nutritional requirements by vein. *Fortschr. Parenteralen Ernahrung, Pallas verlay, Lochan dei Munchen*, **2**, 16

15 Dudrick, S. J., Wilmore, D. W., Vars, H. M. *et al.* (1969). Can intravenous feeding as the sole means of nutrition support growth in the child and restore weight loss in an adult? An affirmative answer. *Ann. Surg.*, **169**, 974

16 Jeejeebhoy, K. N. and Langer, B. (1980). Home parenteral nutrition. *Can. Med. Assoc. J.*, **122**, 143

17 Cahill, G. F. (1970). Starvation in man. *N. Engl. J. Med.*, **282**, 668

18 Harris, J. A. and Benedict, F. G. (1919). *A Biometric Study of Basal Metabolism in Man.* (Washington, DC: Carnegie Institution of Washington, Publication no. 279)

19 Long, C. L., Schaffel, N., Geiger, J. W., Schiller, W. R. and Blackmore, W. S. Metabolic response to injury and illness: estimated energy and protein needs from indirect calorimetry and nitrogen balance. *J. Parent. Ent. Nutr.*, **3**, 452

20 Dahn, M., Bouwman, D. and Kirkpatrick, J. (1979). The sepsis–glucose intolerance riddle: a hormonal explanation. *Surgery*, **86**, 423

21 Kinney, J. M. and Dudrick, S. J. (1970). Trauma workshop report: metabolic response to trauma and nutrition. *J. Trauma*, **10**, 1065

22 Rush, B. F., Richardson, J. D. and Griffen, W. O. (1970). Positive Nitrogen balance immediately after abdominal operations. *Am. J. Surg.*, **119**, 70

23 Shetty, P. S., Jung, R. T., Watrasievicz, K. E. and James, W. P. T. (1979). Rapid turn over transport proteins: an index of sub-clinical protein-energy malnutrition. *Lancet*, **2**, 230

24 MacLean, L. D., Meakins, J. L., Taguchi, K., Duigan, J. P., Dhillon, K. S. and Gordon J. (1975). Host resistance in sepsis and trauma. *Ann. Surg.*, **182**, 207

25 Long, C. L., Haverberg, L. N., Young, V. R., Kinney, J. M., Munro, H. N. and Geiger, J. W. (1975). Metabolism of 3-methylhistidine in man. *Metabolism*, **24**, 929

26 Blackburn, G. L., Bistrian, B. R., Maini, B. S., Schlamm, H. T. and Smith, M. F.

(1977). Nutritional and metabolic assessment of the hospitalized patient. *J. Parent. Ent. Nutr.* **1**, 11

27   Sandler, J. (1980). Specific techniques in delivery of liquid diets. In Deitel, M. (ed.). *Nutrition in Clinical Surgery.* Chapter 5 (Baltimore: Williams & Wilkins)

28   Hoover, H. C., Ryan, J. A., Anderson, E. J. and Fischer, J. E. (1980). Nutritional benefits of immediate post operative jejunal feeding of an elemental diet. *Am. J. Surg.*, **139**, 153

29   Deitel, M. and Syed, A. K. (1974). Elemental diets in management of clinical nutritional problems. *Mod. Med. Can.*, **29**, 271

30   Levine, G. M., Deren, J. J. and Yezdimir, E. (1976). Small bowel resection: oral intake is the stimulus for hyperplasia. *Am. J. Dig. Dis.*, **21**, 542

31   Kay, R. M., Berndl, L. A. and Hladyschersky, I. (1980). In Deitel, M. (ed.). *Nutrition in Clinical Surgery.* Chapter 4. (Baltimore: Williams & Wilkins)

32   Deitel, M. (1976). Nutritional management of external gastrointestinal fistulas. *Can. J. Surg.*, **19**, 505

33   Deitel, M. and Gonzales, M. J. (1979). Intravenous hyperalimentation (IVH) in inflammatory bowel disease (IBD). *J. Parent. Ent. Nutr.*, **3**, 518 (abstr.)

34   Copeland, E. M., Daly, J. M. and Dudrick, S. J. (1977). Nutrition as an adjunct to cancer treatment in the adult. *Cancer Res.*, **37**, 2451

35   Copeland, E. M., MacFadyen, B. V., Lanzotti, V. and Dudrick, S. J. (1975). Intravenous hyperalimentation as an adjunct to cancer chemotherapy. *Am. J. Surg.*, **129**, 167

36   Deitel, M., Alexander, M. and Hew, L. R. (1980). Hyperalimentation and cancer. *Can. J. Surg.*, **23**, 11

37   Filler, R. M. and Eraklis, A. J. (1970). Care of the critically ill child: intravenous alimentation. *Pediatrics*, **46**, 456

38   Health and Welfare Canada (1976). *Dietary Standards for Canada.* Supply and Services Canada, Ottawa

39   Curreri, P. W., Richmond, D., Marvin, J. *et al.* (1974). Dietary requirements of patients with major burns. *J. Am. Diet. Assoc.*, **65**, 415

40   Shenkin, A. and Wretlind, A. (1978). Parenteral nutrition. *World Rev. Nutr. Diet.*, **28**, 1

41   Woods, H. F. and Alberti, K. G. M. M. (1972). Dangers of intravenous fructose *Lancet*, **2**, 1354

42   Long, J. M., Wilmore, D. W., Mason, A. D. and Pruitt, B. A. (1977). Effect of carbohydrate and fat intake on nitrogen excretion during total intravenous feeding. *Ann. Surg.*, **185**, 147

43   Jeejeebhoy, K. N., Anderson, G. H., Nakhooda, A. F., Greenberg, G. R., Sanderson, I. and Marlis, E. B. (1976). Metabolic studies in total parenteral nutrition with lipid in man. Comparison with glucose. *J. Clin. Invest.*, **57**, 125

44   Gazzaniga, A. B., Bartlett, R. H. and Shobe, J. B. (1975). Nitrogen balance in patients receiving either fat or carbohydrate for total intravenous nutrition. *Ann. Surg.*, **182**, 163

45   MacFadyen, B. V., Dudrick, S. J., Tagudar, E. P., Maynard, A. T., Law, D. K. and Rhoads, J. E. (1973). Triglyceride and free fatty acid clearances in patients receiving complete parenteral nutrition using a ten per cent soybean oil emulsion. *Surg. Gynecol. Obstet.*, **137**, 813

46   Askanazi, J., Carpentier, Y. A., Elwyn, D. H., Nordenstrom, J., Jeevanandam, M., Rosenbanon, S. H., Gump, F. E. and Kinney, J. M. (1980). Influence of total parenteral nutrition on fuel utilization in injury and sepsis. *Ann. Surg.*, **191**, 40

47   Wiese, H. F., Hansen, A. E. and Adam, D. J. D. (1958). Essential fatty acids in infant nutrition. 1. Linoleic acid requirement in terms of serum di-, tri-, and tetraenoic acid levels. *J. Nutr.*, **66**, 345

48   Paulsrud, J. R., Pensler, L., Whitten, C. F., Stewart, S. and Holman, R. T. (1972). Es-

sential fatty acid deficiency in infants induced by fat-free intravenous feeding. *Am. J. Clin. Nutr.*, **25**, 897

49   Goodgame, J. T., Lowry, S. F. and Brennan, M. F. (1978). Essential fatty acid deficiency in total parenteral nutrition: Time course of development and suggestions for therapy. *Surgery*, **84**, 271

50   O'Neill, J. A., Caldwell, M. D. and Meng, H. C. (1977). Essential fatty acid deficiency in surgical patients. *Ann. Surg.*, **185**, 535

51   Faulkner, W. J. and Flint, L. M. Jr (1977). Essential fatty acid deficiency associated with total parenteral nutrition. *Surg. Gynecol. Obstet.*, **144**, 665

52   Zlotkin, S. H. and Anderson, G. H. (1980). Amino acid requirements and sources during total parenteral nutrition. In Deitel, M. (ed.). *Nutrition in Clinical Surgery*, Chapter 8 (Baltimore: Williams & Wilkins)

53   Elman, R. (1947). *Parenteral Alimentation in Surgery*. (New York: Paul B. Hoeber)

54   Blackburn, G. L., Flatt, J. B., Cowes, G. H. A. and O'Donnell, T. E. (1973). Peripheral intravenous feeding with isotonic amino acid solutions. *Am. J. Surg.*, **125**, 447

55   Deitel, M., Sauvé, Sr. F., Alexander, M. A., Degani, C. F. and Anand, P. K. (1977). A crystaline amino acid solution for total parenteral nutrition. *Can. J. Hosp. Pharm.*, **30**, 175

56   Anderson, G. H., Patel, D. G. and Jeejeebhoy, K. N. (1974). Design and evaluation by nitrogen balance and blood aminograms of an amino acid mixture for total parenteral nutrition of adults with gastrointestinal diseases. *J. Clin. Invest.*, **53**, 904

57   Christensen, H. N., Lynch, E. L. and Power, J. H. (1946). The conjugated nonprotein amino acids in plasma. III. Peptidemia and hyperpeptidemia as a result of intravenous administration of partially hydrolysed casein (Amigin). *J. Biol. Chem.*, **166**, 649

58   Rose, W. C., Wixom, R. L., Lockhart, H. B. and Lambert, G. F. (1955). The amino acid requirements of man. XV. The valine requirement: summary and final observations. *J. Biol. Chem.*, **217**, 987

59   FAO/WHO (1973). Joint Expert Committee on Energy and Protein Requirements. *World Health Organization Technical Report*, series no. 522, Geneva

60   Long, C. L., Zikria, B. A., Kinney, J. M. and Geiger, J. W. (1974). Comparison of fibrin hydrolysate and crystaline amino acid solutions in parenteral nutrition. *Am. J. Clin. Nutr.*, **27**, 163

61   Johnson, J. O., Albritton, W. L. and Sunshine, P. (1972). Hyperammonaemia accompanying parenteral nutrition in newborn infants. *J. Pediatr.*, **81**, 154

62   Bergstrom, K., Blomstrand, R. and Jacobson, S. (1972). Longterm complete intravenous nutrition in man. *Nutr. Metabol.*, **14**, (Suppl.), 118

63   Heird, W. C., Dell, R. B., Driscoll, J. M., Grehin, B. and Winters, R. W. (1972). Metabolic acidosis resulting from intravenous alimentation mixtures containing synthetic amino acids. *N. Engl. J. Med.*, **287**, 943

64   Heird, W. C., Nicholson, J. F., Driscoll, J. M., Schullinger, J. N. and Winters, R. W. (1972). Hyperammonaemia resulting from intravenous alimentation using a mixture of synthetic L-amino acids: a preliminary report. *J. Pediatr.*, **81**, 162

65   Gelbart, S. M., Reinhardt, G. F. and Greenlee, H. B. (1973). Multiplication of nosocomial pathogens in intravenous feeding solutions. *Appl. Microbiol.*, **26**, 874

66   Sheldon, G. F. and Grzyb, S. (1975). Phosphate depletion and repletion: relation to parenteral nutrition and oxygen transport. *Ann. Surg.*, **182**, 683

67   Craddock, P. R., Yawata, Y., Van Santen, L., Gilberstadt, S., Silvis, S. and Jacob, H. S. (1974). Acquired phagocytic dysfunction. A complication of the hypophosphataemia of parenteral hyperalimentation. *N. Engl. J. Med.*, **290**, 1403

68   Munro, H. N. (1980). The Ninth Edition of Recommended Dietary Allowances, in *Nutrition and the M.D.*, VI, no. 2

69   Vasquez, R. M. (1980). Vitamin requirements in parenteral nutrition. In Deitel, M.,

(ed.). *Nutrition in Clinical Surgery*. Chapter 10 (Baltimore: Williams & Wilkins)

70 Jeejeebhoy, K. N. (1976). Total parenteral nutrition. In *Ann. Coll. Phys. Surg. Can.*, (Oct.) 287

71 Underwood, E. J. (1977). *Trace Elements in Human and Animal Nutrition* (4th edn). (New York: Academic Press)

72 Sandstead, H. H., Burk, R. F., Booth, G. H. and Darby, W. J. (1970). Current concepts on trace minerals. Clinical considerations. *Med. Clin. N. Am.*, **54,** 1509

73 Fraker, P. J., Haas, S. M. and Luecke, R. W. (1977). Effect of zinc deficiency on the immune response of the young adult A/J mouse. *J. Nutr.*, **107,** 1889

74 Fleming, C. R., Hodges, R. E. and Hurley, L. S. (1976). A prospective study of serum copper and zinc levels in patients receiving total parenteral nutrition. *Am. J. Clin. Nutr.*, **29,** 70

75 Okada, A., Takagi, Y., Itakura, T., Satani, M., Manabe, H., Lida, Y., Tanigaki, T., Iwasaki, M. and Kasahara, M. (1976). Skin lesions during intravenous hyperalimentation: zinc deficiency. *Surgery*, **80,** 629

76 Jeejeebhoy, K. N., Chu, R., Marliss, E. B., Greenberg, G. R. and Bruce-Robertson, A. (1975). Chromium deficiency, diabetes and neuropathy, reversed by chromium infusion in a patient on total parenteral nutrition (TPN) for 3½ years. *Clin. Res.*, **23,** 636A

77 Wolman, S. L., Anderson, G. H., Marliss, E. B. and Jeejeebhoy, K. N. (1979). Zinc in total parenteral nutrition: requirements and metabolic effects. *Gastroenterology*, **76,** 458

78 Sauvé, Sr. F. (1972). Preparation of solutions for hyperalimentation. *Can. J. Hosp. Pharm.*, **25,** 60

79 Beck, W. C. (1974). The use of clean work stations in preparing sterile solutions. *Am. J. I.V. Therapy*, **1,** 46

80 Deitel, M. and Kaminsky, V. (1974). Osmolality of hyperalimentation solution infused into the superior vena cava. *Can. J. Surg.*, **17,** 310

81 Deitel, M. and McIntyre, J. A. (1971). Radiologic confirmation of site of central venous pressure catheters. *Can. J. Surg.*, **14,** 42

82 Dudrick, S. J., Groff, D. B. and Wilmore, D. W. (1969). Long-term venous catheterization in infants. *Surg. Gynecol. Obstet.*, **129,** 805

83 Broviac, J. W., Cole, J. J. and Scribner, B. H. (1973). A silicone rubber atrial catheter for prolonged parenteral alimentation. *Surg. Gynecol. Obstet.*, **136,** 602

84 Dudrick, S. J., Englert, D. M., VanBuren, C. T., Rowlands, B. J. and MacFadyen, B. V. (1979). New concepts of ambulatory home hyperalimentation. *J. Parent. Ent. Nutr.*, **3,** 72

85 Prian, G. W. and VanWay, C. W. (1978). The long arm silastic catheter: a critical look at complications. *J. Parent. Ent. Nutr.*, **2,** 124

86 Freeman, J. B. and MacLean, L. D. (1971). Intravenous hyperalimentation: a review. *Can. J. Surg.*, **14,** 180

87 Holland, R. R., Lamoureux, J. L. and Todd, D. W. (1973). Filter system for intravenous alimentation (letter to the editor). *N. Engl. J. Med.*, **289,** 487

88 Deitel, M., Sanderson, I. and Petsoulas, T. (1973). A system of intravenous hyperalimentation. *Intern. Surg.*, **58,** 670

89 Sanderson, I. and Deitel, M. (1973). Intravenous hyperalimentation without sepsis. *Surg. Gynecol. Obstet.*, **136,** 577

90 Curry, C. R. and Quie, P. G. (1971). Fungal septicemia in patients receiving parenteral hyperalimentation. *N. Engl. J. Med.*, **285,** 1221

91 Ryan, J. A., Abel, R. M., Abbott, W. M., Hopkins, C. C., Chesney, T. M., Colley, R., Phillips, K. and Fischer, J. E. (1974). Catheter complications in total parenteral nutrition: a prospective study of 200 consecutive patients. *N. Engl. J. Med.*, **290,** 757

92 Goldmann, D. A. and Maki, D. C. (1973). Infection control in total parenteral nutri-

tion. *J. Am. Med. Assoc.*, **223**, 1360

93 Brennan, M. F., O'Connell, R. C., Rosol, J. A. and Kundsin, R. (1971). The growth of candida albicans in nutritive solutions given parenterally. *Arch. Surg.*, **103**, 705

94 Deitel, M., Kaminsky, V. M. and Fuksa, M. (1975). Growth of common bacteria and candida albicans in 10% soybean oil emulsion. *Can. J. Surg.*, **18**, 531

95 Sanderson, I. and Deitel, M. (1974). Insulin response in patients receiving concentrated infusions of glucose and casein hydrolysate for complete parenteral nutrition. *Ann. Surg.*, **179**, 387

96 Kaminski, M. V. Jr (1978). A review of hyperosmolar hyperglycemic nonketotic dehydration (HHND): etiology, pathophysiology and prevention during intravenous hyperalimentation. *J. Parent. Ent. Nutr.*, **2**, 690

97 Hays, D. M., Kaplan, M. S., Mahour, G. H., Strauss, J. and Huxtable, R. F. (1972). High-calorie infusion therapy following surgery in low birth weight infants: metabolic problems encountered. *Surgery*, **71**, 834

98 Smith, A. R., Rossi-Fanelli, F., Freund, H. and Fischer, J. E. (1979). Sulfur-containing amino acids in experimental hepatic coma in the dog and the monkey. *Surgery*, **85**, 677

99 Fischer, J. E., Funovics, J. M., Aguirre, A., James, J. H., Kean, J. M., Wesdorp, R. I. C., Yoshimura, N. and Westman, T. (1975). The role of plasma amino acids in hepatic encephalopathy. *Surgery*, **78**, 276

100 Abel, R. M. (1976). Parenteral nutrition in the treatment of renal failure. In Fischer, J. (ed.). *Total Parenteral Nutrition*, pp. 143–70. (Boston: Little, Brown & Co.)

101 Freund, H., Yoshimura, N., Lunetta, L. and Fischer, J. E. (1978). Role of branched chain amino acids in decreasing muscle catabolism in vivo. *J. Parent. Ent. Nutr.*, **2**, 48A

8
Drug treatment of peptic ulcer disease

D. C. CARTER and D. H. OSBORNE

INTRODUCTION

Peptic ulceration results from an imbalance between gastric acid/pepsin secretion and the ability of the mucosa of the upper gastrointestinal tract to withstand peptic digestion. Excessive secretion can be incriminated in many patients with duodenal ulceration and in the rare Zollinger-Ellison syndrome, whereas many patients with gastric ulcer have normal or reduced levels of secretion, suggesting that defective mucosal defences are of prime importance in gastric ulceration. Nevertheless, the dictum 'no acid – no ulcer' remains valid in that peptic ulcer is truly exceptional in the absence of acid and pepsin secretion.

Failure to define the basic pathophysiological disturbances responsible for peptic ulceration has restricted therapy to attempts to reduce gastric acidity and pepsin secretion, and/or strengthen mucosal defences against autodigestion. Recent developments in our understanding of the mechanisms regulating gastric secretion have allowed anti-secretory therapy to be placed on a more rational basis, while improved understanding of the nature of mucosal defences has opened the road to exciting advances in this area of therapeutic endeavour. Some of these important conceptual advances will be reviewed briefly before considering ulcer therapy.

219

IMPORTANT CONCEPTS IN THE TREATMENT OF PEPTIC ULCERATION

The role of acid and pepsin as ulcerogens

Separation of the roles of acid and pepsin in ulcerogenesis is well-nigh impossible. Pepsin is only active in an acid milieu and, in general, secretion of acid and pepsin is linked so that their outputs rise and fall in parallel. High concentrations of acid can cause experimental damage in the absence of pepsin, probably by protein denaturation of the gastrointestinal lining. For example, Goldberg and colleagues[1] found that acid solutions at pH 1.0 could cause severe oesophagitis, the severity of which was not increased by pepsin. Less concentrated solutions (pH 1.6 or 2.0) produced oesophagitis only in the presence of pepsin, and at these pH levels peptic digestion was probably responsible. In man, gastric and duodenal pH may at times be low enough to allow damage by acid alone, but as pepsin is also present under these conditions, there is no doubt that proteolysis by pepsin plays the major role in mucosal ulceration.

Pepsins are stored and secreted as inactive pepsinogens, and there are two immunologically distinct groups of pepsinogens in human gastric mucosa[2,3]. On exposure to acid solution (pH <5), fragments cleave from the pepsinogen molecule to leave pepsins of molecular weight of about 35 000. The pH for optimal peptic activity varies according to substrate and environmental conditions, but in general there are two optima, one around pH 2 and the other near pH 4. All pepsins are inactivated irreversibly at neutral or slightly alkaline pH.

Regulation of gastric acid secretion

Three endogenous chemicals have strong claims as physiological stimulants of acid secretion. A physiological role for gastrin and acetylcholine is established, but that of histamine has been controversial. Histamine is readily detectable in human gastric mucosa and is located almost exclusively in mast cells[4], the highest concentrations of which are found in the lamina propria adjacent to parietal cells[5]. It is tempting to speculate that histamine serves as a 'paracrine' regulator of acid secretion, the term 'paracrine' implying a chemical messenger secreted by cells in the immediate vicinity of the target cell (Figure 1). Such messengers might serve to modulate the effects of conventional hormones (blood-borne or endocrine messengers) and neurocrine messengers such as acetylcholine.

The well-known final common pathway hypothesis[6,7] envisaged histamine as the final common mediator used by all parietal cell stimu-

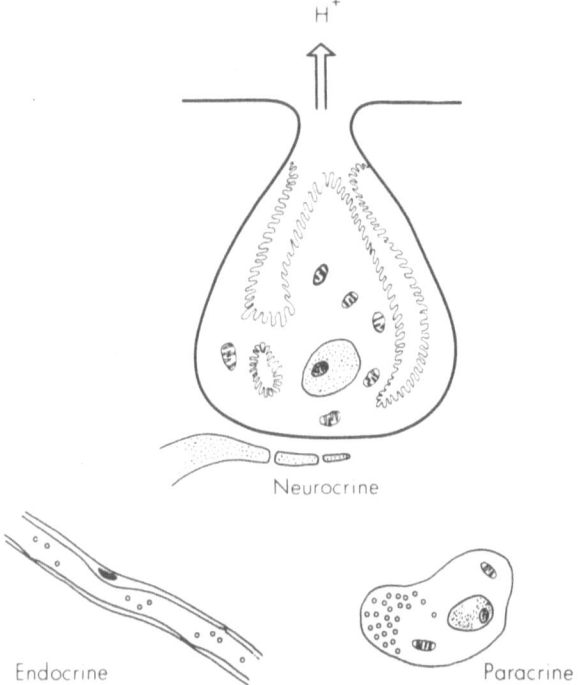

Figure 1 Methods of delivery of chemical messengers regulating acid secretion by the parietal cell

lants. For example, gastrin and acetylcholine were thought incapable of activating the parietal cell directly; each was obliged to stimulate the cell indirectly through the agency of histamine. The advent of the histamine H_2 receptor antagonists provided evidence which at first sight supported this hypothesis. These specific histamine antagonists not only inhibited acid secretion induced by histamine, but were also found to be effective against secretion induced by gastrin, vagal stimulation and food[8-10]. However, as Grossman and Konturek[8] pointed out, the anticholinergic drug atropine also inhibits acid secretion induced by gastrin or histamine in addition to inhibiting secretion induced by cholinergic stimuli. They argued that if inhibition of gastrin-induced secretion by H_2 receptor antagonists is evidence that gastrin acts by releasing histamine, then inhibition of gastrin-induced secretion by atropine is also evidence that it acts by releasing acetylcholine. Arguing that gastrin is unlikely to act through both agencies, they proposed a model in which the parietal cell has separate receptors for gastrin, acetylcholine and histamine.

According to their thesis, blockade of one receptor could also affect the properties of the other types of receptor and so render all three stimulants less effective.

This thesis has received considerable support from studies conducted in isolated parietal cells. Soll[11,12] has presented evidence that oxygen uptake can be taken as a valid index of the response of such isolated cells to secretagogues. Histamine, gastrin and carbamylcholine each stimulated oxygen uptake independently, implying a separate parietal cell receptor for each agent. The maximal response to histamine was less than the maximal response to histamine combined with gastrin or carbamylcholine, reinforcing the conclusion that these two compounds do not depend on histamine for their stimulatory effect. Finally, Soll showed that carbamylcholine could be blocked by atropine but not by metiamide (histamine H_2 receptor antagonist) and histamine could be blocked by metiamide but not by atropine, whereas gastrin was not blocked by either antagonist (Figure 2). The specificity of metiamide and atropine in this system is used by Soll to explain their apparent lack of specificity *in vivo*, if one assumes that the *in vivo* action of any secretagogue represents the outcome of interaction between that agent and a background 'tonic' effect of other endogenous secretagogues. For example, cimetidine blocks only histamine receptors on the parietal cell, but by removing a tonic effect of histamine it renders the cell less susceptible to stimulation by gastrin or acetylcholine. The concept can also be applied to explain the efficiency of surgical vagotomy as a means of reducing gastric secretion. Vagotomy removes acetylcholine as a parietal cell stimulant and in doing so renders the cell less amenable to stimulation by gastrin or histamine.

Isolated parietal cell systems are also being used to elucidate the intracellular mechanisms which regulate gastric secretion. The available evidence suggests that histamine increases cyclic AMP levels in mammalian parietal cells, whereas gastrin and carbachol do not[13]. Further study is required to define the role of cyclic nucleotides as intracellular regulators of secretion.

The gastric mucosal barrier

Healthy gastric mucosa has a great capacity to resist free ionic diffusion between gastric lumen and extracellular fluid. The gastric mucosal barrier can be defined broadly as that property of the mucosa which resists H^+ back-diffusion and ulceration. Under normal circumstances little H^+ ion escapes from the lumen despite a lumen:blood concentration gradient of the order of $3\,000\,000:1$.

According to Hollander[14] this barrier has two components: a protective superficial layer of mucus (mucus barrier) and the underlying

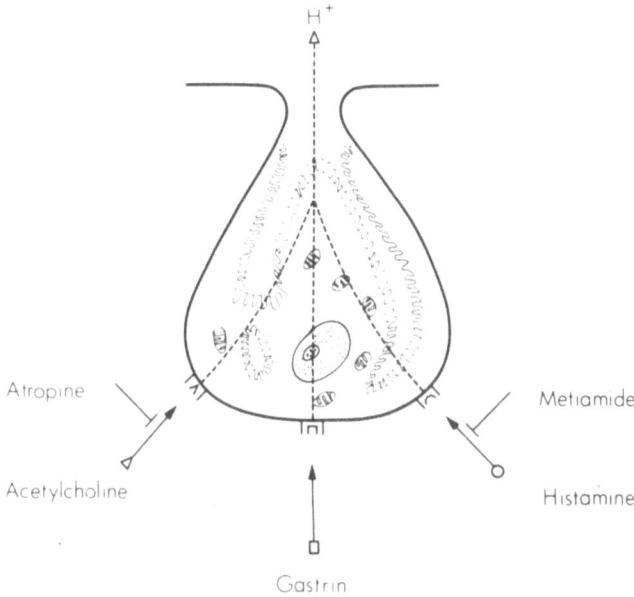

Figure 2 Interplay between agonists and antagonists at parietal cell receptor sites as suggested by studies in isolated parietal cells[11,12]. According to this concept, acetylcholine, gastrin and histamine each have separate receptors. Atropine antagonizes only acetylcholine receptors, and H_2 receptor antagonists (metiamide) antagonize only histamine receptors

surface layer of columnar epithelium lining the gastric lumen (mucosal barrier). Mucus has only a limited capacity to buffer and neutralize acid, but due to its lattice-like architecture may act as a series of unstirred layers which retard mixing of luminal acid with the alkaline secretions of the surface epithelium (Figure 3). The viscous and gel-forming properties of mucus depend on the polymeric structure of undegraded glycoprotein, and proteolysis as with pepsin, splits the glycoprotein molecule with concomitant loss of these properties[15]. Although the exact role of mucus in mucosal protection against autodigestion is uncertain, it seems likely that integrity of the surface mucus gel is an important defensive factor.

The mucosal barrier to potentially damaging agents is formed by the trilaminar lipoprotein membrane of the surface epithelium. The list of agents capable of damaging the mucosa includes bile salts, non-steroidal anti-inflammatory compounds such as aspirin, and alcohol. In general, substances which are ionized at acid (intragastric) pH are

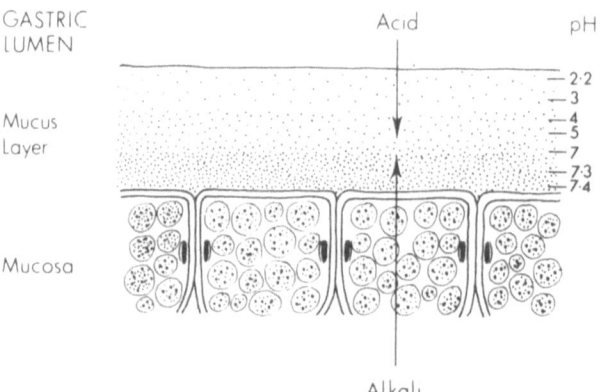

Figure 3 Concept of the mucus barrier. The lattice-like architecture of gastric mucus serves as a series of unstirred layers which retard mixing of luminal acid with the alkaline secretion of surface epithelial cells. The pH values suggested are *not* based on actual measurement, but are included to indicate the nature of the concept

poorly absorbed by the mucosa whereas un-ionized fat-soluble materials penetrate the cell membrane readily. For example, Davenport[16] has proposed that aspirin enters the gastric mucosa by non-ionic diffusion when luminal pH is less than its pK_a (3.5), only to ionize and become trapped within the cell and go on to disturb osmotic, buffering and metabolic functions. Continuing damage leads to disruption of the apical cell membrane and cell extrusion. This damage is accompanied by increased H^+ back-diffusion from the lumen, increased movement of Na^+ from extracellular fluid (ECF) into the gastric lumen, and a fall in transmucosal electrical potential difference (PD) as the various ions move more freely down their concentration gradients (Figure 4). Diffusion of acid between epithelial cells is barred by the tight junctions which bind their contiguous borders. These complexes are relatively resistant to most damaging agents and remain intact after disruption of the apical cell membrane[17,18].

Forte and colleagues[18] have detailed the ultrastructural changes in gastric mucosa exposed to bile salt. The cell surface becomes ruffled and pitted due to swelling of the underlying organelles, the cell membrane disrupts, and the apical portion of the cell is extruded leaving a hollow membranous shell to which fragments of cytoplasm adhere. Further damage leads to cell extrusion and exposure of the basement membrane. These authors suggest that the basement membrane might constitute a second line of defence ('secondary barrier') which reinforces

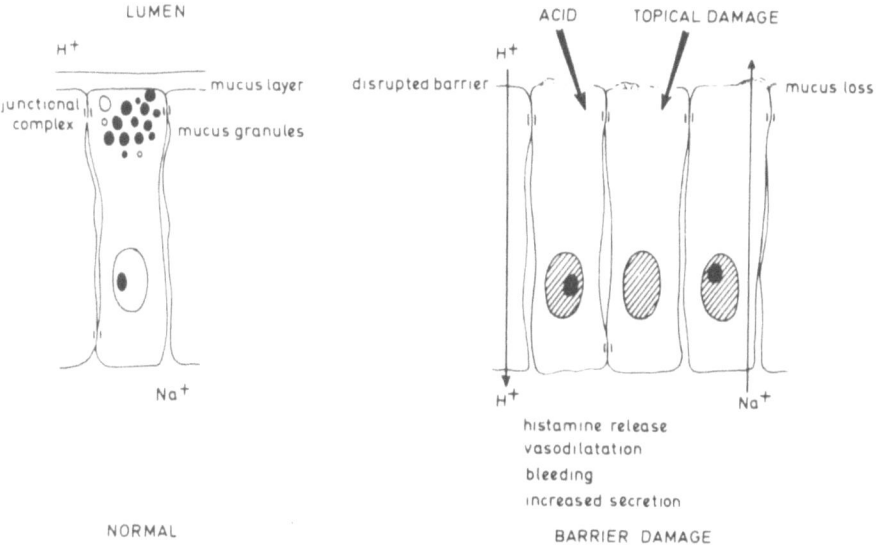

Figure 4 Concept of the gastric mucosal barrier, under normal circumstances and after damage by topical agents such as bile salt. Barrier damage allows H^+ and Na^+ to move freely down their concentration gradients in the directions indicated. The possible consequences of H^+ back-diffusion are outlined

the 'primary barrier' formed by the apical cell membrane. Graded damage to the primary barrier would allow increased ionic diffusion, fall in transmucosal PD, and in its most severe form, loss of plasma protein filtering across a still intact basement membrane. Damage to the secondary barrier would allow large amounts of plasma and red cells to escape into the gastric lumen. This concept of a series of functional and morphological barriers rather than a single all-or-none structure would allow interplay between damaging agents and mucosal defences to result in a spectrum of mucosal damage ranging from mild gastritis to frank ulceration.

Continued gastric mucosal barrier integrity depends on provision of adequate gastric mucosal blood flow and maintenance of cellular metabolism. Silen and his group[19-21] have demonstrated that gastric mucosa which is resting or inhibited is more susceptible to injury by influxing acid than mucosa which is actively secreting. Furthermore, agents such as carbonic anhydrase inhibitors which upset cellular acid–base balance can cause mucosal ulceration without increasing rates of acid back-diffusion. The hypothesis proposed is that secreting mucosa copes with influxing acid by virtue of HCO_3^- generated within the cell as part of the 'alkaline tide', whereas non-secreting mucosa, denied this defence, ulcerates readily when exposed to similar amounts of acid.

The importance of gastric mucosal blood flow is attested by the demonstration that standard rates of acid back-diffusion do not cause ulceration in dogs unless the animals are also subjected to haemorrhagic shock[22,23]. In the same context, Whittle[24] has shown that topical acid–bile salt solution increases H^+ back-diffusion across rat gastric mucosa, but at the same time increases mucosal blood flow and rarely causes ulceration. Administration of indomethacin during exposure to the same acid–bile salt mixture does not alter the rate of acid back-diffusion, but reduces mucosal blood flow and leads to a marked increase in ulcer formation.

In addition to maintaining intracellular metabolism and acid–base balance, the mucosal microcirculation may also serve to 'sweep away' excess H^+ diffusing into the mucosa from the gastric lumen. Cheung and Porterfield[25] have shown that intravenous bicarbonate infusion protects against mucosal damage by acid–bile salt solutions in dogs. The protection afforded is not due to reduction in the amount of H^+ entering the tissues, and presumably relates to the enhanced ability of the mucosa to buffer and dispose of influxing acid.

The duodenal mucosal barrier

The duodenal mucosal barrier has received less attention than its gastric counterpart. The pH of the post-bulbar duodenum is normally between 6.5 and 7.5, and even after food the pH of the second part of duodenum is beneath pH 3 less than 1% of the time. Bulbar pH is more variable and frequently falls beneath pH 3 as acid empties from the stomach[26]. The duodenum disposes of luminal H^+ by a number of mechanisms, the most important of which is neutralization by HCO_3^- in the alkaline secretions of the pancreas, liver and Brunner's glands. The duodenal mucosa can also remove acid by absorption from the lumen, although the factors governing rates of absorption in health and disease are not known[27,28]. It is uncertain whether luminal bile salt concentration affects H^+ absorption, but the duodenal mucosa appears resistant to bile salt concentrations which increase H^+ back-diffusion in the stomach.

Cell kinetics and ulcer healing

Half a million cells are lost from the gastric mucosa each minute by the normal processes of wear and tear. The rate of cell replacement normally equals that of cell loss and the mucosa remains in dynamic equilibrium. The mucous neck cells at the isthmus of the gastric glands are the progenitors of surface epithelial cells, oxyntic and peptic cells, and may even give rise to endocrine polypeptide cells. Maturing surface cells increase their mucus content as they migrate on to the luminal surface. They are replaced every 4–8 days, in contrast to the parietal cells which have a turnover time of the order of 1–3 years[29]. Bursts of cell regeneration follow feeding, but the mechanisms governing mitosis are far from clear.

Mucosal erosion occurs when cell loss exceeds replacement. Damaging agents cause cell death and desquamation, and may impair binding between adjacent surface cells. Erosions and shallow ulcers heal within 24–48 h when the mucosa is capable of normal rates of regeneration. The denuded area is first covered by mucus, and new surface cells migrate from surrounding mucosa to cover the gap and leave no discernible scar.

More severe injury such as that seen in chronic gastric ulceration is associated with penetration of the basement membrane and lamina propria, allowing acid and pepsin access to the relatively acellular submucosa. Collagen liquefaction follows and complete regeneration is impossible when destruction extends to underlying muscle; some degree of fibrous scarring is inevitable. The healing of gastric ulceration can be divided into four stages on the basis of endoscopy, stereoscopic microscopy and histology[30]. An initial healing stage of epithelial ingrowth is followed by a proliferative healing stage, palisade scar stage and final cobblestone scar stage. The ulcer crater disappears during the palisade scar stage and is replaced by palisade-like epithelium gathered radially toward a centre point. Hyperplasia of capillaries in the regenerating tissue causes the scar to be red during this stage and immature pseudo-pyloric glandular tissue appears in the epithelium. The cobblestone scar is associated with fading of the red flare to form a white scar, but pseudo-pyloric glandular structures remain a marked feature. The importance of this classification lies in the fact that healing must not be considered complete once the ulcer crater disappears. The risk of ulcer recurrence is increased if therapy is withdrawn on attaining the palisade (red) scar stage, rather than persisting until the cobblestone (white) scar stage is reached[31].

CLASSIFICATION OF DRUGS USED IN PEPTIC ULCER DISEASE

The interplay between acid/pepsin secretion and mucosal defences is shown diagrammatically in Figure 5. The vast majority of agents used to treat peptic ulcer can be considered conveniently under three headings: those which inhibit secretion, those which neutralize secreted acid and reduce peptic activity, and those which protect the mucosa. It is not our intention to produce an exhaustive list of all compounds which have been used or may be used in ulcer therapy, but to employ this three-part classification to discuss the implications of modern medical management and highlight areas in which advances may be anticipated. All of the drugs to be considered have been used in the United Kingdom but may not be freely available in North America.

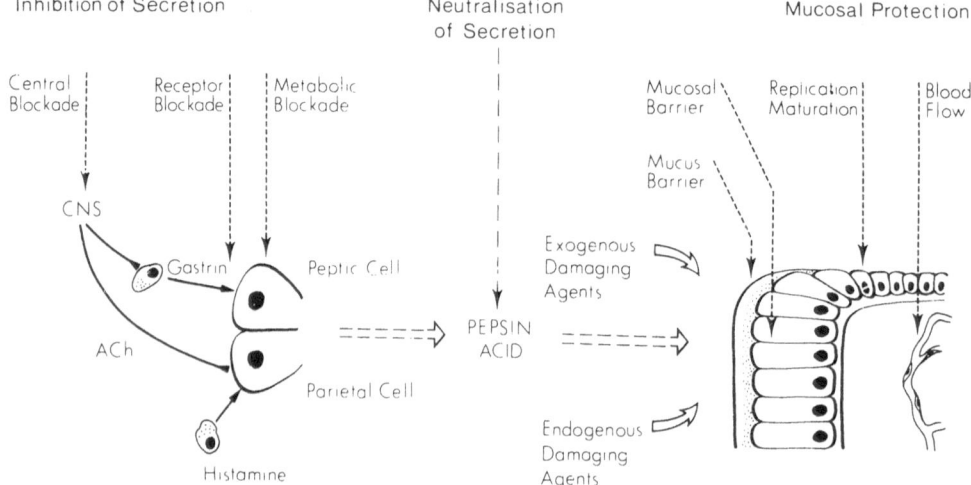

Figure 5 Diagrammatic representation of the interplay between gastric secretion and factors sustaining the mucosal defences against peptic digestion. Drugs used to treat peptic ulcer may act by inhibition of secretion, by neutralization of secretion, or by mucosal protection

DRUGS USED TO INHIBIT SECRETION

Drugs acting centrally

The antidepressant trimipramine (Surmontil) has been found to promote the healing of gastric and duodenal ulcers in 4-week trials in Norway[32,33]. It is not clear whether this effect relates to its relatively weak antisecretory activity, to a sedative effect, to relief of depression, or even to an effect on H_2 receptors in the central nervous system.

Other drugs acting on the central nervous system such as the non-sedative hypothalamic neuroleptic, sulpiride[34], are said to speed healing of duodenal ulcers without affecting gastric acid secretion.

Further controlled studies are needed to evaluate the role of centrally acting drugs in ulcer therapy.

Drugs acting by receptor blockade

Anticholinergic therapy

Anticholinergic drugs competitively inhibit acetylcholine at post-ganglionic nerve endings and smooth muscle. Naturally occurring belladonna alkaloids such as atropine and hyoscyamine are readily absorbed from the gastrointestinal tract, whereas synthetic quaternary ammonium compounds such as poldine and propantheline are less lipid-soluble and less well absorbed. These compounds reduce gastric acidity by vagal blockade and are potent inhibitors of basal, nocturnal and stimulated secretion[35,36]. Debate centres around whether clinically useful inhibition can be achieved without dose-limiting side-effects due to generalized parasympathetic blockade. Such effects include reduced salivation, impaired visual accommodation, intestinal atony and urinary retention. According to Ivey[37], many of these drugs have to be given in maximal doses recommended by the manufacturer, and in some cases up to ten times this dose, before even basal acid secretion is affected. On the other hand, Feldman and colleagues[38] have shown recently that low doses (15 mg) of propantheline reduce acid secretion just as well as near-toxic doses (48 mg) in ulcer patients. However, the consensus view is that undesirable side-effects impose major restrictions on the use of anticholinergic therapy.

Ivey[37] has reviewed the extensive literature dealing with ulcer healing and anticholinergic therapy. The results are conflicting with respect to both symptom relief and ulcer healing, but the majority of studies using maximum tolerated doses failed to show significant benefit. Admittedly, many studies were not adequately controlled and were carried out before the advent of endoscopy. Nevertheless, there is insufficient evidence to recommend continued use of anticholinergics now that inhibitors are available which are not subject to dose-limiting side-effects. Anticholinergic drugs have been shown to increase the inhibitory effect of H_2 receptor antagonists[39] but such combination therapy has not found application in clinical practice[40].

Antigastrin therapy

Attempts to reduce gastric acidity by preventing gastrin release or by blocking gastrin receptors with secretin[41], have proved unsuccessful in clinical practice. Somatostatin is a product of gastrointestinal APUD cells which may prove to have a paracrine role as a regulator of gastric secretion. Somatostatin infusion inhibits both gastrin and gastric acid secretion[42], and a synthetic octapeptide is now available. Somatostatin may prove useful as a means of elucidating the basic pathophysiological mechanisms responsible for peptic ulceration, and preliminary results indicate that it may control peptic ulcer bleeding in patients considered unsuitable for surgery[43].

Antihistamine therapy

The advent of histamine H_2 receptor antagonists has made a major impact on the medical management of peptic ulcer disease. Three compounds have been studied extensively; burimamide was used to characterize H_2 receptors pharmacologically[44], the more potent inhibitor metiamide was investigated clinically until its use was restricted by reports of transient granulocytopenia[45], while cimetidine has emerged as a safe effective inhibitor for clinical use[46]. A number of other potent H^2 receptor antagonists such as ranitidine[47], are now available but the continuing success of cimetidine has not necessitated their clinical use.

Actions of cimetidine

As with its forerunners, cimetidine is a competitive antagonist of histamine at H_2 receptors with no significant interaction with catecholamine β receptors, histamine H_1 receptors or muscarinic receptors[44,46]. Studies in isolated parietal cells indicate that H_2 receptor antagonists act there by specific antagonism of histamine, and that their ability to block secretion induced by gastrin or cholinergic stimuli is a result of withdrawing a tonic effect of histamine on the parietal cell response to these other agents[11,12].

Cimetidine is effective when given orally or intravenously, and is a potent inhibitor of acid and pepsin secretion induced by histamine, gastrin, vagal stimulation or feeding[9,10,46]. Basal and nocturnal secretion are both inhibited, and a bedtime dose of cimetidine reduces nocturnal secretion by 80% in duodenal ulcer patients[10]. Reduction in acid secretion is achieved by a fall in volume and a profound fall in acid concentration[10], and although this effect persists for hours, the compound is most effective when given three times a day with meals and on retiring. The recommended dose is 200 mg with meals and 400 mg at bedtime, but dosage can be increased if need be. A course of full-dose treatment usually lasts for 4–6 weeks and may be followed by an extended period of low-dose maintenance therapy (see below).

Therapeutic uses of cimetidine

Duodenal ulceration – The results of a number of endoscopically con-

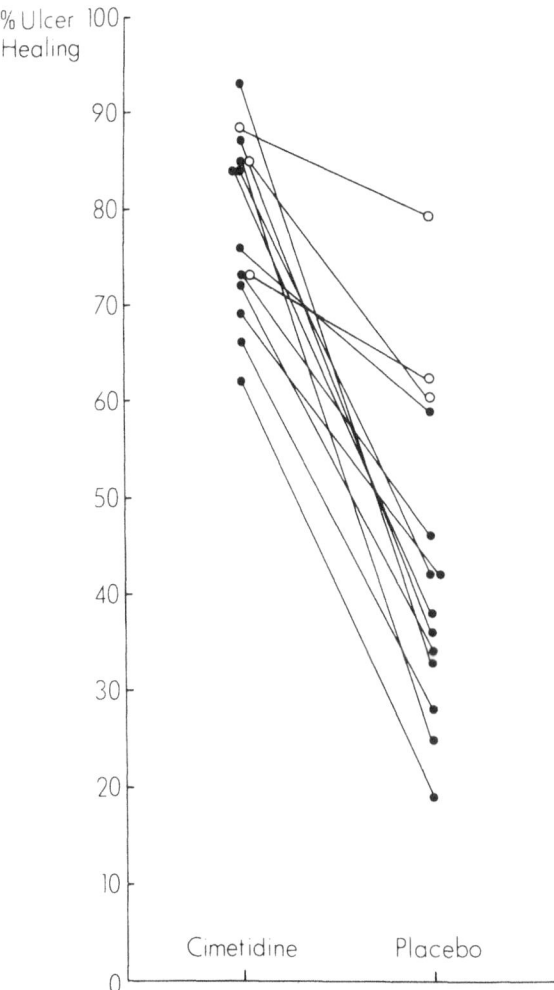

Figure 6 Proportion of patients showing healing of duodenal ulcer in endoscopically controlled trials comparing cimetidine with placebo. Trials showing significant benefit for cimetidine are drawn with closed circles (●——●; reference nos. 48, 49, 50, 51, 53, 54, 55, 56, 58, 59), whereas trials showing no significant benefit for cimetidine are drawn with open circles (○——○; reference nos. 52, 57, 61)

trolled trials of cimetidine are shown in Figure 6. More than 1000 patients were involved in these trials and 76% of cimetidine-treated patients healed their ulcers as opposed to 44% of patients receiving placebo[48-61]. All but three studies showed that the therapeutic advantage attributable to cimetidine was statistically significant, and failure to achieve statistical significance in these three trials is probably due to the high healing rates in patients receiving placebo (62%[52], 79%[57], and 60%[61]). Ulcer healing is exponential and the proportion of ulcers healed at various stages in therapy is shown in Figure 7.

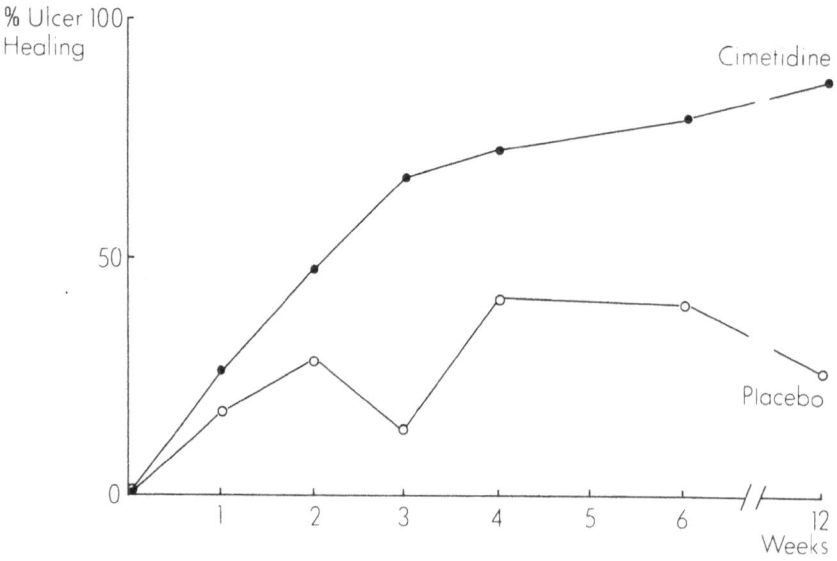

Figure 7 Proportion of patients showing healing of duodenal ulcer at varying times after commencing cimetidine or placebo in double-blind controlled studies. Data drawn from those collated by Winship[122]

It is not clear why some ulcers fail to heal on a standard course of cimetidine. The drug may be less successful in patients with a high pretreatment acid output[52,55], but factors which do not appear to influence response include age, sex, duration of symptoms, smoking habits and alcohol consumption[62].

The use of cimetidine maintenance therapy is controversial. Once healing has been achieved by a standard course of therapy, some 65–90% of patients can be kept free of relapse for 6–12 months if placed on maintenance therapy consisting of 400 mg b.d. or a single nocturnal dose of 400 or 800 mg[63–69]. This contrasts with ulcer recurrence rates of around 80% in patients receiving placebo rather than maintenance cimetidine. There is no evidence that long-term cimetidine ultimately reduces the risk of ulcer recurrence; indeed the rate of recurrence is the same in patients completing a year of maintenance therapy as in those placed on placebo after a 4–6-week course of full-dose cimetidine[66] (Figure 8). Maintenance therapy may prove valuable in patients who refuse ulcer surgery or in whom the risks of surgery are greater than normal. For the majority of ulcer patients we would recommend surgery when ulceration fails to heal on a standard course of full-dose cimetidine or in whom ulceration recurs after such a course has been completed. We do not employ maintenance therapy, believing that in the main it merely defers surgery in patients prone to ulcer recurrence. This is by no means a universal view and many physicians advocate maintenance therapy routinely[70].

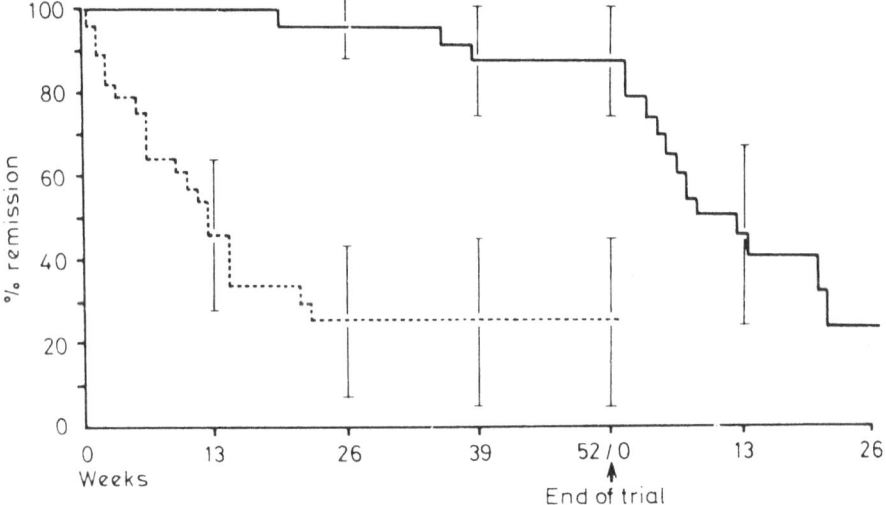

Figure 8 Life-table analysis showing estimated % probability (± 2 SE) of continued remission during and after cimetidine treatment for 1 year (solid line) and during placebo treatment for 1 year (broken line), as published by Gudmand-Høyer *et al.*[66] (by permission of the Editor, *British Medical Journal*)

Gastric ulceration – Cimetidine has proved less effective in gastric than in duodenal ulcer, reflecting the fact that agencies other than acid and pepsin secretion are concerned in gastric ulcerogenesis. The results of seven endoscopically controlled gastric ulcer trials are available, three of which showed significant benefit for cimetidine whereas four did not[71–77]. Overall, cimetidine patients had an ulcer healing rate of 70%

compared to 45% in patients receiving placebo, although it should be stressed that patients were usually given free access to antacids for symptom relief regardless of the trial options drawn.

On balance it seems reasonable to conclude that cimetidine is a safe and effective drug for use in gastric ulceration, provided that customary precautions are taken to ensure that the gastric lesion is benign peptic ulcer and not ulcerating cancer. In one controlled trial, 21 of 27 patients receiving cimetidine had ulcer healing after 6 weeks as opposed to 14 of 27 patients receiving carbenoxolone[78]. Although these differences were not significant, the authors concluded that cimetidine was at least as effective as carbenoxolone for benign gastric ulcer and produced fewer side-effects. It is our practice to employ cimetidine rather than carbenoxolone in this disease, advocating ulcer surgery if healing has not progressed significantly after a 6-week course.

Recurrent ulceration after surgery – When ulceration recurs after gastrectomy or vagotomy the usual cause is inadequate reduction of acidity. Cimetidine might therefore be expected to promote healing of recurrent ulcers but there are few data to substantiate this expectation. For example, Kennedy and Spencer[79] found that seven of 12 recurrent ulcer patients given cimetidine had ulcer healing at 6 weeks compared to five of 12 placebo controls. They concluded that if cimetidine is to be used for recurrent ulceration, larger doses and longer courses may be needed for ulcer healing. In common with most surgeons we would not advocate cimetidine as an alternative to re-operation, although the drug may prove useful in preparation for further surgery or when re-operation is contraindicated.

Gastro-oesophageal reflux – Since the severity of reflux oesophagitis can be related directly to the duration of high intraluminal acidity[80], inhibition of acid secretion by cimetidine is a rational form of treatment. Contrary to early expectations, cimetidine does not increase pressure in the lower oesophageal sphincter[81,82], but this need not detract from its value in reflux oesophagitis. One multicentre controlled trial[83] found that cimetidine significantly decreased antacid consumption and the severity and frequency of heartburn. In this and other trials[84], cimetidine-treated patients showed no more endoscopic evidence of improvement than placebo controls, although other workers have reported endoscopic evidence of benefit after cimetidine[85]. When used in patients with tight oesophageal stricture, long-term cimetidine did not reduce the frequency of dilatation relative to control patients[85].

Thus cimetidine may be of value in patients with gastro-oesophageal reflux but it remains to be seen whether it is any more effective than intensive antacid therapy.

Acute gastrointestinal bleeding – On theoretical grounds, inhibition of acid and pepsin secretion by H_2 receptor antagonists might be expected to prove useful in prevention and management of bleeding from gastritis and stress ulceration. There has been considerable debate as to whether these compounds have any additional beneficial properties involving mucosal cytoprotection. For example, Ivey and colleagues[86] found that cimetidine increased transmucosal PD in man and suggested that this might reflect 'tightening' of the gastric mucosal barrier and increased resistance to injury. While injury to the barrier is generally attended by a fall in transmucosal PD, there are no grounds for suggesting that cimetidine-associated increases in PD are anything more than a reflection of inhibition of gastric secretion. Studies of transmucosal ion flux in dogs have failed to show any potentially beneficial effects of H_2 receptor antagonists on acid back-diffusion induced by topical bile salt[87,88], although cimetidine appears to reduce ion flux induced by topical aspirin in rats[89]. This question of cimetidine's ability to protect rats against aspirin-induced gastric mucosal injury has proved particularly controversial. One group of workers report that the protective effect of cimetidine was lost in the presence of exogenous acid, indicating that its ability to prevent erosion is due solely to inhibition of secretion and not to any additional cytoprotective property[90]. On the other hand, others have found that cimetidine still prevents mucosal damage in the presence of exogenous acid[89,91], and present evidence that cimetidine shares the cytoprotective properties of prostaglandin and probanthine in this experimental model[92]. The significance of these findings in human peptic ulcer disease is uncertain, and the mechanism whereby antisecretory drugs might confer cytoprotection is far from clear.

Histamine release has been implicated in the pathophysiology of mucosal inflammation following damage to the gastric mucosal barrier. The compound is a potent vasodilator and its effects on the gastrointestinal vasculature are thought to be mediated by both H_1 and H_2 receptors, the H_1 effect predominating[93]. Rees and colleagues[88] examined the effect of H_1 and H_2 receptor antagonists on ion flux induced by topical bile salt in dogs. Neither metiamide (H_2 antagonist) nor mepyramine (H_1 antagonist) prevented bile salt-induced ion flux when given singly, but were effective when given in combination. This finding awaits substantiation but any application of this type of combination therapy in man has been prevented by the toxic doses of H_1 receptor antagonist required. Owen and colleagues[94] have shown that cimetidine reduces acute gastric bleeding in rats when blood is reinfused following mucosal damage by exposure to exogenous acid during gastric ischaemia. As inhibition of acid secretion cannot account for this effect, and as the effect can be demonstrated after mucosal injury has occurred, the authors suggest that cimetidine may act by antagonizing histamine-induced vasodilatation at the sites of gastric injury and thereby reducing bleeding. There is clear evidence that H_2 receptor antagonists reduce the incidence of gastrointestinal bleeding following renal transplantation[95] and in patients with fulminant hepatic failure[96]. However, antacid therapy is also of value in preventing acute haemorrhage in critically ill and burned patients[97,98], and one recent study has indicated that cimetidine (300 mg 6-hourly) was less effective than maintaining intragastric pH above 3.5 by high-dose antacids[99]. Uncontrolled trials suggest that H_2 receptor antagonists are effective in the control of established gastrointestinal bleeding secondary to erosive gastritis[100,101]. The efficacy of cimetidine in controlling bleeding from frank peptic ulceration is less certain. One controlled trial suggests that cimetidine prevents further bleeding from gastric but not duodenal ulcers[102], whereas a number of recent trials have failed to show any significant benefit in cimetidine-treated patients[43,103,104]. It has been our practice to prescribe cimetidine (300–400 mg 6-hourly) routinely in all critically ill patients and in those known to be bleeding from erosive gastritis. In the light of recent reports of the advantages of intensive antacid therapy, we would now supplement cimetidine by 2-hourly antacid instillation (30 ml alternately of aluminium hydroxide and magnesium trisilicate) in patients judged to be at particular risk of developing acute mucosal bleeding. We remain unconvinced of the value of cimetidine in preventing further bleeding from frank gastric or duodenal ulceration, but in the absence of significant undesirable side-effects, can see no objection to routine prescription of the drug in an attempt to speed ulcer healing.

Zollinger–Ellison syndrome – Cimetidine has proved an effective alternative to total gastrectomy in the management of patients with the Zollinger–Ellison syndrome. The collected experience from the United States involving 61 patients showed that two-thirds of the patients responded to a dose of 300 mg 6-hourly although others required doses of up to 600 mg 6-hourly[105]. Pain was relieved in all cases and ulcer healing, where documented, was greater than 95% at 3 months. At the time of reporting, 48 patients were still on the drug, three who had been well controlled were treated surgically, five had died from reasons unrelated to therapy, and five had significant problems. Our own limited experience of H_2 receptor antagonists in management of the Zollinger–Ellison syndrome is also favourable. We have used metiamide to control acid hypersecretion prior to total gastrectomy in one patient, and have since employed cimetidine as an alternative to total gastrectomy for periods now extending to 2 years.

Side-effects of cimetidine

Cimetidine is generally accepted as a safe drug. Review of clinical trial data indicates that withdrawal from protocol occurred with the same frequency (1.3%) in cimetidine-treated patients as in controls. There were no striking differences in the pattern of minor symptoms which did not cause withdrawal from therapy[106].

Granulocytopenia – Granulocytopenia with metiamide is now thought to be a consequence of the thiourea moeity in its side-chain. Cimetidine is a non-thiourea antagonist in which the imidazole ring is attached to a cyanoguanidine group. Unlike metiamide, cimetidine does not cause granulocytopenia in test animals and is not taken up by bone marrow cells. Admittedly there have been isolated reports of transient marrow depression during cimetidine therapy[107,108] but this complication appears to be extremely rare and the association is of uncertain significance. It is reassuring that granulocytopenia attributed to metiamide has improved after commencing treatment with cimetidine[109].

Endocrine side-effects – An anti-androgenic effect has been demonstrated in some animal species but blood levels of testosterone, luteinizing hormone and FSH remained normal in patients receiving the drug for 6 weeks[110]. Gynaecomastia has been reported infrequently during therapy[111] and may relate to cimetidine's ability to raise serum prolactin levels[112].

It is of interest that cimetidine may reduce abnormal circulating parathormone levels in patients with primary but not secondary hyperparathyroidism[113], and it may be that cimetidine blocks the synthesis or release of parathormone. The significance of this controversial finding remains uncertain.

Drug interaction – Cimetidine prolongs prothrombin time in patients on oral anticoagulants[114], and may potentiate the sedative effect of benzodiazepines such as diazepam[115].

Gastric side-effects – There have been conflicting reports concerning the effect of cimetidine on intrinsic factor secretion by the parietal cell[116,117], but it is uncertain whether long-term therapy will have any significant effect on vitamin B_{12} absorption.

There is no evidence that cimetidine inhibits acid secretion by a primary blockade of gastrin release from the antrum, but on theoretical grounds it might be expected that suppression of acid secretion would allow serum gastrin concentrations to rise to levels greater than normal after feeding. Witzel and colleagues[118] have shown that a 14-day course of metiamide increases parietal cell mass and maximal acid output in rats, and there has been anxiety that cimetidine might cause hypergastrinaemia and a similar trophic effect on the parietal cell mass in man. Sewing and associates[119] found that 1 month of cimetidine did increase meal-stimulated gastrin concentrations in ulcer patients, but others have failed to show any consistent effect on gastrin levels[120,121]. There is certainly no evidence to suggest that cimetidine therapy increases human parietal cell mass or leads to rebound acid hypersecretion on stopping therapy[122].

It is now realized that gastric resection for peptic ulcer increases the long-term risk of gastric cancer, and vagotomy may also be associated with increased risk. The gastric flora and its metabolic activity are largely determined by intragastric pH[123], and cimetidine is known to cause major increases in total bacterial counts and counts of nitrate-reducing organisms[124]. In theory, such changes could increase the risk of gastric cancer after long-term cimetidine therapy and the issue must remain under scrutiny. Elder and colleagues[125] suggest that nitrosation of cimetidine could result in formation of a chemical carcinogen, and question whether the association of gastric cancer and cimetidine therapy in three of their patients was fortuitous. While it seems inherently unlikely that cimetidine was responsible for development of cancer in these patients, there can be no doubt that patients with dyspepsia must be evaluated fully before commencing cimetidine. The risk is greatest in patients with gastric ulcer and the importance of endoscopy and multiple biopsy cannot be overemphasized.

Drugs acting by metabolic blockade

There is still uncertainty regarding the exact nature of the intracellular mechanisms which regulate gastric secretion. It has been known for many years that carbonic anhydrase inhibitors such as acetazolamide (Diamox) can reduce acid secretion by impairing the hydration of carbon dioxide to carbonic acid, but there is little prospect of harnessing such activity for clinical use in peptic ulceration. A more promising line of attack concerns the role of cyclic nucleotides such as adenosine-3',5'-monophosphate (cyclic AMP) in intracellular metabolism. The formation of cyclic AMP from ATP is catalysed by the enzyme, adenylate cyclase, and there is an increasing body of evidence that histamine stimulates gastric acid secretion by activating fundic mucosal adenylate cyclase[126,127]

Prostaglandins and inhibition of gastric secretion

A wide variety of body tissues can synthesize prostaglandins (PGs) from free fatty acid precursors such as arachidonic acid. The gastrointestinal tract is no exception and gastric mucosa has the ability to synthesize PGs, notably those of the E series and the most recently recognized compound, prostacyclin[128]. Attempts to influence gastric secretion by administration of naturally occurring PGE and PGA compounds yielded inconsistent or unimpressive results, although some degree of inhibition of acid secretion was detected when the compounds were administered by constant intravenous infusion[129,130]. These compounds had little or no clinical potential, but the synthesis of methylated analogues of PGE_2 opened exciting new avenues for clinical research. These analogues differ from their parent compound in that they are not susceptible to rapid enzymic degradation, and this extended half-life is reflected in their potency as inhibitors of basal and stimulated gastric secretion in animals and man[131-133]. Depending on the choice of analogue, inhibition can be achieved by oral or intravenous administration for periods of some 4 h. The compounds protect against peptic ulceration in a variety of animal models[131], and preliminary trials suggest that they may be effective in the treatment of peptic ulcer in man[134,135].

Mode of action of PGs

The ability of PGs to protect against peptic ulceration is attributable only in part to their potency as inhibitors of gastric secretion. Great interest centres on mucosal cytoprotection by these compounds, and this topic will be considered subsequently (p.245). Concerning their antisecretory activity, the mechanism responsible is still uncertain. PGE compounds inhibit secretion induced by histamine or gastrin but not by cyclic AMP or its analogues[136,137], leading to the hypothesis that they block histamine-stimulated acid secretion by preventing cyclic AMP formation. A drawback to this hypothesis has been the observation that fundic mucosal adenylate cyclase activity is stimulated both by histamine and by inhibitors of acid secretion such as PGs or secretin[138,139].

Much of the confusion may stem from the fact that experiments using intact gastric mucosa or broken cell preparations involve heterogeneous cell populations, and that parietal cell responses may be masked by those of other cell types. Using isolated canine fundic mucosal cells, Wollin and colleagues[127] have shown that histamine stimulates cyclic AMP production in parietal cells, whereas secretin stimulates cyclic AMP production in chief cells. PGE_2 stimulation of cyclic AMP production could not be localized to any single cell type, but occurred primarily in non-parietal cells. It may now be proposed that there are two distinct cyclic AMP systems in gastric mucosa; a histamine-sensitive system located primarily in parietal cells, and a PGE_2-sensitive system located mostly in non-parietal cells. This hypothesis does not preclude an inhibitory effect of PGs on histamine-stimulated cyclic AMP production by parietal cells as the concentration of PGE_2 may be critical. Concentrations of PGE_2 beneath the range required for stimulation of *mucosal* cyclic AMP production have been shown to specifically inhibit histamine-stimulated cyclic AMP production by fractions rich in *parietal* cells[140]. Thus it may be that direct activation of mucosal adenylate cyclase by PGE_2 is a pharmacological activity, and that concentrations of the order achieved *in vivo* serve to reduce acid secretion by preventing histamine stimulation of cyclic AMP production within parietal cells.

Clinical trials of PGs

Prostaglandins have not yet been applied widely to the problem of human peptic ulcer disease. In a small clinical trial from Singapore[134], the 15(R) methylated analogue of PGE_2 promoted the healing of gastric ulcer, while in another small trial from Poland[135], two methylated analogues of PGE_2 were thought to favour the healing of duodenal but not gastric ulcer. Undesirable side-effects of the analogues include a tendency to cause diarrhoea, and in the Polish trial, endoscopy after 2 weeks of PG therapy revealed an appearance suggesting active gastritis.

Further controlled clinical trials will be required before the therapeutic role of PGs in ulcer disease can be defined.

DRUGS USED TO NEUTRALIZE SECRETED ACID AND REDUCE PEPTIC ACTIVITY

Antacid therapy

Antacids have been the traditional mainstay of ulcer therapy and were prescribed in an endeavour to neutralize secreted acid and thereby inactivate pepsin. Conventional teaching held that while antacids were effective in affording pain relief, they did not speed the healing of duodenal or gastric ulcer. This teaching requires re-appraisal in the light of recent experience.

Mode of action of antacids

All antacids react with hydrochloric acid to form a salt and water, e.g.

$$Al(OH)_3 + 3\,HCl \rightarrow AlCl_3 + 3\,H_2O$$

The various antacids differ greatly in their capacity to neutralize acid but in theory an intragastric pH greater than pH 5 would completely prevent peptic activity and favour ulcer healing.

Clinical pharmacology

In the fasting state, rapid gastric emptying leads to rapid loss of antacid from the stomach, much of it unchanged. Antacids should be taken after meals and the optimal time of administration is at 1 *and* 3 h after eating[141]. Intragastric titration studies in duodenal ulcer patients have shown that there is a steady state of acid secretion following a meal. Over the first 1–2 h much of the acidity is buffered by meal protein but gastric acidity rises sharply thereafter. Administration of antacid 1 h after the meal offsets this late increase and further benefit is obtained by a dose of antacid at 3 h.

With regard to dosage, Fordtran and colleagues[142] showed that five-fold reduction in gastric acidity for 2 h in duodenal ulcer patients required administration of some 156 mmol of antacid. Depending on the preparation selected, this implied an amount of antacid varying from 22 to 371 ml. Physicians have traditionally prescribed 15–30 ml of antacid regardless of potency and it is hardly surprising that antacids were thought not to influence ulcer healing.

Choice of antacid

So-called long-acting preparations do not appear to have particular benefit in that they are lost by gastric emptying. Antacid tablets are less effective than liquids, probably due to failure of the tablet to disintegrate and disperse rapidly. If patient preference decrees use of tablets they should be crushed, sucked or chewed thoroughly.

Sodium bicarbonate is a potent antacid but cannot be recommended in view of its tendency to produce alkalosis, promote fluid retention, and empty rapidly from the stomach. Calcium-containing antacids are also potent but are contraindicated because they may stimulate gastrin release and acid secretion, cause hypercalcaemia, and cause the milk–alkali syndrome.

Aluminium hydroxide and magnesium salts are the preferred ant-acids and form the basis of most proprietary preparations. Differences in manufacturing methods result in marked differences in potency due to differing solubilities of aluminium salts. Magnesium salts are virtually insoluble in water but still seem to react promptly with acid. Magnesium compounds have a cathartic effect whereas aluminium salts tend to constipate. Functional bowel problems can be avoided by judicious combination of the two types of antacid.

Efficacy of antacid therapy

A number of controlled studies have examined the ability of antacids to relieve ulcer pain[143–147]. In contrast to classical teaching, antacids were no more effective than placebo in relieving the symptoms of duodenal ulcer, although one trial reported that calcium carbonate gave effective relief in outpatients with gastric ulcer[146]. The striking feature of all such studies is the degree of benefit afforded by placebo.

On the question of ulcer healing, Peterson and his colleagues[147] have shown recently that a MgAlOH mixture (Mylanta II) in doses of 1008 mmol/day (210 mg/day) was significantly better than placebo in promoting the healing of duodenal ulcer. The authors suggest at least three reasons why they found antacids effective while others had not. Firstly, the use of high dosage, secondly the avoidance of calcium-containing antacid, and finally the use of endoscopy rather than symptoms or radiology to assess healing. Other recent controlled trials[148,34] suggest that smaller doses of antacid may retain these benefits, but given good patient compliance and lack of side-effects there is no reason to restrict dosage. A clear message emerging from the recent crop of endoscopically controlled ulcer trials is that persistence of symptoms does not necessarily reflect persisting ulceration, and conversely that loss of symptoms does not always denote healing. Demonstration that antacids may influence ulcer healing has led to their comparison with histamine H_2 receptor antagonists. Deering and Malagelada[149] found that Maalox (30 ml, 1 and 3 h after food) and cimetidine (400 mg after food) were equally effective in reducing the acid secretory response to feeding. In terms of ulcer healing, Ippoliti and colleagues[150] found no significant differences between intensive antacid therapy and cimetidine after a 4-week course of treatment.

One must conclude that antacid therapy cannot now be dismissed on the basis of previous inadequate trials, and that used correctly these drugs should retain a useful place in the therapeutic armamentarium.

Antipeptic agents

Amylopectin sulphate

This synthetic sulphated polysaccharide has antipeptic properties, the exact nature of which are unclear. Amylopectin may bind directly to pepsin, or combine with mucus or the mucosa to protect against proteolysis. Early reports[151] that amylopectin was of benefit in promoting duodenal ulcer healing have not been confirmed[152,153] and the agent is not used widely.

Sucralfate

Basic aluminium sucralfate also inhibits pepsin activity while increasing gastric pH. In acid gastric juice the compound forms an adhesive paste resistant to attack by hydrogen ion and this property may have therapeutic significance. Sucralfate has been assessed primarily in terms of its ability to heal gastric ulcers and reports of its efficacy are conflicting[31,154].

DRUGS WHICH PROTECT THE GASTROINTESTINAL MUCOSA

Carbenoxolone

Liquorice root and its extracts have enjoyed a long-standing reputation as folk-lore remedies for dyspepsia. It is now appreciated that the benefits of such preparations are due to a glycyrrhizic acid fraction, and carbenoxolone is a synthetic derivative of this acid. Carbenoxolone is a lipophilic compound with a high affinity for biological membranes and plasma proteins, and has been shown to promote the healing of gastric ulcers.

The manner in which carbenoxolone acts is not clear, but it appears to strengthen mucosal defences rather than prevent gastric secretion. Effects attributed to carbenoxolone include increased synthesis and secretion of mucus[155,156], reduced rates of epithelial cell loss[157,158], diminished rates of acid back-diffusion[159], and inhibition of luminal peptic activity[160]. The relative significance of these potential modes of action is uncertain but the beneficial effects of improved mucus production on surface cell survival is probably the key factor. The earliest clinical trials showed that carbenoxolone accelerated healing of gastric ulcers in ambulatory outpatients[161], and this finding has been confirmed in subsequent trials employing both radiological and endoscopic control regardless of whether the patients were hospitalized[162–165]. A 4–6-week course of therapy is recommended with a dose of 100 mg three times a day during the first week falling to 50 mg three times a day thereafter. The proportion of patients showing ulcer healing ranges from 36 to 67% on this regime, and healing does not appear to be related to ulcer size or the patient's age and sex. Healing rates may improve if treatment is prolonged but this benefit is probably obtained only at the expense of an increased incidence of side-effects[166].

Once therapy has been discontinued, recurrence rates are comparable in patients treated initially by carbenoxolone and those given placebo. Maintenance treatment does not appear to be of value[167]. As in the treatment of all forms of gastric ulcer, endoscopy and multiple biopsy is essential to exclude malignancy prior to therapy and should be repeated at 4–6 weeks to assess ulcer healing.

Carbenoxolone and duodenal ulcer

A 'positioned release' capsule (duogastrone), which was intended to swell in gastric juice and rupture in the pylorus, was designed to deliver carbenoxolone in maximum concentration to the duodenal cap. It is debatable whether such delayed release in fact takes place. Earlier studies using radiological or clinical assessment failed to show any consistent benefit for duogastrone in duodenal ulcer. However, five recent endoscopically controlled trials using duogastrone in doses of 50 mg four times a day all showed that the drug was significantly better than placebo when given for 4–6 weeks[168-172]. These trials involved some 300 patients and healing rates ranged from 60 to 75% in duogastrone-treated patients as opposed to 19 to 48% in controls.

Side-effects of carbenoxolone

Carbenoxolone has a structural resemblance to the corticosteroids and therapy may be complicated by its mineralocorticoid properties. Side-effects include salt and water retention, oedema, hypokalaemia and even hypertension. The effects are dose-related, occur more frequently when treatment is prolonged, and may necessitate cessation of treatment. The elderly are particularly prone to troublesome side-effects, and this may relate to reduced rates of plasma clearance and higher serum concentration of drug. In contrast to its beneficial action on ulcer healing, which is attributed to the drug penetrating gastric mucosa, all of the undesirable metabolic effects are mediated systemically. Oral potassium supplements are used to counter hypokalaemia, while a thiazide diuretic can be used to reduce salt and water retention. Spironolactone should not be used as it may hinder ulcer healing.

We no longer employ carbenoxolone in the treatment of gastric or duodenal ulcer in view of its ability to produce side-effects in some 25% of patients. This view is by no means universal and the drug is still prescribed widely.

Deglycyrrhizinized liquorice

Liquorice extract from which all but a small fraction of glycyrrhizinic acid has been removed is available without additives (Ulcedal) or with added alkali and frangula bark (Caved-S). The resulting compounds have no mineralocorticoid activity and do not incur the troublesome side-effects encountered with carbenoxolone. Contrary to earlier reports, none of the recent controlled trials have found deglycyrrhizinized liquorice to be of value in either gastric or duodenal ulceration[173,174].

Tri-potassium di-citrato bismuthate

The bismuth preparation De-Nol is thought to combine with proteins to form a chelate at acid pH and so form a protective layer which promotes healing of peptic ulcers. It is claimed that bismuth has a particular affinity for granulation tissue and that a bismuth–protein coagulum covers ulcer craters to protect them from acid–pepsin digestion. Colloidal bismuth also has pepsin-binding properties but does not appear to inhibit acid or pepsin secretion.

Endoscopically controlled trials in duodenal ulceration have shown significant benefit for De-Nol with ulcer healing in 74–97% of patients[175-180], and there is evidence that the preparation is of benefit in patients with gastric ulcer[181,182].

De-Nol is a liquid preparation with an ammoniacal odour that some patients find unacceptable: 5 ml of the complex is diluted 1 in 4 with water and taken ½ h before meals and at night, and the complex is taken for at least 28 days. Significant side-effects have not been reported but some patients complain of blackening of the tongue and passage of dark stools. De-Nol is not recommended for patients with renal disease.

Geranyl farnesylacetate

Geranyl farnesylacetate (Gefarnate) is a synthetic isoprenoid which chemically resembles the terpine side-chains of natural vitamin K. Its mode of action is unclear but it has been suggested that the compound has a direct effect on gastric cells which regenerate more rapidly and become enriched with enzyme granules. Benefit has been reported in controlled trials of Gefarnate in gastric ulcer[183,184], but the compound has not been used widely and its therapeutic place has not been established.

Prostaglandins

A number of prostaglandin compounds reduce indomethacin-induced damage to the small intestinal mucosa in experimental animals[185] and it was in this context that Robert first applied the term 'cytoprotection'[186]. Non-steroidal anti-inflammatory compounds (NOSAC) such as aspirin and indomethacin are also ulcerogenic to gastric mucosa, and PGs have been shown to inhibit NOSAC-induced gastric ulceration in the rat[187,188]. This protective effect is seen with doses of PGE_2 analogues which do not inhibit gastric secretion[189], and with other PGs which do not have antisecretory activity[187]. Cytoprotection is not confined to prevention of damage by NOSACs and PGs protect against damage induced by a wide variety of agents including alcohol, HCl (in concentrations four times that found in gastric juice), 0.2 mmol/l NaOH, hypertonic salt solution and boiling water[190]. As mentioned above, there is debate as to whether cimetidine also has cytoprotective activity in gastric mucosa[90,91], but cimetidine does not share the cytoprotective action of PGs with regard to indomethacin-induced small bowel ulceration in rats[191].

The mechanisms responsible for cytoprotection are unknown. The fact that prostaglandin synthetase inhibitors cause gastric mucosal damage suggests that PGs may play a normal role in protecting the gastric mucosa against injury. Mechanisms suggested include an effect on gastric mucosal blood flow[192], stimulation of active transport of sodium[193], and stimulation of mucus and non-parietal cell secretion[194,195]. There can be no doubt that elucidation of the mechanism underlying cytoprotection would present a major step forward in the treatment of peptic ulceration, and would undoubtedly throw light on the basic pathophysiological disturbances leading to ulcer formation.

CONCLUSIONS

The past decade has witnessed a truly remarkable transformation in the management of peptic ulceration. Major advances in the basic sciences have increased our understanding of the mechanisms responsible for gastric secretion and mucosal defence against injury. In large measure, these advances have stemmed from the development of compounds such as the H_2 receptor antagonists and prostaglandins, and have led to the availability of new effective agents for clinical use. The advent of endoscopy has allowed a more objective assessment of ulcer healing and the widespread use of controlled trials has resulted in valid appraisal of new candidate compounds in the peptic ulcer diathesis.

Inhibition of gastric secretion by H_2 receptor antagonists is now accepted as a safe, effective form of therapy; antacids have emerged with a new lease of life as useful agents; and a number of mucosal protectants such as carbenoxolone and De-Nol have promoted ulcer healing without inhibition of gastric secretion. Of the compounds awaiting full clinical evaluation, the prostaglandins offer an exciting prospect of a two-pronged attack on ulcer disease by inhibition of secretion and by cytoprotection. Despite these advances, surgery remains the one definitive means of reducing acid/pepsin secretion and is likely to retain a major role in the treatment of relapsing and complicated ulcer disease.

References

1 Goldberg, H. I., Dodds, W. J., Gee, S., Montgomery, C. and Zboralske, F. F. (1969). Role of acid and pepsin in acute experimental esophagitis. *Gastroenterology*, **56**, 223

2 Samloff, I. M. (1971). Pepsinogens, pepsins and pepsin inhibitors. *Gastroenterology*, **60**, 586

3 Samloff, I. M., Secrist, D. M. and Passaro, E. (1975). A study of the relationship between serum group I pepsinogen levels and gastric acid secretion. *Gastroenterology*, **69**, 1196

4 Håkanson, R., Lilja, B. and Owman, Ch. (1969). Cellular localisation of histamine and monoamines in the gastric mucosa of man. *Histochemie*, **18**, 74

5 Räsänen, T. (1958). Tissue eosinophils and mast cells in the human stomach wall in normal and pathological conditions. *Acta Pathol. Microbiol. Scand.*, 129 (Suppl.)

6 MacIntosh, F. C. (1938). Histamine as a normal stimulator of gastric secretion. *Q. J. Exp. Physiol.*, **28**, 87

7 Code, C. F. (1965). Histamine and gastric secretion: a later look, 1955–1965. *Fed. Proc.*, **24**, 1311

8 Grossman, M. I. and Konturek, S. J. (1974). Inhibition of acid secretion in dog by metiamide, a histamine antagonist acting on H_2 receptors. *Gastroenterology*, **67**, 517

9 Carter, D. C., Forrest, J. A. H., Logan, R. A., Ansell, I., Lidgard, G., Heading, R. C. and Shearman, D. J. C. (1976). Effect of the histamine H_2-receptor antagonist, Cimetidine, on gastric secretion and serum gastrin during insulin infusion in man. *Scand. J. Gastroenterol.*, **11**, 565

10 Richardson, C. T. (1978). Effect of H_2 receptor antagonists on gastric acid secretion and serum gastrin concentration. *Gastroenterology*, **74**, 366

11 Soll, A. H. (1978). The actions of secretagogues on oxygen uptake by isolated mammalian parietal cells. *J. Clin. Invest.*, **61**, 370

12 Soll, A. H. (1978). The interaction of histamine with gastrin and carbamylcholine on oxygen uptake by isolated mammalian parietal cells. *J. Clin. Invest.*, **61**, 381

13 Soll, A. H. and Wollin, A. (1979). Histamine and cyclic AMP in isolated canine parietal cells. *Am. J. Physiol.*, **237**, 444

14 Hollander, F. (1954). The two-component mucous barrier: its activity in protecting gastroduodenal mucosa against peptic ulceration. *Arch. Intern. Med.*, **93**, 107

15 Pearson, J., Allen, A. and Venables, C. (1980). Gastric mucus: isolation and polymeric structure of the undegraded glycoprotein: its breakdown by pepsin. *Gastroenterology*, **78**, 709

16 Davenport, H. W. (1967). Salicylate damage to the gastric mucosal barrier. *N. Engl. J. Med.*, **276**, 1307

17 Hingson, D. J. and Ito, S. (1971). Effect of aspirin and related compounds on the fine structure of mouse gastric mucosa. *Gastroenterology*, **61**, 156

18 Forte, T. M., Silen, W. and Forte, J. C. (1976). Ultrastructural lesions in gastric mucosa exposed to deoxycholate: implications toward the barrier concept. In Kasbekar, D. K., Sachs, G. and Rehm, W. S. (eds.). *Gastric Hydrogen Ion Secretion*, pp. 1–28. (New York: Marcel Dekker Inc.)

19 O'Brien, P. and Silen, W. (1976). Influence of acid secretory state on the gastric mucosal tolerance to back diffusion of H^+. *Gastroenterology*, **71**, 760

20 Smith, P., O'Brien, P., Fromm, D. and Silen, W. (1977). Secretory state of gastric mucosa and resistance to injury by exogenous acid. *Am. J. Surg.*, **133**, 81

21 Silen, W. (1977). New concepts of the gastric mucosal barrier. *Am. J. Surg.*, **133**, 8

22 Ritchie, W. P. (1975). Acute gastric mucosal damage induced by bile salts, acid and ischaemia. *Gastroenterology*, **68**, 699

23 Ritchie, W. P. and Shearburn, E. W. (1976). Acute gastric mucosal ulcerogenesis is dependent on the concentration of bile salt. *Surgery*, **80**, 98

24 Whittle, B. J. R. (1977). Mechanisms underlying gastric mucosal damage induced by indomethacin and bile salts and the actions of prostaglandins. *Br. J. Pharmacol.*, **60**, 455

25 Cheung, L. Y. and Porterfield, G. (1979). Protection of gastric mucosa against acute

ulceration by infusion of sodium bicarbonate. *Am. J. Surg.*, **137**, 106

26 Rhodes, J. and Prestlich, C. J. (1966). Acidity at different sites in the proximal duodenum of normal subjects and patients with duodenal ulcer. *Gut*, **7**, 509

27 Dorricott, N. J., Fiddian-Green, R. G. and Silen, W. (1975). Mechanisms of acid disposal in canine duodenum. *Am. J. Physiol.*, **228**, 269

28 Wormsley, K. C. (1971). Reactions to acid in the intestine in health and disease. *Gut*, **12**, 67

29 Lipkin, M. (1977). Growth kinetics of normal and premalignant gastrointestinal epithelium. In Drewinho, B. and Humphrey, R. M. (eds.). *Growth Kinetics and Biochemical Regulation of Normal and Malignant Cells*, pp. 569–589. (Baltimore: Williams & Wilkins)

30 Miyake, T., Suzaki, T. and Oishi, M. (1980). Correlation of gastric ulcer healing features by endoscopy, stereoscopic microscopy and histology and a reclassification of the epithelial regenerative process. *Dig. Dis. Sci.*, **25**, 8

31 Miyake, T., Ariyoshi, J., Suzaki, T., Oishi, M., Sakai, M. and Ueda, S. (1980). Endoscopic evaluation of the effect of sucralfate therapy and other clinical parameters on the recurrence rate of gastric ulcers. *Dig. Dis. Sci.*, **25**, 1

32 Wetterhus, A., Aubert, E., Berg, C. E., Bjerkeset, T., Halvorsen, L., Hovdenak, N., Myren, J., Roland, M., Sigstad, H. and Guldahl, M. (1977). The effect of trimipramine (Surmontil) on symptoms and healing of peptic ulcer. A double blind study. *Scand. J. Gastroenterol.*, **12** (Suppl.), 33

33 Valnes, K., Myren, J. and Qvigstad, T. (1978). Trimipramine in the treatment of gastric ulcer. *Scand. J. Gastroenterol.*, **14**, 497

34 Lam, S. K., Lam, C. C., Lai, C. C., Yeung, C. K., Yam, L. Y. C. and Wong, W. S. (1979). The treatment of duodenal ulcer with antacid and sulpiride. *Gastroenterology*, **76**, 315

35 Dotevall, G., Schroder, G. and Walan, A. (1965). Effect of poldine glycopyrrolate and 1-hyoscyamine on gastric secretion of acid in man. *Acta Med. Scand.*, **177**, 169

36 Barman, M. L. and Larson, R. K. (1963). The effect of glycopyrrolate on nocturnal gastric secretion in peptic ulcer patients. *Am. J. Med. Sci.*, **246**, 325

37 Ivey, K. J. (1975). Anticholinergics: do they work in peptic ulcer? *Gastroenterology*, **68**, 154

38 Feldman, M., Richardson, C. T., Peterson, W. L., Walsh, J. H. and Fordtran, J. S. (1977). Effect of low dose propantheline on food stimulated gastric acid secretion. *N. Engl. J. Med.*, **297**, 1427

39 Venables, C. W., Stephen, J. G., Blair, E. L., Reed, J. D. and Saunders, J. D. (1978). Cimetidine in the treatment of duodenal ulceration and the relationship of this therapy to surgical management. In Wastell, C. and Lance, P. (eds.). *Cimetidine Westminster Hospital Symposium*, p. 13 (Edinburgh, London, New York: Churchill Livingstone)

40 Pounder, R. E., Hunt, R. H., Vincent, S. H., Milton-Thompson, G. J. and Misiewicz, J. J. (1977). 24 hour intragastric acidity and nocturnal acid secretion in patients with duodenal ulcer during oral administration of cimetidine and atropine. *Gut*, **18**, 85

41 Henn, R. M., Selcon, S., Sturdevant, R. A. L., Isenberg, J. I. and Grossman, M. I. (1976). Experience with synthetic secretin in the treatment of duodenal ulcer. *Am. J. Dig. Dis.*, **21**, 921

42 Bloom, S. R., Mortimer, C. H., Thorner, M. O., Besser, G. M., Hall, R., Gomez-Pan, A., Roy, V. M., Russell, R. C. G., Coy, D. H., Kastin, A. J. and Schally, A. V. (1974). Inhibition of gastrin and gastric acid secretion by growth-hormone release-inhibiting hormone. *Lancet*, **2**, 1106

43 Kayasseh, L., Gyr, K., Keller, V., Stalder, G. A. and Wall, M. (1980). Somatostatin and cimetidine in peptic-ulcer haemorrhage. A randomised controlled trial. *Lancet*, **1**, 844

44 Black, J. W., Duncan, W. M., Durrant, C. J., Ganellin, C. R. and Parsons, M. E. (1972). Definition and antagonism of histamine H_2 receptors. *Nature (London)*, **236**, 385

45 Forrest, J. A. H., Shearman, D. J. C., Spence, R. and Celestin, L. R. (1975). Neutropenia associated with metiamide. *Lancet*, **1**, 392

46 Brimblecombe, R. W., Duncan, W. A. M., Durant, G. J., Emmett, J. C., Ganellin, C. R. and Parsons, M. E. (1975). Cimetidine – a non thiourea H_2 receptor antagonist. *J. Int. Med. Res.*, **3**, 86

47 Woodings, E. P., Dixon, G. T., Harrison, C., Carey, P. and Richards, D. A. (1980). Ranitidine – a new H_2-receptor antagonist. *Gut*, **21**, 187

48 Albano, O., Barbara, L., Miglioli, M., Porro, G. B., Petrillo, M., Blasi, A., Marletta, F., Cheli, R., Giacosa, A., Coltorti, M., Del Vecchio Blanco, C., Dobrilla, G., Valentini, M., Scura, L., Cavallini, G., Verme, G. and Pera, A. (1978). Trattamento ra breve termine con cimetidina nell ulcera duodenale. Risultati di una recerca polycentrica contrullata. In P. Lucchelli (ed.). *Cimetidina: Farmacologie e Clinica*, p. 149. (Milano: Smith, Kline & French)

49 Bank, S., Barbezat, G. O., Novis, B. H., Ou Tim, L., Odes, H. S., Helman, C., Narunsky, L., Duys, P. and Marks, I. N. (1976). Histamine H_2 receptor antagonists in the treatment of duodenal ulcer. *S. Afr. Med. J.*, **50**, 1781

50 Bardhan, K. D., Saul, D. M., Edwards, J. L., Smith, P. M., Fettes, M., Forrest, J., Heading, R. C., Logan, R. F. A., Dronfield, M. W., Langman, M. S., Larkworthy, W., Haggie, S. J., Wyllie, J. H., Corbett, C., Duthie, H. L., Fussey, I. V., Holdsworth, C. D., Balmforth, G. V. and Maruyama, T. (1979). Comparison of two doses of cimetidine and placebo in the treatment of duodenal ulcer: a multicentre trial. *Gut*, **20**, 68

51 Porro, G. B., Cheli, R., Dobrilla, G., Verme, G., Molinari, F., Pera, A., Petrillo, M. and Valentini, M. (1978). Treatment of active duodenal ulcer with oral cimetidine: a multicentre controlled endoscopic trial. *Digestion*, **17**, 383

52 Binder, H. J., Cocco, A., Crossley, R. J., Finkelstein, W., Font, R., Freidman, G., Groarke, J., Hughes, W., Johnson, A. F., McGuigan, J. E., Summers, R., Vlahievic, R., Wilson, E. C. and Winship, D. H. (1978). Cimetidine in the treatment of duodenal ulcer. *Gastroenterology*, **74**, 380

53 Bodemar, G. and Walan, A. (1976). Cimetidine in the treatment of active duodenal and prepyloric ulcers. *Lancet*, **2**, 161

54 Gray, G. R., McKenzie, I., Smith, I. S., Crean, G. P. and Gillespie, G. (1977). Oral cimetidine in severe duodenal ulceration. *Lancet*, **1**, 4

55 Hetzel, D. J., Hansky, J., Shearman, D. J. C., Korman, M. G., Hecker, R., Taggart, G. J., Jackson, R. and Gabb, B. W. (1978). Cimetidine treatment of duodenal ulceration. Short term clinical trial and maintenance study. *Gastroenterology*, **74**, 389

56 Lambert, R., Bader, J. P., Bernier, J., Bertrand, J., Betourne, C., Gastard, J., Laverdant, C., Ribet, A., Sahel, J. and Toulet, J. (1977). Treatment of gastric and duodenal ulcers with cimetidine. *Gastroenterol. Clin. Biol.*, **1**, 855

57 Malchow, H., Sewing, K. F., Albinus, M., Horn, B., Schomerus, H. and Dolle, W. (1978). In-patient treatment of peptic ulcer with cimetidine 1. Effect on the healing of duodenal ulcer. *Dtsch. Med. Wochenschr.*, **103**, 149

58 Moshal, M. G., Spitaels, J. M. and Bhoola, R. (1977). Treatment of duodenal ulcers with cimetidine. *S. Afr. Med. J.*, **52**, 760

59 Northfield, T. C. and Blackwood, W. S. (1977). Controlled clinical trial of cimetidine for duodenal ulcer. In Burland, W. L. and Simkins, M. A. (eds.). *Cimetidine: Proceedings of the Second International Symposium on Histamine H_2 Receptor Antagonists*, pp. 272–273. (Amsterdam, Oxford: Excerpta Medica)

60 Petrillo, M., Prada, A., Grossi, E. and Bianchi Porro, G. (1978). Traitamento con cimetidina del' ulcera duodenale attiva. *Rec. Prog. Med.* (In press)

61 Semb, L. S., Berstad, A., Myren, J., Foss, Chr. J., Carlsen, E. and Kruse-Jensen, A. (1977). A double blind multicentre comparative study of cimetidine and placebo in short-term treatment of active duodenal ulceration. In Burland, W. L. and Simkins, M. A. (eds.). *Cimetidine: Proceedings of the Second International Symposium on Histamine H_2 Receptor Antagonists*, pp. 248–253. (Amsterdam, Oxford: Excerpta Medica)

62 Wyllie, J. H. (1978). Experience of controlled comparative trials in patients with duodenal ulcer. In Creutzfeldt, W. (ed.). *Cimetidine. Proceedings of an International Symposium on Histamine H_2 Receptor Antagonists*, pp. 202–216. (Amsterdam: Excerpta Medica)

63 Bardhan, K. D. (1978). Cimetidine in duodenal ulceration. In Wastell, C. and Lance, P. (eds.). *Cimetidine. The Westminster Hospital Symposium*, pp. 31–55. (Edinburgh: Churchill Livingstone)

64 Bodemar, G. and Walan, A. (1978). Maintenance treatment of recurrent peptic ulcer by cimetidine. *Lancet*, **1**, 403

65 Blackwood, W. S., Maudgal, D. P. and Northfield, T. D. (1978). Prevention by bedtime Cimetidine of duodenal ulcer relapse. *Lancet*, **1**, 626

66 Gudmand-Høyer, E., Birger-Jensen, K., Krag, E., Rask-Madsen, J., Ranbek, I., Rune, S. J. and Wulff, H. J. (1978). Prophylactic effect of Cimetidine in duodenal ulcer disease. *Br. Med. J.*, **1**, 1095

67 Gray, G. R., Smith, I. S., Mackenzie, I. and Gillespie, G. (1978). Long-term Cimetidine in the management of severe duodenal ulcer dyspepsia. *Gastroenterology*, **74**, 397

68 Hetzel, D. J., Shearman, D. J. C., Hansky, J., Korman, M. G., Hecker, R., Jackson, R., Garb, B. W. and Sheers, R. (1978). Maintenance of remission of duodenal ulcer by Cimetidine: a double-blind controlled trial. *Gut*, **19**, A442

69 Dronfield, M. W., Batchelor, A. J., Larkworthy, W. and Langman, M. J. S. (1979). Controlled trial of maintenance cimetidine treatment in healed duodenal ulcer: short and long-term effect. *Gut*, **20**, 526

70 Baron, J. H., Alexander-Williams, J. and Bennett, J. R. (1979). Cimetidine and duodenal ulcer. *Br. Med. J.*, **1**, 169

71 Dyck, W. P., Belsito, A., Fleshler, B., Liebermann, T. R., Dickinson, P. B. and Wood, J. M. (1978). Cimetidine and placebo in the treatment of benign gastric ulcer. A multicenter double blind study. *Gastroenterology*, **74**, 410

72 Bader, J. P., Morin, T., Bernier, J. J., Bertrant, D. J., Betourne, C., Gastard, J., Lambert, R., Ribet, A., Sarles, H. and Toulet, J. (1977). Treatment of gastric ulcer by Cimetidine. A multicentre trial. In Burland, W. L. and Simkins, M. A. (eds.). *Cimetidine: Proceedings of the Second International Symposium on Histamine H_2 Receptor Antagonists*, pp. 287–297. (Amsterdam: Excerpta Medica)

73 Frost, F., Rahbek, I., Rune, S. J., Birger Jensen, K., Gudmand-Høyer, E., Krag, E., Rask-Madsen, J., Wulff, J. R., Garbol, J., Gotlied Jensen, K., Hojlund, M. and Nissen, V. R. (1977). Cimetidine in patients with gastric ulcer: a multicentre controlled trial. *Br. Med. J.*, **2**, 795

74 Englert, E. Jr, Freston, J. W., Graham, D. Y., Finkelstein, W., Kruss, D. M., Priest, R. J., Raskin, J. B., Rhodes, J. B., Rogers, A. I., Wenger, J., Wilcox, L. L. and Crossley, R. J. (1978). Cimetidine, antacid and hospitalisation in the treatment of benign gastric ulcer. A multicenter double blind study. *Gastroenterology*, **74**, 416

75 Ciclitira, P. J., Machell, R. J., Farthing, M. J., Dick, A. P. and Hunter, J. G. (1977). Experience with cimetidine in the treatment of gastric ulceration. *Gut*, **18**, 419

76 Sewing, K. F., Malchow, H., Albinus, M., Horn, B., Schomerus, H. and Dolle, W. (1978). Cimetidin in der stationaren behandlung des peptischen ulcus. II Doppelblind-studie bei ulcus ventriculi. *Dtsch. Med. Wochenschr.*, **103**, 152

77 Smith, P. M., Edwards, J. L. and Aubrey, D. A. (1978). Gastric secretory studies and cimetidine treatment in gastric ulcers. In Wastell, C. and Lance, P. (eds.). *Cimetidine. The Westminster Hospital Symposium*, pp. 258–272. (Edinburgh: Churchill Livingstone)

78 La Brooy, S. J., Taylor, R. M., Hunt, R. M., Golding, P. L., Laidlaw, J. M., Chapman,

R. G., Pounder, R. E., Vincent, S. M., Colin-Jones, D. G., Milton-Thompson, G. J. and Misiewicz, J. J. (1979). Controlled comparison of cimetidine and carbenoxolone sodium in gastric ulcer. *Br. Med. J.*, **1**, 1308

79 Kennedy, Y. and Spencer, A. (1978). Cimetidine for recurrent ulcer after vagotomy or gastrectomy: a randomised controlled trial. *Br. Med. J.*, **1**, 1242

80 Atkinson, M. and Van Gelder, A. (1977). Esophageal intraluminal pH recording in the assessment of gastro-esophageal reflux and its consequences. *Am. J. Dig. Dis.*, **22**, 365

81 Osborne, D. H., Lennon, J., Henderson, M., Lidgard, G., Creel, R. and Carter, D. C. (1977). Effect of cimetidine on the human lower oesophageal sphincter. *Gut*, **18**, 99

82 Kravits, J. J., Snape, W. J. and Cohen, S. (1978). Effect of histamine and histamine antagonists on human lower esophageal sphincter function. *Gastroenterology*, **74**, 435

83 Behar, J., Brand, D. L., Brown, F. C., Castell, D. O., Cohen, S., Crossley, R. J., Pope II, C. E. and Winans, C. S. (1978). Cimetidine in the treatment of symptomatic gastroesophageal reflux. *Gastroenterology*, **74**, 441

84 Powell-Jackson, P., Barkley, H. and Northfield, T. C. (1978). Effect of cimetidine in symptomatic gastro-oesophageal reflux. *Lancet*, **2**, 1068

85 Ferguson, R., Dronfield, M. W. and Atkinson, M. (1979). Cimetidine in treatment of reflux oesophagitis with peptic stricture. *Br. Med. J.*, **2**, 472

86 Ivey, K. J., Baskin, W. and Jeffrey, G. (1975). Effect of cimetidine on gastric potential difference in man. *Lancet*, **2**, 1072

87 O'Brien, P. E. and Carter, D. C. (1975). Effect of gastric secretory inhibitors on the gastric mucosal barrier. *Gut*, **16**, 437

88 Rees, W. D. W., Rhodes, J., Wheeler, M. H., Meek, E. M. and Newcombe, R. G. (1977). Role of histamine receptors in the pathophysiology of gastric mucosal damage. *Gastroenterology*, **72**, 67

89 Bommelaer, G. and Guth, P. H. (1979). Protection by histamine receptor antagonists and prostaglandin against gastric mucosal disruption in the rat. *Gastroenterology*, **77**, 303

90 Carmichael, H. A., Nelson, L. M. and Russell, R. I. (1978). Cimetidine and prostaglandin: evidence for different modes of action on the rat gastric mucosa. *Gastroenterology*, **74**, 1229

91 Kauffman, G. L. and Grossman, M. I. (1978). Prostaglandin and cimetidine inhibit the formation of ulcers produced by parenteral salicylates. *Gastroenterology*, **75**, 1099

92 Guth, P. H., Aures, D. and Paulsen, G. (1979). Topical aspirin + HCl lesions in the rat: cytoprotective effect of prostaglandin, cimetidine and probanthine. *Gastroenterology*, **76**, 88

93 Owen, D. A. A. and Parsons, M. E. (1974). Histamine receptors in the cardiovascular system of the cat. *Br. J. Pharmacol.*, **51**, 123

94 Owen, D. A. A., Parsons, M. E., Farrington, H. E. and Blakemore, R. (1979). Reduction by cimetidine of acute gastric hemorrhage caused by reinfusion of blood after exposure to exogenous acid during gastric ischemia in rats. *Gastroenterology*, **77**, 979

95 Jones, R. H., Rudge, C. J., Bewick, M., Parsons, V. and Weston, M. J. (1978). Cimetidine: prophylaxis against upper gastrointestinal haemorrhage after renal transplantation. *Br. Med. J.*, **1**, 398

96 Macdougall, B. R. D., Bailey, R. J. and Williams, R. (1977). H₂ receptor antagonists and antacids in the prevention of acute gastrointestinal haemorrhage in fulminant hepatic failure, two controlled trials. *Lancet*, **1**, 617

97 McAlhany, J. C. Jr, Czaja, A. J. and Pruitt, B. A. Jr (1976). Antacid control of complications from acute gastroduodenal disease after burns. *J. Trauma*, **16**, 645

98 Hastings, P. R., Skillman, J. J., Bushnell, L. S. and Silen, W. (1978). Antacid titration in the prevention of acute gastrointestinal bleeding, a controlled randomised study in 100 critically ill patients. *N. Engl. J. Med.*, **298**, 1041

99   Priebe, H. J., Skillman, J. J., Bushnell, L. S., Long, P. C. and Silen, W. (1980). Antacid versus cimetidine in preventing acute gastrointestinal bleeding. *N. Engl. J. Med.*, **302**, 426

100 Macdonald, A. S., Steele, B. J. and Bottomley, M. G. (1976). Treatment of stress induced gastrointestinal haemorrhage with metiamide. *Lancet*, **1**, 68

101 Dunn, D. H., Fischer, R. C., Silvis, S. E., Onstad, G. R., Howard, R. J. and Delaney, J. P. (1978). The treatment of hemorrhagic gastritis with cimetidine. *Surg. Gynecol. Obstet.*, **147**, 737

102 Hoare, A. M., Bradby, G. V. H., Hawkins, C. F., Kang, J. Y. and Dykes, P. W. (1979). Cimetidine in bleeding peptic ulcer. *Lancet*, **2**, 671

103 La Brooy, S. J., Misiewicz, J. J., Edwards, J., Smith, P. M., Haggie, S. J., Libman, L., Sarner, M., Wyllie, J. N., Croker, J. and Cotton, P. (1979). Controlled trial of cimetidine in upper gastrointestinal haemorrhage. *Gut*, **20**, 892

104 Pickard, R. G., Sanderson, I., South, M., Kirkham, J. S. and Northfield, T. C. (1979). Controlled trial of cimetidine in acute upper gastrointestinal bleeding. *Br. Med. J.*, **1**, 661

105 McCarthy, D. M. (1978). Report on the United States experience with cimetidine in Zollinger–Ellison syndrome and other hypersecretory states. *Gastroenterology*, **74**, 453

106 Kruss, D. M. and Littman, A. (1978). Safety of cimetidine. *Gastroenterology*, **74**, 478

107 Druart, F., Frocrain, C., Metois, P., Martin, J. and Matuchansky, C. (1979). Association of cimetidine and bone marrow suppression in man. *Dig. Dis. Sci.*, **24**, 730

108 Ufberg, M. H., Brooks, C. M., Bosawac, P. R. and Kintzel, J. E. (1977). Transient neutropenia in a patient receiving cimetidine. *Gastroenterology*, **73**, 635

109 Burland, W. L., Sharpe, P. C., Colin-Jones, D. G., Turnbull, P. R. G. and Bowskill, P. (1975). Reversal of metiamide-induced agranulocytosis during treatment with cimetidine. *Lancet*, **2**, 1085

110 Sharpe, P. C. and Hawkins, B. W. (1977). Long term treatment with cimetidine. In Burland, W. L. and Simkins, M. A. (eds.). *Cimetidine: Proceedings of the Second International Symposium on Histamine H$_2$ Receptor Antagonists*, pp. 358–366. (Amsterdam, Oxford: Excerpta Medica)

111 Spence, R. W. and Celestin, L. R. (1979). Gynaecomastia associated with cimetidine. *Gut*, **20**, 154

112 Carlson, H. E. and Ippoliti, A. (1977). Cimetidine, an H$_2$-antihistamine, stimulates prolactin in man. *J. Clin. Endocrinol. Metab.*, **45**, 367

113 Sherwood, J. K., Ackroyd, F. W. and Garcia, M. (1980). Effect of cimetidine on circulating parathyroid hormone in primary hyperparathyroidism. *Lancet*, **1**, 616

114 Serlin, M. S., Sibeon, R. G., Mossman, S., Breckenridge, A. M., Williams, J. R. B., Atwood, J. L. and Willoughby, J. N. T. (1979). Cimetidine: interaction with oral anticoagulants in man. *Lancet*, **1**, 319

115 Klotz, N. and Reimann, I. (1980). Delayed clearance of diazepam due to cimetidine. *N. Engl. J. Med.*, **302**, 1012

116 Fielding, L. P., Chalmers, D. M., Stafford, D. M. and Levi, J. (1977). Cimetidine and intrinsic factor secretion. In Burland, W. L. and Simkins, M. A. (eds.). *Cimetidine: Proceedings of the Second International Symposium on Histamine H$_2$ Receptor Antagonists*, pp. 184–186. (Amsterdam, Oxford: Excerpta Medica)

117 Sharpe, P. C., Mills, J., Horton, M. A., Hunt, R. H., Vincent, S. H. and Milton-Thompson, G. J. (1979). Is intrinsic factor really affected by cimetidine? *Br. Med. J.*, **2**, 1251

118 Witzel, L., Halter, F., Olah, A. J. and Häcki, W. H. (1977). Effects of prolonged metiamide medication on the fundic mucosa. A secretory and histomorphometric study in the rat. *Gastroenterology*, **73**, 797

119 Sewing, K. F., Haggie, L., Ippoliti, A. F., Isenberg, J. I., Samloff, I. M. and Sturdevant, R. A. L. (1978). Effect of one month treatment with cimetidine on gastric secre-

tion and serum gastrin and pepsinogen levels. *Gastroenterology*, **74**, 376

120 Spence, R. W., Celestin, L. R., McCormick, D. A. and Owens, C. J. (1977). The effect of 3 months treatment with cimetidine on basal and 'oxo'-stimulated serum gastrin. In Burland, W. L. and Simkins, M. A. (eds.). *Cimetidine: Proceedings of the Second International Symposium on Histamine H₂ Receptor Antagonists*, pp. 163–174. (Amsterdam, Oxford: Excerpta Medica)

121 Bank, S., Barbezat, G. O., Vinik, A. J., Halter, F. and Helmann, C. A. (1977). Cimetidine and serum gastrin levels in man. In Burland, W. L. and Simkins, M. A. (eds.). *Cimetidine: Proceedings of the Second International Symposium on Histamine H₂ Receptor Antagonists*, pp. 155–162. (Amsterdam, Oxford: Excerpta Medica)

122 Winship, D. H. (1978). Cimetidine in the treatment of duodenal ulcer. Review and commentary. *Gastroenterology*, **74**, 402

123 Ruddell, W. S. J., Bone, E. S., Hill, M. S., Blendis, L. M. and Walters, C. L. (1976). Gastric juice nitrite. A risk factor for cancer in the hypochlorohydric stomach? *Lancet*, **2**, 1037

124 Ruddell, W. S. J., Axon, A. T. R., Findlay, J. M., Bartholomew, B. A. and Hill, M. J. (1980). Effect of cimetidine on gastric bacterial flora. *Lancet*, **2**, 672

125 Elder, J. B., Ganguli, P. C. and Gillespie, I. E. (1979). Cimetidine and gastric cancer. *Lancet*, **2**, 1005

126 Dousa, T. P. and Dozois, R. R. (1977). Interrelations between histamine, prostaglandins and cyclic AMP in gastric secretion: a hypothesis. *Gastroenterology*, **73**, 904

127 Wollin, A., Soll, A. H. and Samloff, I. M. (1979). Action of histamine, secretin and PGE₂ on cyclic AMP production by isolated canine fundic mucosal cells. *Am. J. Physiol.*, **237**, 437

128 Moncada, A., Salmon, J. A., Vane, J. R. and Whittle, B. J. R. (1978). Formation of prostacyclin (PGI₂) and its product 6-oxo-PGF₁α by the gastric mucosa of several species. *J. Physiol. (Lond.)*, **275**, 4P

129 Classen, M., Koch, H., Deyhle, P., Weidenhiller, S. and Demling, L. (1970). Wirking von Prostaglandin E₁ ant die basale magensekretion des Menschen. *Klin. Wochenschr.*, **48**, 876

130 Wilson, D. E., Phillips, C. and Levine, R. A. (1971). Inhibition of gastric secretion in man by prostaglandin A₁. *Gastroenterology*, **61**, 201

131 Robert, A., Schultz, J. R., Nezamis, J. E. and Lancaster, C. (1976). Gastric antisecretory and antiulcer properties of PGE₂, 15-methyl PGE₂, and 16,16-dimethyl PGE₂. Intravenous, oral and intrajejunal administration. *Gastroenterology*, **70**, 359

132 Karim, S. M. M., Carter, D. C., Bhana, D. and Ganesan, P. A. (1973). Effect of orally administered prostaglandin E₂ and its 15-methyl analogues on gastric secretion. *Br. Med. J.*, **1**, 143

133 Carter, D. C., Karim, S. M. M., Bhana, D. and Ganesan, P. A. (1973). Inhibition of human gastric secretion by prostaglandins. *Br. J. Surg.*, **60**, 828

134 Fung, W. P. and Karim, S. M. M. (1976). Effect of 15(R) methyl prostaglandin E2 on the healing of gastric ulcers. A double blind endoscopic study. *Med. J. Austr.*, **2**, 127

135 Gibinski, K., Rybicka, J., Mikos, E. and Nowak, A. (1977). Double-blind clinical trial on gastroduodenal ulcer healing with prostaglandin E₂ analogues. *Gut*, **18**, 636

136 Way, L. and Durbin, R. P. (1969). Inhibition of gastric acid secretion in vitro by prostaglandin E₁ (letter to the Editor). *Nature (London)*, **221**, 874

137 Main, I. H. M. and Whittle, B. J. R. (1974). Prostaglandin E₂ and the stimulation of rat gastric acid secretion by dibutryl cyclic 3', 5'-AMP. *Eur. J. Pharmacol.*, **26**, 204

138 Thompson, W. K., Chang, L. K., Rosenfeld, G. C. and Jacobsen, E. D. (1977). Activation of rat gastric mucosal adenyl cyclase by secretory inhibitors. *Gastroenterology*, **72**, 251

139 Wollin, A., Code, C. F. and Dousa, T. P. (1976). Interaction of prostaglandins and histamine with enzymes of cyclic AMP metabolism from guinea pig gastric mucosa.

J. Clin. Invest., **57**, 1548

140   Soll, A. H. (1978). Prostaglandin inhibition of histamine-stimulated aminopyrine uptake and cyclic AMP generation by isolated canine parietal cell (abstr.). *Gastroenterology*, **74**, 1146

141   Fordtran, J. S. and Collyns, S. A. H. (1966). Antacid pharmacology in duodenal ulcer: effect of antacids on post cibal gastric acidity and peptic activity. *N. Engl. J. Med.*, **274**, 921

142   Fordtran, J. S., Morawski, S. G. and Richardson, C. T. (1973). In vivo and in vitro evaluation of liquid antacids. *N. Engl. J. Med.*, **288**, 923

143   Doll, R., Price, A. V., Pygott, F. and Sanderson, P. H. (1956). Continuous intragastric milk drip in treatment of uncomplicated gastric ulcer. *Lancet*, **1**, 70

144   Butler, M. L. and Gersh, H. (1975). Antacids vs placebo in hospitalised gastric ulcer patients. A controlled therapeutic study. *Am. J. Dig. Dis.*, **20**, 803

145   Sturdevant, R. A. L., Isenberg, J. I., Secrist, D. and Ansfield, J. J. (1977). Antacid and placebo produced similar pain relief in duodenal ulcer patients. *Gastroenterology*, **72**, 1

146   Hollander, D. and Harlan, J. (1973). Antacids vs. placebos in peptic ulcer. *J. Am. Med. Assoc.*, **226**, 1181

147   Peterson, W. L., Sturdevant, R. A. L., Frankl, H. D., Richardson, C. T., Isenberg, J. I., Elashoff, J. D., Sones, J. Q., Gross, R. A., McCallum, R. W. and Fordtran, J. S. (1977). Healing of duodenal ulcer with an antacid regimen. *N. Engl. J. Med.*, **297**, 341

148   Marks, I. N. (1979). Healing of peptic ulcers on conventional antacid therapy with or without butriptyline. *S. Afr. Med. J.*, **55**, 331

149   Deering, T. B. and Malagelada, J-R. (1977). Comparison of an H_2 receptor antagonist and a neutralising antacid on post prandial acid delivery into the duodenum in patients with duodenal ulcer. *Gastroenterology*, **73**, 11

150   Ippoliti, A. F., Sturdevant, R. A. L., Isenberg, J. I., Binder, M., Camacho, R., Cano, R., Cooney, C., Kline, M. M., Koretz, R. L., Meyer, J. H., Samloff, I. M., Schwabe, A. D., Strom, E. A., Valenzuela, J. E. and Wintroub, R. H. (1978). Cimetidine versus intensive antacid therapy for duodenal ulcer. *Gastroenterology*, **74**, 393

151   Sun, D. C. H. and Ryan, M. L. (1970). A controlled study on the use of propantheline and amylopectin sulphate (SN-263) for recurrence in duodenal ulcer. *Gastroenterology*, **58**, 756

152   Baron, J. H., Gribble, R. J. N., Holdstock, D. J. and Misiewicz, J. J. (1977). A double blind controlled trial of amylopectin sulphate (Depepsen) in the symptomatic treatment of duodenal ulcer. *Gut*, **18**, 723

153   Landecker, K. D., McCallum, E. M., Fevre, D. I., Green, P. H. R., Kasumi, A. and Piper, D. W. (1976). Effect of sodium amylosulfate (Depepsen) on the healing of duodenal ulcer. *Gastroenterology*, **71**, 723

154   Mayberry, J. F., Williams, R. A., Rhodes, J. and Lawrie, B. W. (1978). A controlled trial of sucralfate in the treatment of gastric ulcer. *Br. J. Clin. Pract.*, **32**, 291

155   Shillingford, J. S., Lindup, W. E. and Parke, D. V. (1974). The effects of carbenoxolone on the synthesis of gastric glycoproteins in the rat and ferret. *Biochem. Soc. Trans.*, **2**, 1104

156   Parke, D. V. and Symons, A. M. (1977). The biochemical pharmacology of mucus. In Elstein, M. and Parke, D. V. (eds.). *Mucus in Health and Disease*, pp. 423–441. (London: Plenum)

157   Lipkin, M. (1971). In defence of the gastric mucosa. *Gut*, **12**, 559

158   Croft, D. N. (1978). Gastric epithelial cell dynamics and the healing of gastric ulcers using carbenoxolone. In Avery-Jones, F., Langman, M. J. S. and Mann, R. D. (eds.). *Peptic Ulcer Healing. Recent Studies on Carbenoxolone*, pp. 9–19. (Lancaster: MTP Press)

159   Domschke, S., Domschke, W. and Demling, L. (1975). Effect of intravenous prednisolone on net ion fluxes across human gastric mucosa: antagonism by carbenoxolone

sodium. In Avery-Jones, F. and Parke, D. V. (eds.). *Fourth Symposium on Carbenoxolone*, pp. 75–86. (London: Butterworths)

160   Taylor, W. H., Walker, V. and Roberts, N. B. (1978). Pepsins, pepsinogens, and carbenoxolone. In Avery-Jones, F., Langman, M. J. S. and Mann, R. D. (eds.). *Peptic Ulcer Healing. Recent Studies on Carbenoxolone*, pp. 33–46. (Lancaster: MTP Press)

161   Doll, R., Hill, I. D., Hutton, C. F. and Underwood, D. J. (1962). Clinical trial of triterpenoid liquorice compound in gastric and duodenal ulcer. *Lancet*, **2**, 793

162   Cocking, J. B. and McCraig, J. N. (1969). Effect of low dosage of carbenoxolone sodium on gastric ulcer healing and acid secretion. *Gut*, **10**, 219

163   Gilbert, J. A. L. (1976). Multi-centre Canadian double blind study of carbenoxolone (Biogastrone) in the treatment of gastric ulcer. In Black, I. T. (ed.). *North American Symposium on Carbenoxolone*, pp. 85–92. (Amsterdam: Excerpta Medica)

164   Lorber, S. H. (1976). U.S. trial of carbenoxolone (Biogastrone) in gastric ulcer. In Black, I. T. (ed.). *North American Symposium on Carbenoxolone*, pp. 93–97. (Amsterdam: Excerpta Medica)

165   Hampel, K. E., Billoch, C., Dannenmeier, H. D., Fintelmann, V., Fischer, R., Schmid, E., Treske, U. and Walz, A. (1972). Therapie des Ulcus ventriculi et duodeni mit carbenoxolon–Natrium (Doppel blind versuch). *Munch. Med. Wochenschr.*, **114**, 925

166   Horwich, L. and Galloway, R. (1965). Treatment of gastric ulcer with carbenoxolone sodium. Clinical and radiological evaluation. *Br. Med. J.* **2**, 1274

167   Langman, M. J. S. (1978). Carbenoxolone in the treatment of chronic gastric ulcer. In Avery-Jones, F., Langman, M. J. S. and Mann, R. D. (eds.). *Peptic Ulcer Healing. Recent Studies on Carbenoxolone*, pp. 59–69. (Lancaster: MTP Press)

168   Sahel, J., Sarles, H., Boisson, J., Bonnet-Eymard, J., Cornet, A., Delmont, J., Dubarry, J., Dupuy, R., Gisselbrecht, R., Monges, H., Ribet, A., Roberti, A., Valla, A., Weill, J. P. and Cros, R. C. (1977). Carbenoxolone sodium capsules in the treatment of duodenal ulcer. An endoscopic controlled trial. *Gut*, **18**, 717

169   Nagy, G. S. (1978). Evaluation of carbenoxolone sodium in the treatment of duodenal ulcer. *Gastroenterology*, **74**, 7

170   Davies, W. A. and Reed, P. I. (1977). Controlled trial of Duogastrone in duodenal ulcer. *Gut*, **18**, 78

171   Archambault, A., Farley, A., Gosselind, D., Martin, F. and Birkett, J. P. (1978). Evaluation of Duogastrone (carbenoxolone sodium) for the treatment of duodenal ulcer: a multicentre study. *Can. Med. J.*, **117**, 1155

172   Young, G. P., St John, D. J. B. and Coventry, D. A. (1978). A double-masked endoscopic evaluation of carbenoxolone sodium in duodenal ulcer: further evidence for a beneficial effect. In Avery-Jones, F., Langman, M. J. S. and Mann, R. D. (eds.). *Peptic Ulcer Healing. Recent Studies on Carbenoxolone*, pp. 117–125. (Lancaster: MTP Press)

173   Larkworthy, W., Holgate, P. F. L., McIlmurray, M. B. and Langman, M. J. (1977). Deglycyrrhizimised liquorice in duodenal ulcer. *Br. Med. J.*, **2**, 1123

174   Hollanders, D., Green, G., Woolf, I. L., Boyes, B. E., Wilson, R. Y., Cowley, D. J. and Dymock, I. W. (1978). Prophylaxis with deglycyrrhizinised liquorice in patients with healed gastric ulcer. *Br. Med. J.*, **1**, 148

175   Moshal, M. G. (1975). The treatment of duodenal ulcers with TDB: a duodenoscopic double-blind cross-over investigation. *Postgrad. Med. J.*, **51** (Suppl.), 36

176   Salmon, P. R. (1975). Evaluation of TDB in the treatment of duodenal ulcer employing endoscopic selection and follow-up. *Postgrad. Med. J.*, **51** (Suppl.), 26

177   Shreeve, D. R. (1975). A double-blind study of tri-potassium di-citrato bismuthate in duodenal ulcer. *Postgrad. Med. J.*, **51** (Suppl.), 33

178   Lee, S. P. and Nicholson, G. I. (1977). Increased healing of gastric and duodenal ulcers in a controlled trial using tripotassium dicitrato-bismuthate. *Med. J. Austr.*, **1**, 808

179 Goughlin, G. P., Kupa, A. and Alp, M. H. (1977). The effect of tri-potassium di-citrato bismuthate (De-Nol) on the healing of chronic duodenal ulcers. *Med. J. Aust.*, **1**, 294

180 Poulantzas, J., Polymerpoulos, P. S. and Papasomatious, A. (1978). A double-blind evaluation of the effect of tri-potassium di-citrato bismuthate in peptic ulcers. *Br. J. Clin. Pract.*, **32**, 147

181 Brogden, R. N., Pinder, R. M., Sawyer, P. R., Speight, T. M. and Avery, G. S. (1976). Tri-potassium di-citrato bismuthate: a report of its pharmacological properties and therapeutic efficacy in peptic ulcer. *Drugs*, **12**, 401

182 Gilliland, I., Read, A. E. and Wright, T. (1975). Tri-potassium di-citrato bismuthate. *Postgrad. Med. J.*, **51** (Suppl.)

183 Newcomb, P. B., Stone, W. D., Richardson, P. C., Smith, P. M., Gent, A. and Donovan, B. (1976). A double blind trial of gefarnate and placebo in the treatment of gastric ulcer. *Practitioner*, **217**, 435

184 Truelove, S. C. and Rocca, M. (1976). Treatment of chronic gastric ulcer with gefarnate: a long-term controlled therapeutic trial. *Curr. Med. Res. Opin.*, **4**, 218

185 Robert, A. (1975). An intestinal disease produced experimentally by a prostaglandin deficiency. *Gastroenterology*, **69**, 1045

186 Robert, A. and Asano, T. (1977). Resistance of germ-free animals to intestinal lesions produced by indomethacin. *Prostaglandins*, **14**, 333

187 Robert, A. (1976). Antisecretory, antiulcer, cytoprotective and diarrheogenic properties of prostaglandins. *Adv. Prostagland. Thrombox. Res.*, **2**, 507

188 Robert, A. (1977). Effect of prostaglandins on gastrointestinal function. In Borti, F., Samuelsson, B. and Velo, G. P. (eds.). *Prostaglandin and Thromboxanes*, pp. 287–313. (New York: Plenum)

189 Whittle, B. J. R. (1976). Relationship between the prevention of rat gastric erosions and the inhibition of acid secretion by prostaglandins. *Eur. J. Pharmacol.*, **40**, 233

190 Robert, A., Nezamis, J. E., Lancaster, C. and Hanchar, A. J. (1979). Cytoprotection by prostaglandins in rats: prevention of gastric necrosis produced by alcohol, HCl, NaOH, hypertonic NaCl and thermal injury. *Gastroenterology*, **77**, 433

191 Kauffman, G. L., Foley, K. T. and Grossman, M. I. (1979). Cimetidine does not inhibit indomethacin-induced small bowel ulceration in the rat. *Proc. Soc. Exp. Biol. Med.*, **161**, 512

192 Main, I. H. M. and Whittle, B. J. R. (1974). Prostaglandin and prostaglandin synthetase inhibition in gastrointestinal function and disease. In Robinson, H. J. and Vane, J. R. (eds.). *Prostaglandin Synthetase Inhibitors*, pp. 363–372. (New York: Raven Press)

193 Chaudhury, T. K. and Jacobson, E. D. (1978). Prostaglandin cytoprotection of gastric mucosa. *Gastroenterology*, **74**, 59

194 Bolton, J. P. and Cohen, M. M. (1978). Stimulation of non-parietal cell secretion in canine Heidenhain pouches by 16,16-dimethyl prostaglandin E_2. *Digestion*, **17**, 291

195 Bolton, J. P., Palmer, D. and Cohen, M. M. (1978). Stimulation of mucus and non-parietal cell secretion by the E_2 prostaglandins. *Dig. Dis.*, **23**, 359

9
Recent realizations in the surgical treatment of ascites

H. H. LEVEEN

INTRODUCTION

Ascites, the excessive accumulation of fluid in the peritoneal cavity, has been a focus for attention and concern since the time of Hippocrates. His intuition (discussed by Atkinson in 1956)[1] that the liver becomes full of liquid that overflows into the peritoneal cavity, swelling the belly and causing death, has been confirmed. The most common aetiology is as a sequel of alcoholic cirrhosis, which is in itself a growing problem. Ascites adversely influences the prognosis of alcoholic cirrhosis. More than 30 years have passed, but the fatality rate has not been appreciably reduced since Ratnoff and Patek reported in 1942[2] that 50% of patients were dead 6 months after the onset of ascites.

Use of the peritoneovenous shunt to divert ascitic fluid from the swollen abdomen to the venous circulation has become a standard form of therapy for ascites throughout the world (Figure 1). This therapy extends the lifespan of patients with ascites. The idea that peritoneal fluid should be returned to the circulatory system is physiologically reasonable because such fluid originates in the circulation. This review summarizes features of ascites, explains the one-way, pressure-sensitive valve that is used in the peritoneovenous shunt, and discusses the indications, methods, results, and complications of this surgery in the management of ascites.

257

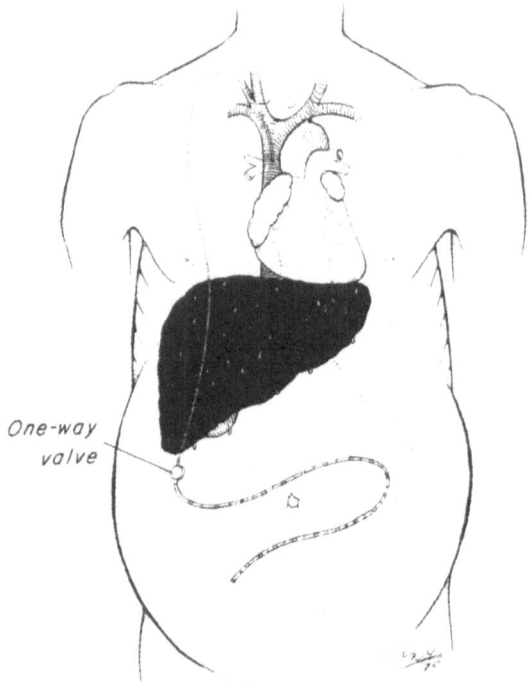

Figure 1   A schematic drawing shows the one-way ascites valve connecting the peritoneal cavity with the superior vena cava via a silicone tube inserted into the jugular vein

CAUSES OF ASCITES

Cirrhosis

Excessive alcohol consumption and viral hepatitis are the most common causes of cirrhosis in the Western hemisphere.

Alcohol

Facts on alcoholism from the National Council on Alcoholism include the estimate that 10 million people in the United States suffer from the disease, and that it is a serious problem even among teenagers. It is becoming more frequent in the inner cities with the introduction of inexpensive wine with a 20% alcohol content. Perhaps one in twelve alcoholics goes on to develop cirrhosis[3]. Cirrhosis is the leading cause of death in alcoholics, and the Council estimates that it causes over 30 000 deaths per year in the United States. The risk of developing cirrhosis increases 25-fold when an individual consumes over 160 g of alcohol per day, and according to Pequignot[4] a daily consumption of 180 g for 25 years will induce cirrhosis. It is difficult to estimate what percentage of people with cirrhosis progress to develop ascites.

As the damaged liver becomes cirrhotic, there is an increase in the resistance to the flow of blood, especially in the venous system. Venous dilatation progresses through the capillaries and into the arterial system. Arteriovenous shunts are thus formed and cause a reversal of portal blood flow and a progressively rising portal hypertension. Blood from the splanchnic bed is then shunted through various communications in and outside the liver, so that much of the portal vein blood bypasses circulation through the liver. In ascites the obstruction to venous flow has been shown to be mainly post-sinusoidal, while in oesophageal varices without ascites the obstruction is mainly pre-sinusoidal.

Chronic viral hepatitis

Cirrhosis can progress from viral hepatitis due to type B and non-A–non-B viruses, but not type A virus. For type B virus chronic viral hepatitis appears, on the average, 3 months after contact. Chronic viral hepatitis appears microscopically as intralobular and limiting plate necrosis. Marked inflammatory changes occur in the portal areas, followed by necrosis and loss of normal architecture. Fibrosis and nodular regeneration lead to compression of portal and hepatic venous tributaries and to portal hypertension, and shunting of blood from the splanchnic bed through venous communications inside and outside the liver.

Other causes of cirrhosis

Other causes of cirrhosis are less frequent but should be kept in mind; they can usually be distinguished from viral hepatitis by immunological or other tests. These include infections by other viruses, toxic drug reactions, parasites, schistosomiasis, cancer chemotherapy, Wilson's disease, iron overload, cancer, chemotherapy, and α-1-antitrypsin deficiency. Occasionally the disease is cryptogenic.

Other causes and types of ascites

Other causes of ascites include Budd–Chiari syndrome, and other types of ascites include chylous ascites, malignant ascites, postoperative ascites, nephrogenic ascites, cardiogenic ascites, and nutritional ascites.

Budd–Chiari Syndrome

The Budd–Chiari syndrome is often a fatal condition. It arises from obstruction to hepatic vein outflow at any point from the efferent vein of the lobule to the point of entry of the inferior vena cava into the right atrium. It is often caused by hepatic vein thrombosis or by thrombosis of the inferior vena cava at the level of the hepatic veins. In turn, the cause for thrombosis is often an abnormal clotting tendency such as is seen in polycythaemia vera and paroxysmal nocturnal haemoglobinuria, and in certain patients taking oral contraceptives[5-7].

Partial occlusion of the inferior vena cava above the liver is the standard method of producing ascites in an experimental animal. Lower[8] in 1679 ligated the inferior vena cava in the dog, causing ascites. This classical work has served as a prototype for inducing experimental ascites ever since. Occasionally, hepatic tumours will compress the hepatic veins and produce the Budd–Chiari syndrome. A web-like obstruction can also occur and has been successfully dealt with surgically. This obstruction can often be diagnosed by Doppler ultrasonography.

Angiography including a cavagram is most important in the diagnostic work-up of the Budd–Chiari syndrome. Some patients resolve their problem spontaneously but life-threatening situations should be treated promptly by insertion of a peritoneovenous (PV) shunt.

Isovolaemic haemodilution by removal of red cells and their replacement with plasma has proved most beneficial in obstruction to venous outflow. Lowering the haematocrit to levels of 25–30% appreciably lowers blood viscosity and thus relieves congestion.

Chylous ascites

In chylous ascites, the peritoneal fluid is milky white. This is due to the presence of fat in the peritoneal fluid that is normally absorbed from the gastrointestinal tract through the lymphatic system. A rupture of one of the lymphatics causes chylosis. Rupture of a large lymphatic duct will produce a continuous leak of lymph if there is obstruction of the thoracic duct due to carcinoma, trauma, tuberculosis, parasites, or lymphoma. The nephrotic syndrome and lymphangiectasia are less common causes. Wasting and malnutrition can be severe, and mortality rates due to the underlying disorder exceed 40%. The condition responds promptly to insertion of a PV shunt.

Malignant ascites

The abdominal visceral serosa and fine mesothelial lining of the periton-eal cavity are vulnerable to tumour implantation from the ovary, alimen-tary tract, and remote sites. Tumour implantation in these sites stimulates the production of ascitic fluid. The peritoneal fluid resembles an exudate more than a transudate and has a high protein content.

Not all cases of ascites occurring in cancer patients are caused by malignant implantation in the peritoneal cavity. Cirrhosis, congestive heart failure, renal disease, and extensive liver metastases that can cause compression of hepatic veins may also account for ascites for-mation[9].

The prognosis for patients with malignant ascites is grave. Most die within 6 months after the onset of ascites. Patients are made more com-fortable by insertion of a PV shunt, and survival is favourably influenced.

Postoperative ascites

Occasionally, surgery on cirrhotic patients with portal hypertension is followed by intractable ascites. This occurs most especially after retro-peritoneal dissection or after operations for oesophageal varices, many of which involve dissection of the posterior wall of the lesser sac. A major lymphatic duct is cut, but remains unnoticed at laparotomy and ascites occurs. These openings would seal spontaneously with fibrin clots in normal patients but lymphorrhagia persists in the presence of portal hypertension, because lymph flow is increased in cirrhosis and the ducts are distended and under pressure. The fluid is often turbid because of high protein and fat content, and it mimics chylous ascites since it contains fat, but the fluid is usually not as milky white. Insertion of PV shunts in some such cases has been lifesaving. Loss of fluid and protein into the peritoneal cavity can be so copious that the situation resembles a body burn with a rising haematocrit and a falling plasma volume.

Nephrogenic ascites

Despite the use of haemodialysis, refractory ascites occurs in 5–15% of patients with chronic renal failure. The cause is unknown. Biopsies of liver and peritoneum are not revealing. The ascitic fluid has a high protein content and resembles an exudate. The condition responds to insertion of a PV shunt.

Cardiogenic ascites

Primary heart disease, such as tricuspid valve disease, constrictive pericarditis, and chronic right heart failure can cause cardiogenic ascites. Patients with cirrhosis may also have heart disease, and in such cases it may be difficult to distinguish between ascites secondary merely to right-sided congestive heart failure, or due to both heart and liver disease.

Nutritional ascites

Nutritional ascites is a serious problem in areas where kwashiorkor and malnutrition are frequently encountered. It has never been seen by the author, but he has been told the disease is common in areas of Asia and Africa and patients respond favourably to insertion of a PV shunt.

PATHOPHYSIOLOGY OF ASCITES

General features

The exchange of fluid across the peritoneal surface and intestines in ascites conforms to Starling's hypothesis. The fluid is driven from the vessels because of the hydrostatic pressure in the portal vein and the oncotic pressure of the ascitic fluid. These pressures are opposed by the intraperitoneal hydrostatic pressure and the plasma oncotic pressure.

It has been estimated that 60% of ascitic fluid is derived from the liver surface while 40% has its origin from other abdominal viscera. The liquid that is shed from the liver's surface has a higher protein concentration because the liver capillaries are permeable to protein. The high protein content of the ascitic fluid initially tends to stabilize the ascites. It also accounts for the severe protein depletion which is brought about by repeated paracentesis.

Portal hypertension and hypoalbuminaemia occurring independently in cirrhosis do not readily correlate with the appearance of ascites. Ascitic fluid accumulates readily when these two factors are combined[10]. Serum albumin is commonly reduced in cirrhosis associated with ascites, and there is a better correlation between the presence of ascites and the serum albumin concentration than there is between the presence of ascites and the portal vein pressure.

The rate and the extent of ascitic fluid accumulation is modified by the site of the venous occlusion. Postsinusoidal obstruction, occurring in nodular compression around the central vein in cirrhosis, central vein thrombosis, Budd–Chiari syndrome, and right-sided heart failure, is much more likely to result in ascites than presinusoidal obstruction or portal vein thrombosis. The hepatic vasculature is said to be different in patients with ascites.

The accumulation of excessive fluid in the peritoneal cavity brings on typical pathophysiological changes. Patients with ascites are more likely to develop other complications, such as bleeding from oesophageal varices. The presence of massive ascites can restrict respiratory function. The large amount of fluid in the peritoneal cavity adversely affects appetite leading to malnourishment and a lowered resistance to infection.

Features of renal pathophysiology in ascites

Death from ascites is most commonly linked to renal failure; indeed, some investigators have found that almost every patient dying from advanced cirrhosis is terminally uraemic and oliguric[11]. That renal tubular reabsorption of sodium chloride plays a central role in the pathogenesis of intractable ascites has been recognized since 1948[12]. Avid sodium retention has been ascribed as a principal cause of ascites by Lieberman et al.[13]. Whether or not azotaemia is present, increased tubular absorption of sodium chloride in ascitic patients is usually associated with a fall in renal blood flow and an increase in renal vascular resistance[14,15]. Indeed, the relationship between reduced renal perfusion and increased salt reabsorption is so critical to kidney failure in patients with ascites that Baldus and others have categorized ascites into three stages, depending on renal perfusion[14-18].

More recent studies indicate that even the sodium retention in the initial phase of ascites formation may be due to a redistribution of blood volume with a diminished effective plasma volume. The effective plasma volume is that critical volume which stimulates volume receptors to notify the body that volume is adequate. Since so little is known about the position and nature of these receptors, it is obvious that it is difficult to determine what an effective blood volume really is. Immersion of the body suddenly increases blood volume, and if the stimulus for sodium retention in cirrhotics is the loss of effective blood volume, immersion should counteract it and indeed it does[19]. An ineffective blood volume is a potent stimulus for the hyperaldosteronism observed in ascites. Since the stimulus is an ineffective blood volume it makes little sense to thwart this compensatory mechanism by diuretic therapy. It makes good sense to permanently expand the plasma volume with a PV shunt. It also explains the unsustained response to interrupted infusions of ascitic fluid, and the sustained response following a PV shunt. Laragh[20] has shown that the hyperaldosteronism observed in cirrhotic ascites is probably the result of renin stimulation from diminished renal perfusion.

The stages in Baldus' classification[14] which usefully divides cirrhotics according to their renal function are as follows:

Class I. Cirrhosis with simple ascites – renal salt clearance relatively normal with a minimal reduction in renal perfusion.

Class II. Cirrhosis with ascites refractory to diuretics and medical management – avid increase in sodium reabsorption with decreased renal perfusion and glomerular filtration rate.

Class III. Cirrhosis with refractory ascites and azotaemia – severely decreased renal perfusion and glomerular filtration rate.

Because absorption in the proximal tubule is obligatory, a substantial reduction in the glomerular filtration rate causes the proximal tubule to reabsorb most of the water and salt that enters it. This situation leaves little urine for facultative reabsorption by distal tubules. Because diuretics act chiefly on the distal tubules, they can have little or no influence on urinary salt and water excretion unless there is a supply of distal tubular urine. This explains why some patients become refractory to such therapy – an indication of serious impairment in renal function and a warning of an impending functional renal failure, unfortunately referred to as the hepatorenal syndrome (HRS).

HRS is characterized by oliguria, azotaemia, and urine with very low sodium content. The low urinary salt concentration is evidence of excellent tubular function, and proves that active tubular necrosis has not yet occurred. The low sodium values are even further diminished by an overactive renin–angiotensin system, which acts on the distal tubules.

Azotaemia is an urgent indication for the inserion of a PV shunt in patients with ascites. The tubules still function when the urinary sodium concentration is less than 10 mEq/l. Nonetheless, functional renal failure rapidly progresses to acute tubular necrosis. The oliguria persists or worsens and the urinary sodium concentration rises to above 25 mEq/l, indicating that the tubules are damaged and can no longer absorb sodium from the glomerular filtrate. Azotaemia may precipitate ammonia intoxication and coma in cirrhotic patients. Such cases of encephalopathy respond favourably to a reduction in blood urea nitrogen, which occurs with the return of kidney function. Kidney function is restored by a properly functioning PV shunt.

PROGNOSIS OF ASCITES

Ascites is a problem extending beyond its effect on the patient's appearance. It is a sign of approaching end-stage liver disease with a poor prognosis. Treatment of cirrhosis has advanced over the last 30 years, and there have been improvements in nutritional supplementation, control of massive oesophageal varices and hepatic coma, and the use of salt restriction and diuretics in controlling ascites. Even so, mortality rates from haemorrhage, ascites, hepatic coma, renal failure, and infection in cirrhosis reported by Garceau et al.[21] in 1963 were similar to those reported 20 years previously by Ratnoff and Patek[2].

Cure of massive ascites is unlikely unless the liver disease is reversible, as in the cases of ascites associated with acute viral hepatitis. Newly introduced therapeutic measures have always attracted initial attention, but have failed the test of time. Aggressiveness and zeal in the medical treatment of ascites has tended to shorten rather than prolong patient survival.

SEQUELAE OF ASCITES

Some of the pathophysiological disturbances that result from ascites have already been discussed. The profound changes in kidney function have been outlined, and it has already been indicated that renal failure is the usual cause of death in cirrhotic ascites.

Malnutrition

Extensive ascites causes malnutrition that is not secondary to liver damage but to ascites itself. When the Budd–Chiari syndrome is induced by caval occlusion in dogs with normal liver function, they undergo marked wasting of subcutaneous fat and eventually of protein mass. A diminished food intake produces an inversion of the plasma protein albumin-globulin ratio similar to that which is encountered in cirrhosis. In essence, this situation represents an end-stage in starvation (Figure 2). In the terminal phase of starvation the urinary nitrogen output suddenly increases, indicating that all the subcutaneous fat which was available for energy needs has been fully utilized and is now exhausted, making it necessary for the body to metabolize protein for its energy needs. It is an autocannibalistic stage which heralds that the end is near. Because some patients with ascites suffer from caloric malnutrition, it is evident they may also be in the end-stages of starvation, possibly merely due to a diminished food intake. Patients suffer a loss of vitality and have a marked predisposition to infection.

Mechanical sequelae

Hydrothorax

There are mechanical sequelae arising from the pressure and thinning of the abdominal wall. One of the most serious is the development of

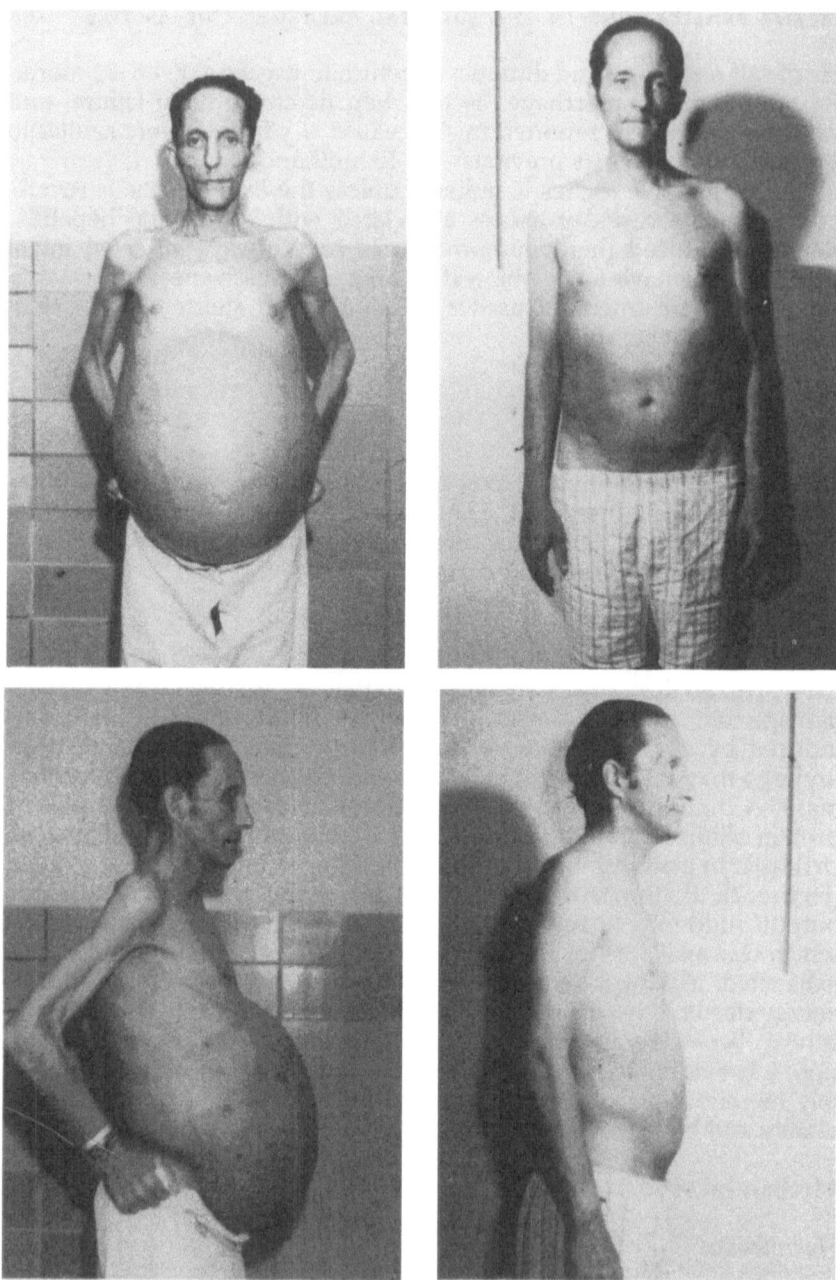

Figure 2 A malnourished thin patient is shown prior to PV shunt and 1½ years following the shunt. The patient is well 6 years after the shunt

hydrothorax, which occurs in 5.4% of cirrhotics with ascites[22]. Before the development of the PV shunt, patients in this condition seldom left the hospital alive.

The hydrothorax is caused by a small defect in the diaphragm separating the peritoneal cavity and the thoracic cavity. This usually occurs on the right but may occur on the left. Tiny holes sometimes occur in the diaphragms of normal people. This explains why pneumothorax has occasionally occurred after the Fallopian tubes were insufflated with air as a test for tubal patency.

Usually these small defects are covered with a thin layer of pleuroperitoneal membrane. The peritoneal fluid pressure causes a bleb to form on the superior surface of the diaphragm. This bleb eventually ruptures, producing a one-way valve that pumps fluid from the peritoneal cavity into the thorax. Radio-iodinated albumin injected into the pleural cavity does not appear in the peritoneal cavity, but when injected into the peritoneal cavity does appear in the pleural cavity[22] demonstrating the one-way nature of the fluid flow.

For many years these blebs were not recognized at autopsy. It was only when autopsy was done while maintaining high intraperitoneal water pressure that leaks through the diaphragm were recognized through the opened chest[23]. Ascites is frequently but temporarily alleviated with the drainage of the fluid into the chest: a new absorptive surface is provided for fluid absorption and a new equilibrium is established.

There is a great temptation to insert a chest tube but this should be avoided. The diaphragmatic defect is often small so that movement of fluid from the abdomen into the chest is slow even with the pumping action of the thorax. It must be assumed, however, that a patient with hydrothorax and ascites has a communication rather than two diseases. The treatment is emergency PV shunt followed immediately by thoracentesis. The chest should be tapped dry and a sclerosing agent injected into the thorax to stimulate attachment of visceral and parietal pleura. Both nitrogen mustard and tetracycline (250–500 mg) injection have had good success in our experience. It is futile to inject sclerosing agents before a PV shunt and may even be detrimental. In some patients the hydrothorax requires repeated thoracenteses preoperatively, yet the ascites is so minimal that surgery may have been denied the patient on this account.

Hernia

The increased peritoneal pressure is responsible for another mechanical sequela, hernia. Umbilical hernias are commonplace in ascites patients and should be repaired only after the ascites has been properly treated.

Occasionally these hernias reach sufficient size to rupture. Such patients usually die from peritonitis and must be treated quickly if they are to survive. On an emergency basis, a PV shunt is inserted after all ascitic fluid has been aspirated. The hernial sac and ulcerated skin are excised and the wound is irrigated with gentamycin and closed. Systemic antibiotics are administered and definitive hernia repair is postponed until a later date.

Spontaneous peritonitis

Spontaneous peritonitis occurs in 8% of cirrhotics with ascites[24].

MANAGEMENT OF ASCITES – PREVIOUS TECHNIQUES

Medical management

Salt restriction is the mainstay of medical management. In the past, when salt restriction and bed rest failed, paracentesis was used to bring about relief. With the development of more potent diuretics, the control over fluid and salt balance has become more complex. However, treatment with diuretics may introduce serious complications: hypokalaemia, hyponatraemia, azotaemia, hepatorenal syndrome, and hepatic encephalopathy. The infusion of albumin to induce diuresis in hypoalbuminaemic patients has met with mixed success[25]. The enthusiasm for reinfusion of ascitic fluid has declined[26]. Only those patients who respond to one or two auto-reinfusions of ascitic fluid with a complete and permanent loss of ascites are helped by this treatment. Those who require continuous reinfusions should be treated by insertion of a PV shunt.

Surgical management

Numerous surgical procedures have been tried for the correction of ascites. These were aimed at increasing absorption of ascitic fluid, at reducing portal pressure, or at diverting ascitic fluid into the venous system.

Increasing absorption of ascitic fluid

Drummond and Morison[27] reported the successful application of omentopexy in 1896. The omentum and anterior abdominal wall were abraded and joined together. Other surgeons elaborated on and changed the procedure, whose rationale was based on the belief that new lymphatic vessels would form, draining fluid away from the peritoneal cavity. Limited success with this procedure forced its abandonment. Others[28] inverted a loop of small intestine (ileoentectropy) to increase the surface area available for absorption of ascitic fluid. Half of a small group of patients died within 3 weeks of the operation, although other patients had temporary relief of ascites.

Reducing portal pressure

Hahn is reported to have studied 60 normal dogs with an Eck fistula[29]. The animals died within a few months if all the portal blood was shunted from the liver into the vena cava. This work emphasizes the profound physiological changes associated with total portacaval shunting. Portal vein blood must go through the liver before entering the systemic circulation; diversion of portal vein blood into the systemic circulation produces a porta-prival syndrome[30]. The experience of Welch and co-workers'[31] series of 40 cases with cirrhotic ascites illustrates that the portacaval shunt operation is complicated by high in-hospital mortality and high late mortality, 32.5% and 75% in Welch's group. Even children with normal livers developed encephalopathy as a complication of portacaval shunting for oesophageal varices secondary to portal hypertension produced by cavernous transformation of the portal vein following umbilical vein thrombosis[32].

Diverting ascitic fluid

Generally insertion of the ventriculoperitoneal shunts useful in treating hydrocephalic patients has been unsatisfactory for treating ascites. Smith *et al.*[33] described using a Holter valve in reporting the first successful drainage of ascitic fluid back into the systemic circulation in a patient with refractory ascites. The lack of success in the use of ventriculoperitoneal shunts stimulated our group to develop a special shunt for ascites and a special procedure for its insertion.

DESIGN REQUIREMENTS FOR THE PV SHUNT

Though the concept that peritoneal fluid could be emptied into the venous system was not new, previous venosystemic shunts were plagued by high failure rates. This stimulated us to do an extensive hydrodynamic study to develop the specifications for a successful ascites valve. Earlier workers had not fully appreciated the fluid dynamics that characterize the intrathoracic negative venous pressure and the high positive pressure below the diaphragm. Thus, the use of off-the-shelf ventricular valves was poorly suited to the specific fluid dynamics of ascites. A valve was specially designed to function indefinitely as a PV with a special operation to allow exact intravascular catheter placement in the thorax. The peritoneal cavity must be connected via this special valve to an intrathoracic vein.

Fluid dynamics set valve requirements

The negative intrathoracic pressure, which varies with respiration, is much lower than the intraperitoneal pressure. The pressure in the inferior vena cava approximates the intraperitoneal pressure while the pressure in large intrathoracic veins is close to the negative intrapleural pressure. The primary consideration for a system designed to transport fluid from the peritoneal cavity to a large intrathoracic vein must take into account these pressure differences.

In the supine position, breathing must provide the propulsive force to move ascitic fluid into the venous system. As the diaphragm descends, intraperitoneal pressure rises and intrathoracic pressure falls. During quiet respiration, this pressure difference reaches 4–5 cm of water. This differential gradient must be able to open the valve and allow ascitic fluid to enter the superior vena cava with little resistance to flow offered by the valve. A forced inspiratory effort against a resistance accentuates the pumping forces. On the other hand, sitting up or positive-pressure breathing closes the valve. Constant positive end pressure breathing (PEEP) will maintain the value in the closed position (Figure 3).

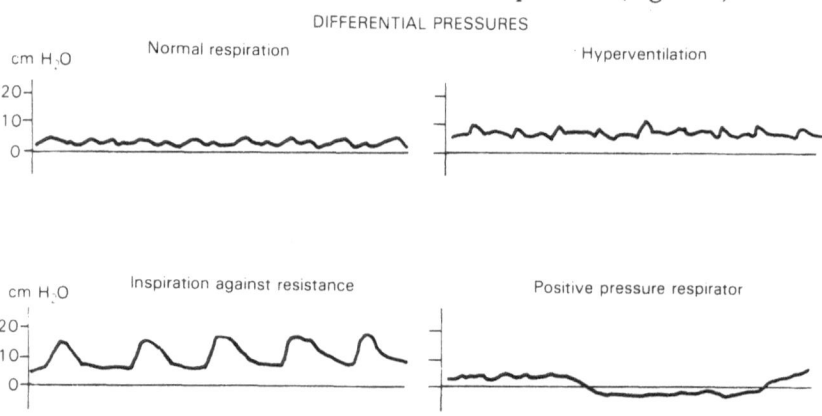

Figure 3 The pressure difference between the peritoneal cavity and the intrathoracic vena cava is widened during inspiration when the descent of the diaphragm raises the intrathoracic pressure. Forceful respirations accentuates the difference and inspiration against resistance further exaggerates the pressure differential. PEEP or positive pressure breathing raises the intrathoracic pressure and prevents the valve from opening

Valve design principles

To insure patency, the valve must remain competent at all pressures. Low pressure competence is difficult to achieve but of primary importance if failure is to be avoided. With the slightest backflow of blood into the venous tubing, clotting will occur and occlude the tubing. The valve must be able to maintain an ascitic fluid–blood interface at the tip of the tube in the vein. The valve must be pressure-sensitive and remain in the open position only when the gradient tension between the abdomen and central venous pressure rises above 3 cm of water. When the central venous pressure is excessively elevated, the valve will close and prevent further flow of ascitic fluid and thus prevent pulmonary oedema and fluid overload. A valve which opens at 3 cm of water introduces a new homeostatic mechanism to allow the proper amount of inflow before closing. A flow-activated valve such as a slit valve does not introduce a new homeostatic pressure system and can bring about fluid overload. The design of a valve which proved best was a disc-type valve where the disc covered a large valve orifice. The disc was suspended over a large polypropylene orifice by silicone rubber struts (Figure 4).

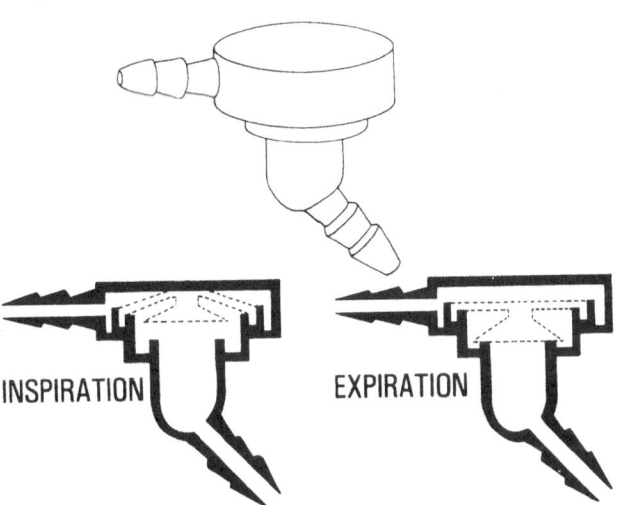

Figure 4   The valve is shown in cross-section. The body of the valve is made of rigid polypropylene. It suspends a bell-like silicone disc over a large orifice. Increased abdominal pressure lifts the disc and opens the valve bending the silicone struts

Valve materials and quality control

Silicone rubber is at present the best though not the ideal material to insert into large blood vessels without risk of causing a high incidence of vascular thrombosis. The successful use of silicone rubber in pacemaker leads and intravenous alimentation has provided broad experience. Although the valve itself is made of silicone, the housing is made of rigid polypropylene that maintains its shape and does not adhere to silicone rubber in the way in which silicone rubber sticks to itself. A spring-loaded ball valve was tried but offers too high a resistance to flow if the ball is small enough to insure low pressure competence. The valve must be enclosed in a rigid housing to avoid temporary incompetence that might occur from distortion of an elastomeric casing.

The valve itself must be detachable from the venous tubing. This is a requirement in the event that the valve fails but the venous tube remains patent. In such a situation, the only surgery that is necessary is removal and replacement of the valve, with the new valve connected to the old venous tube. This is not possible if the valve cannot be detached from the tubing.

The competence and opening pressure of every valve must be tested electronically by the manufacturer. After sterilization, a representative sample must again be tested to insure that sterilization does not distort the valve and impair its competence. Surgeons should inquire about such testing.

The valve that was originally employed[34] was designed for intraperitoneal insertion. This valve was subsequently modified to be inserted extraperitoneally and was introduced by LeVeen et al.[35]. When intraperitoneal valves are used they must be well fixed to the abdominal wall. Several instances have occurred in which the entire valve system migrated into the peritoneal cavity: this cannot happen with extraperitoneal placement.

The valve must not contain pumping devices of any type. Forceful introduction of fluid into the venous limb has caused fatal pulmonary emboli. It is unwise to attempt to flush the system unless a cavogram is done to rule out the presence of thrombi in the vena cava (Figure 5). Also, if the abdominal collecting tube is blocked, use of a bulb-shaped pump will empty ascitic fluid into the venous system but blood will be drawn back into the bulb. The blood will clot in the bulb and render the entire system nonfunctional (Figure 6), making replacement of venous tubing also mandatory.

The valve must offer low resistance to flow when open, since the differential pressures are small. Some patients need not use respiratory exercises in the late postoperative period since the LeVeen valve has a wide orifice over which the valve seats and its resistance to flow once opened is very low. Large differential pressures are therefore not needed to pump fluid. Slit valves and sometimes ball valves do not share these advantages.

Slit valves with pump chambers are especially unsatisfactory. These valves can be incompetent on hydrodynamic tests for 10–15 s after compressing the chamber unless the direction of pressure is exactly parallel to the slit. This of course will lead to repeated embolization of the lung with small clots and will slowly destroy pulmonary function. The two

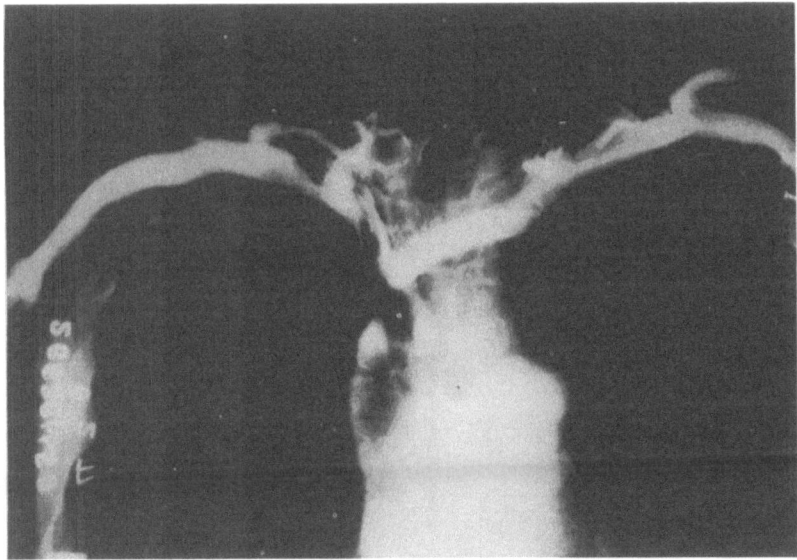

Figure 5 A cavogram performed on a non-functioning shunt shows a large clot in the vena cava. The venous tubing was injected in one such patient and precipitated a fatal pulmonary embolus. Such patients should be treated by thrombolysis or heparin, without attempting to clear the venous tubing of thrombi. See text under the heading 'Valve failure'

sides of a silicone slit valve have a tendency to stick together and do not have precise opening pressures. They require opening pressures, offer high resistance to flow and can become incompetent. Although such valves are commercially available, we abandoned them after animal tests showed them to be unsatisfactory. This was one reason a special ascites valve was developed, rather than adopting existing valves.

If the valve ceases to flow, a systematic investigation must be undertaken to find the cause for failure (see below). Sometimes a fibrin plug is thought to be the cause. Yet such debris must be examined microscopically before a judgment is rendered; often this plug represents an inflammatory exudate. Serious peritonitis will also interrupt flow through the valve. Obviously, neither the patient nor doctor would try to flush infected debris from an occluded valve system if they were aware that the occlusion contained bacteria and was a product of infection.

INDICATIONS FOR INSERTING THE PERITONEOVENOUS SHUNT

The basic and elective indications

The basic indication for insertion of a PV shunt in a cirrhotic patient with massive ascites is the failure of the patient to respond to 2 weeks on a low-salt diet. This indication has evolved from the commonly held

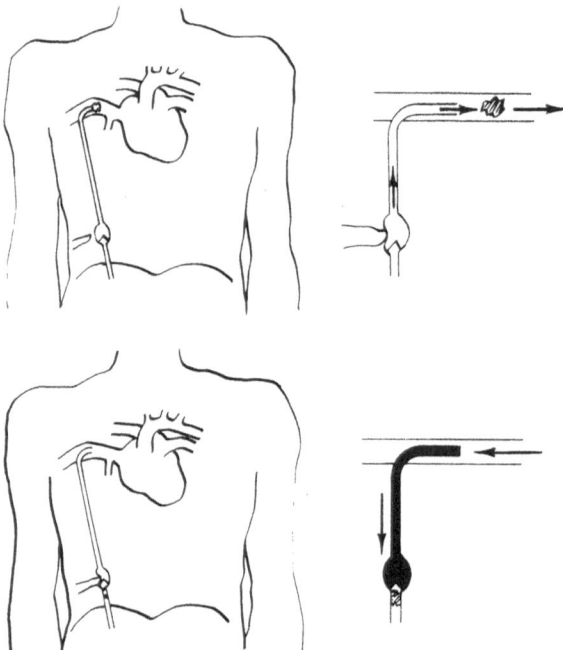

Figure 6   The futility of putting a pump in the venous line is shown. If there is a thrombus in the vena cava a fatal embolus could be dislodged (see Figure 3). If the obstruction is in the peritoneal cavity or in the valve, compression of the bulb will draw back blood rather than suck peritoneal fluid into the bulb. The bulb then becomes hard and incompressible, requiring replacement of the entire valve system rather than just the peritoneal portion

position that only refractory ascites should be considered an indication for insertion of a PV shunt. Studies such as those of Arroyo and Rodes[36] showed an overall in-hospital mortality of 44% in 34 patients with massive ascites that did not respond to a low-salt diet. Observations such as this led to a randomized prospective comparison of medical therapy versus shunt insertion in a group of 22 patients who failed to respond to a low-salt diet. Survival of the surgically treated patients was far longer than that in the medically treated group, where only one patient survived more than a year[37,38]. Survival after insertion of a shunt was so superior to that following medical treatment that the study was interrupted for ethical reasons. The unavoidable conclusion is that the basic indication for insertion of a PV shunt in cirrhotic patients is the failure of the patient to respond to a low-salt diet.

Insertion of the shunt can be recommended for patients who fail to adhere to prescribed therapy, who require repeated admissions to the hospital, or who require repeated paracentesis. Insertion of a shunt and control of ascites may facilitate subsequent intra-abdominal operations such as herniorrhaphy, which may not be treatable unless a shunt has been inserted.

In ascites caused by conditions other than cirrhosis, a PV shunt should be inserted when the ascites is intractable, interferes with nutrition, impairs quality of life or requires repeated paracentesis. These conditions include malignant ascites, chylosis, Budd–Chiari syndrome, nephrogenic ascites, and other rare conditions. Numerous reports have shown that the palliation afforded in malignant ascites is worthwhile and have allayed the fear that the shunt would disseminate malignant cells. Patients with malignant ascites have been made more comfortable and their lives may even have been prolonged. There has not been an increase in the incidence of pulmonary metastases. Most patients with malignant ascites die from cachexia due to ascites rather than from excessive tumour burden. One case of tumour emboli to the lungs with pulmonary distress syndrome has been encountered.

Urgent and absolute indications

Indications for the insertion of a shunt take precedence over relative contraindications. The hepatorenal syndrome is an urgent, absolute indication for insertion of a shunt. Elevated concentrations of blood urea nitrogen and creatinine are indications of impending renal failure that will progress to acute tubular necrosis and death unless a shunt is inserted soon after the condition is discovered. There are numerous accounts in the literature of recovery from hepatorenal syndrome after a PV shunt.

Hydrothorax, as previously described, is a serious complication of ascites since it often seriously compromises respiration and leads to a respiratory cause of death. Because the hydrothorax is caused by a one-way communication between the peritoneal and pleural cavities, the intrapleural pressure eventually rises and a tension hydrothorax can result in a life-threatening mediastinal shift. The intrapleural pressure should be measured before tapping the chest cavity.

Perforation of hernias such as umbilical hernias allows the unsterile outside world to communicate with the peritoneal cavity. This condition is an absolute indication for immediate surgery if death from peritonitis is to be averted.

RELATIVE CONTRAINDICATIONS TO THE USE OF THE PV SHUNT

Hepatic encephalopathy, hepatic coma, alcoholic hepatitis with jaundice, and severe coagulopathy are relative contraindications to inserting a PV shunt. Lack of response to diuretics or the presence of hepatorenal syndrome may be necessary to justify shunt insertion in patients with relative contraindications to the procedure.

Specific criteria for determining contraindications to inserting the shunt include:

(1) Severe alcoholic hepatitis and jaundice with bilirubin levels higher than 8–10 mg/dl.
(2) Encephalopathy, unless secondary to azotaemia.
(3) Preoperative coagulopathy or disseminated intravascular coagulation (DIC) with bleeding which would be aggravated by the insertion of a PV shunt. Such cases can be individualized and may be treatable by epsilon-aminocaproic acid.
(4) Bleeding from oesophageal varices prior to shunt insertion. In this situation patients will rebleed after shunt insertion unless the bleeding has not been from varices, or unless definitive therapy such as portacaval shunt or disconnection has been performed for variceal bleeding. Otherwise, such patients will require procedures both for oesophageal varices and ascites; these have been done simultaneously with success. Although the author feels that the only acceptable portasystemic shunt is one which selectively decompresses oesophageal varices, discussion of this problem is not within the scope of this chapter. In treating cases of acute oesophageal bleeding, the author prefers to perform surgery to interrupt variceal bleeding with simultaneous insertion of a shunt. Four successful operations of this type have been performed[39].
(5) Peritonitis discovered at the time of surgery. The author formerly

believed that occult peritonitis discovered at surgery was a contra-indication for the insertion of a PV shunt. However, such peritonitis has a high mortality not because of sepsis but due to liver failure and renal shutdown. The ascites is markedly aggravated and intensified by the presence of proteinaceous material in the peritoneal cavity. Five patients with peritonitis seen over the past 4 years were treated non-surgically with antibiotics to await resolution of the peritonitis before shunt insertion. All died of liver failure or renal shutdown. Three patients were treated with thorough irrigation of the periton-eal cavity, systemic antibiotics and immediate insertion of a shunt. All of these patients survived. A successful experiment has been done in our laboratory on ascitic dogs with peritonitis and confirms that a shunt can be safely inserted in cases with peritonitis after washing out the peritoneal cavity with antibiotic solution. The reader is referred to the section on infection.

INSERTING A PV SHUNT

Preoperative evaluation and orders

A thorough and comprehensive work-up is designed to determine the extent of derangement in liver function and to determine if cardiac, pul-monary, or renal function is impaired. Physical examination determines if muscle wasting, peripheral oedema, ecchymoses, jaundice, or encephalopathy are present. Studies examining the presence of oeso-phageal varices are appropriate.

Many cirrhotic patients have some type of heart disease[40]. The clinical manifestations of heart disease are often so masked by previous diuretic therapy that the severity of the heart disease is not appreciated pre-operatively. However, the volume expansion brought about by inser-tion of a PV shunt makes this apparent since the ascites may fail to be excreted and the venous pressure unfortunately rises sufficiently to maintain the valve in the closed position. Thus, the patient seemingly has valve failure. The reader is referred to the section on non-functioning shunts for diagnosis of this situation. Patients who are sus-pected of heart disease should receive digitalis preoperatively. All the fluid in the peritoneal cavity must be aspirated and discarded at the time of surgery since the patient will have serious difficulty in excreting even small amounts of fluid.

A preliminary peritoneal tap may be done if there is a question of malignancy or peritonitis; otherwise, a tap is not recommended since it can be followed by infection.

The patient receives a penicillinase–resistant penicillin for a day or two before surgery. Electrolyte imbalances are corrected. The patient is weighed daily and is informed that after the operation he or she will be required to carry out incentive inspiratory exercises while wearing a tight abdominal binder and lying flat in bed.

The surgical procedure

Anaesthesia and fluid administration

Local (0.5% xylocaine) anaesthesia is preferable for patients with cirrhotic ascites. The patient must be sufficiently sedated so as to be spontaneously sleeping but rousable. Tranquillizers and opiates are necessary, and an anaesthetist should be available. Fluids should be administered during surgery. General anaesthesia is possible in the absence of liver failure, but curare should be avoided or counteracted to enable the patient to participate in the patency test near the end of surgery. The valve will not function with the positive pressure breathing required by controlled respiration.

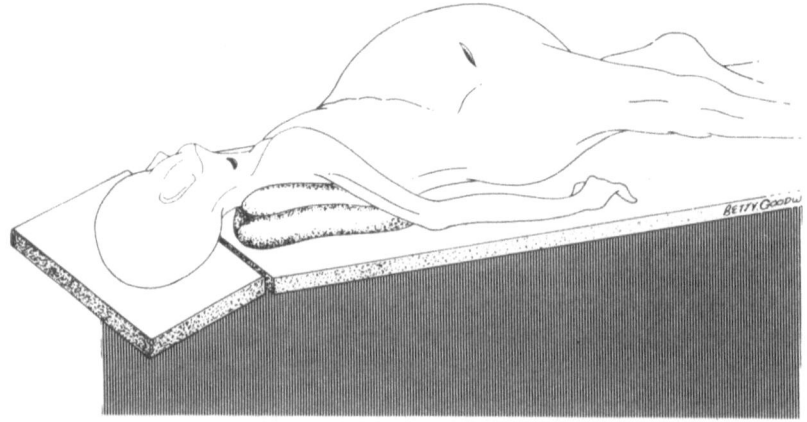

Figure 7   The patient is positioned on the table to slightly extend the neck by elevating the shoulders and dropping the head support. The table is rotated to place the abdominal wound uppermost

Patient position

The patient's position on the operating table is important. The patient is placed supine and a sandbag is placed under the shoulders (Figure 7). The head is extended and rotated slightly to the left, although the head is rotated to the right if the left side is to be chosen for the operation.

The head should not be bent to rest the face on the shoulder, but should be kept in the midline. Bending the head predisposes the venous tube to enter the subclavian vein rather than the vena cava. (See the section on technical failures.) The table should be rotated so that the abdominal incision will be placed uppermost. This avoids spillage of ascitic fluid onto the floor and shoes of the operator.

Abdominal incision

A 2–3 in. (5–7 cm) transverse incision is made over the anterior axillary line and 2–3 in. below the costal margin on the right side (Figure 8). The left side should be chosen if the liver is exceptionally large or if there has been previous right upper quadrant surgery. Previous surgery can obliterate the peritoneal cavity with adhesions and make it impossible to enter the peritoneal cavity with such a small incision. Blind dissection with the finger is hazardous since it can cause bleeding and obstruction of the valve postoperatively.

The exposure is gained through a muscle-splitting incision. The peritoneum, transversalis fascia, and transversus muscle are left as a single layer. This provides greater substance to the layer and facilitates closure of this layer around the stem of the valve since a watertight closure is desirable. A double purse-string, non-absorbable suture is placed with a stab wound in its centre. A pool suction tip is inserted and the peritoneum is emptied of most of the fluid. Cardiac patients and those with nephrogenic ascites cannot excrete large volumes of fluid. Disseminated intravascular coagulation, a postoperative complication whose occurrence is related to the quantity of ascitic fluid introduced into the venous system, has been completely avoided ever since the ascitic fluid has been removed and discarded.

The aspirated fluid should be sent to the laboratory for cytological and chemical studies. The protein content should be determined. Although split products from lysis of fibrin or fibrinogen are usually present, fibrinogen itself is rarely present in peritoneal fluid. If the fluid is turbid, the cause for such cloudiness must be immediately determined. Peritonitis is ruled out by smear and cell count, which reveals peritonitis if the white cell count is more than $1000/cm^3$ with a predominance of polymorphonuclear leukocytes. It is unsafe to introduce turbid fluid into the venous system unless peritonitis has been unquestionably excluded. Turbid fluid containing no polymorphonuclear leukocytes has been encountered in malignant ascites, but the absence of polymorphonuclear leukocytes in this type of case cannot be assumed; absence must be verified by microsopic examination. Such assumption has led to a fatality in one instance.

When large quantities of ascitic fluid are removed at the operating

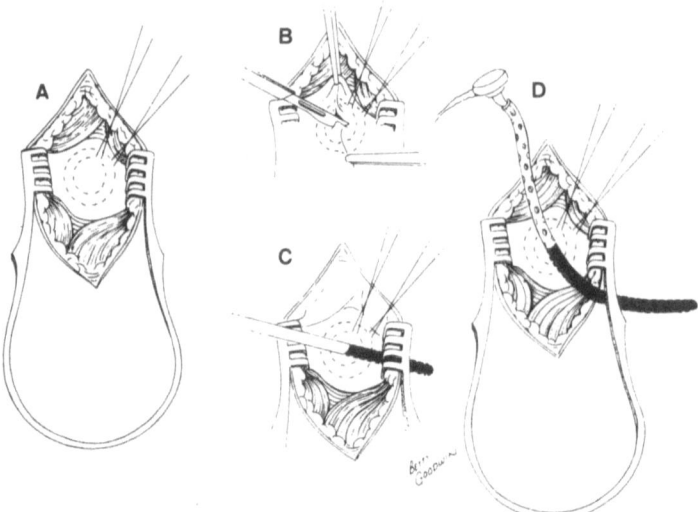

Figure 8 A 2½ in. (6 cm) transverse abdominal incision is made lateral to the rectus sheath and the muscles are split in the direction of their fibres. (**A**) A double purse-string suture is placed in the peritoneum without removing the transversus muscle, and transversalis fascia. (**B**) A stab wound is made in the centre of the purse-string. (**C**) A pool sump suction (abdominal sucker) is inserted into the peritoneal cavity. The fluid is almost completely emptied. If jaundice or turbid fluid is encountered the abdomen should be washed out with Ringers solution containing a small amount of antibiotic. (**D**) After cutting off 3–4 in. (7.5–10 cm) of the perforated collecting tube, the tube is thrust into the peritoneal cavity

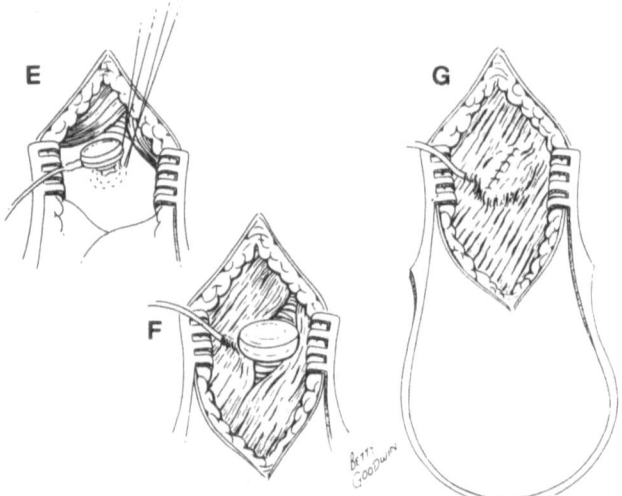

Figure 9 (**E**) The purse string suture is tied around the valve stem. (**F**) The venous tubing is brought into the subcutaneous position through a stab wound in the muscle. (**G**) The muscle is closed over the valve which remains extraperitoneal

table, blood pressure may drop. This is a result of hypovolaemia second-ary to the reduction in the hydrostatic pressure on the splanchnic veins, which allows them to expand and sequester additional blood from the circulation thereby reducing the effective circulating volume. Also, ascitic fluid forms quite rapidly as a result of the reduced intraperitoneal hydrostatic pressure. Plasma and saline should be administered during any extensive removal of fluid to prevent hypovolaemia and to avoid any precipitous fall in blood pressure.

The peritoneal collecting tube should often be shortened to approxi-mately 3 inches (7.5 cm) in length, because it was designed to fit very tall men. Pressure from excess tubing in the peritoneal cavity can cause pain in the lower quadrants, probably due to point pressure on viscera. The collecting tube is inserted into the peritoneal cavity after shortening it. The venous tubing is brought through a stab wound in the muscle, and the incision is closed tightly above the valve with non-absorbable suture after the wound has been thoroughly irrigated with an aminoglycoside antibiotic (Figure 9).

The venous tube should be drawn into the neck wound before final closure of the abdominal wound. Therefore, the incision in the skin and subcutaneous tissue of the neck should be started while the abdominal wall is being closed. Two teams are desired for speed.

Cervical incision

The neck incision is made on the same side as the abdominal incision. Although any large vein can be used to gain access to the superior vena cava, the right internal jugular vein offers the straightest pathway and the lowest possibility of malplacement. The internal jugular vein is exposed between the two heads of the sternocleidomastoid muscle through a transverse skin incision two finger-breadths above the clavicle.

The table is placed in a slight Trendelenburg position to distend the jugular vein before it is explored. The jugular vein should be sufficiently distended that it does not completely collapse on inspiration. This will prevent any sudden air embolus should the vein be inadvertently opened. The vein is cleared for a distance of 3–4 cm.

The venous tubing is brought into the neck at this point. This can be done in several different ways. The author prefers a special tube-passer that should be obtained by hospitals when many shunt insertions or vascular bypasses are performed. The passer consists of a thin, rigid steel tube surrounding a flexible central stylet. The tube-passer is pushed from the abdominal wound into the neck wound (Figure 10). The stylet is grasped and held when it appears in the cervical incision, while the outer rigid tube is removed. This leaves the flexible stylet transversing the subcutaneous tissue. The venous tube is then attached to the abdominal end of the stylet and pulled into the neck. This method is fast, direct and leaves a very small subcutaneous tunnel. This is important since dead space predisposes to infection and accumulation of ascitic fluid alongside the tubing. Bringing the venous tube through the subcutaneous tissue of the chest usually does not require further local anaesthesia if the patient is properly sedated. In females, the breast should be retracted toward the midline and the tube passed lateral to the breast.

An alternative way of bringing the venous tube from the abdomen to the neck begins by passing alligator forceps from the abdominal wound to the neck wound. A heavy suture is pulled down from the neck wound to the abdominal wound (Figure 11). The venous tubing is attached to this heavy suture and the tubing pulled into the neck.[41].

The proper length of venous tubing is measured so that its tip will be just above, or even extended into, the right atrium. The distance from the venotomy site to the second interspace is measured and the venous tubing is cut transversely at that point and the excess discarded (Figure 12). A tapered cut in the venous tube is not recommended. There are fewer complications from clotting if the tube extends into the vena cava or even into the right atrium since blood flow at these points is quite rapid. If the tubing is too short and its tip extends merely into the jugular vein clotting is very frequent. This is the most common error accounting for technical failure.

The venous tubing can be inserted into the jugular vein in various ways. The author prefers to use a newly designed venous introducer fashioned like a pacemaker-lead introducer, but this is not yet commercially available. The simplest method is to ligate the jugular vein with a circumferential absorbable ligature, taking care that the recurrent laryngeal nerve is not included in the tie.

The vein is tied off above and used for traction. A simple loop is placed around the jugular vein below and a longitudinal venotomy is made between the ties. A circumferential absorbable suture secures the tubing to the vein. Alternatively, a simple purse-string can be placed on the surface of the jugular vein through which the tubing can be inserted as shown in Figure 12. The completed operation in schematic is shown in Figure 13.

Patency testing and closure

Before the wounds are closed, 1 cc of methylene blue or indigo carmine dye is injected above the valve with a 25- or 26-gauge needle into the straight part of the tubing. Leakage can develop if the tube is injected at a bend. When the patient takes a deep breath the dye will move out of

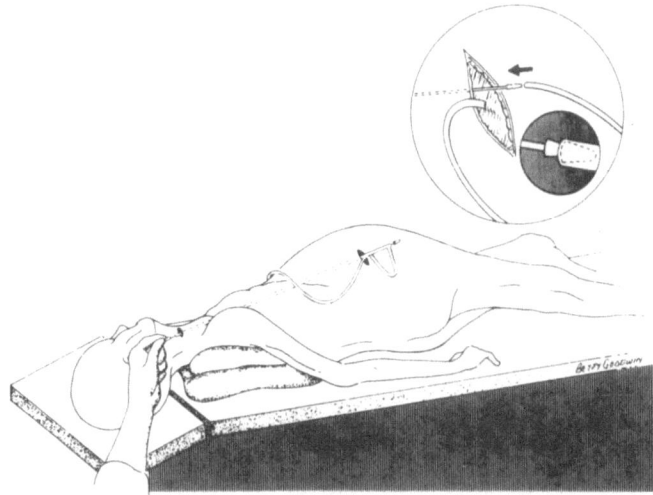

Figure 10   The tube-passer is pushed through the subcutaneous tissue from the abdominal wound to the neck wound. The bullet tip on the flexible stylet is grasped in the neck and the outer rigid tubing is removed, leaving the flexible stylet in the subcutaneous tissue. The venous tubing is attached to a nipple adapter at the end of the stylet and pulled into the neck

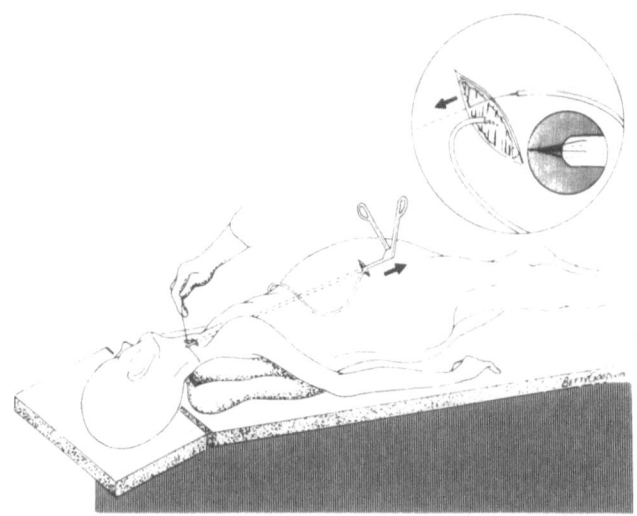

Figure 11   A sigmoidoscopic or bronchial biopsy forceps may be used to pass the venous tubing into the neck. The biopsy forceps is pushed through the subcutaneous tissue from the abdominal to the neck wound. A heavy suture is grasped and pulled down into the abdominal wound. The venous tubing is attached to the suture and pulled into the neck

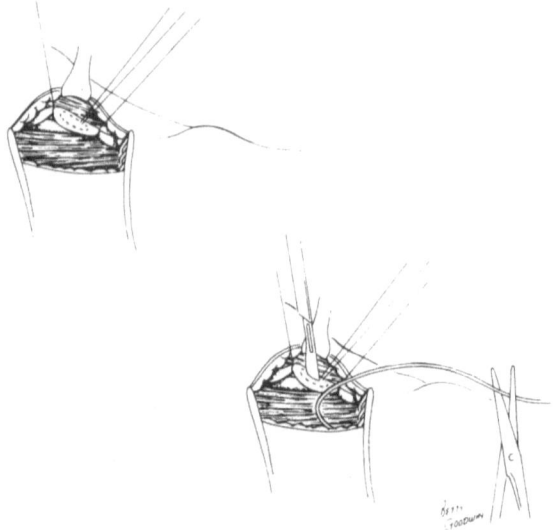

Figure 12   The venous tubing has been pulled into the neck. The jugular vein may be tied off or a purse-string suture applied. The distance from the venotomy to the second inter-space is measured and excess silicone tubing cut off and discarded

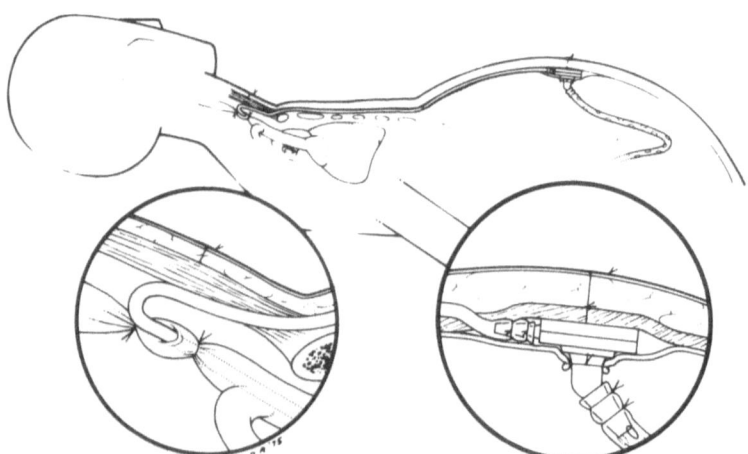

Figure 13   A schematic of the operation is shown. The valve lies extraperitoneally with the collecting tube intraperitoneal. The venous tube extends subcutaneously and enters the internal jugular vein in the neck from whence it extends into the superior vena cava

the tubing and into the vein (Figure 14). This is the last functional test made during surgery, and it is important that the patient be able to breathe spontaneously for it. This explains why curare should be avoided or counteracted if general anaesthesia is used. It may be necessary for the patient to breathe against a forced resistance if the venous pressure is elevated.

If the patency test reveals a working shunt, wounds are irrigated with an aminoglycoside solution (the author prefers Amikacin) and carefully closed. It is imperative that the closure of the abdominal skin wound and skin wound of the neck be watertight. The closure of the skin must be done with utmost care. Any leakage of ascitic fluid can cause fatal sepsis. Leakage should be treated immediately by the placement of sutures. There is often very little or no subcutaneous fat to cover the venous tubing in malnourished patients. Then, even a stitch infection can be fatal. A continuous subcuticular suture of absorbable synthetic material is preferable for the skin closure of both the abdominal and neck wounds. There is no reason for wound sepsis and we have observed none if these precautions are followed. The report of frequent wound infections in the literature is reprehensible and totally preventable[42]. A wound infection has not been encountered in more than 100 consecutive operations in our experience.

Alternative infraclavicular incision for placement of venous tubing

In left-sided placements the venous tubing should be introduced into the left axillary vein. This has been advised by some as a routine on both sides[43]. An incision is made one finger-breadth below and parallel to the deltopectoral groove. The cephalic vein can be avoided by retracting it upwards. The fibres of the pectoralis muscles are split to expose the costocoracoid membrane, which is incised. The pulse of the axillary artery may not be readily palpated until this is done. Although the axillary artery is the key to dissection, it should be palpated but not exposed. The axillary vein lies below and superficial to the artery, and is easily isolated. The distal axillary vein can be ligated without the danger of producing oedema of the arm even if the cephalic vein was unintentionally ligated. No attempt should be made to pass the venous tubing around the bend of the left innominate vein into the superior vena cava. This can cause the tubing to abut against the wall of the contralateral innominate vein and obstruct the outflow, a reason for technical failure. Because the tubing has a radiopaque marker, its position can be ascertained by chest X-ray.

The left axillary vein approach is especially useful for infants and small children. Because the bend into the axillary vein is a gentle 90° curve there is less likelihood of kinking as contrasted to the sharp bend into the internal jugular vein, which is very acute in children.

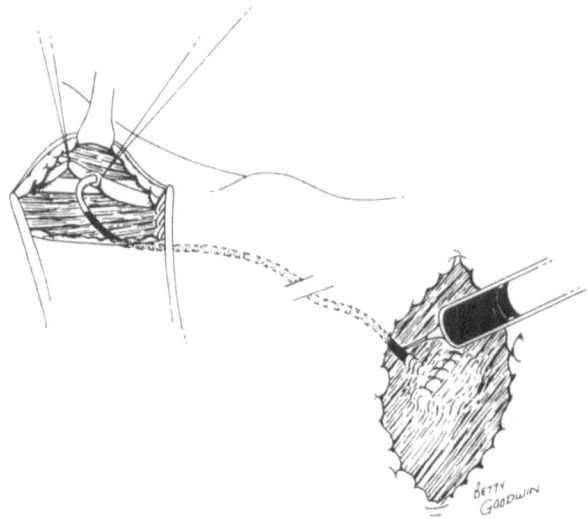

Figure 14   Methylene blue or indigo carmine is injected into the venous tubing with a 25-
or 26-gauge needle. A forced inspiration should empty the dye from the tubing

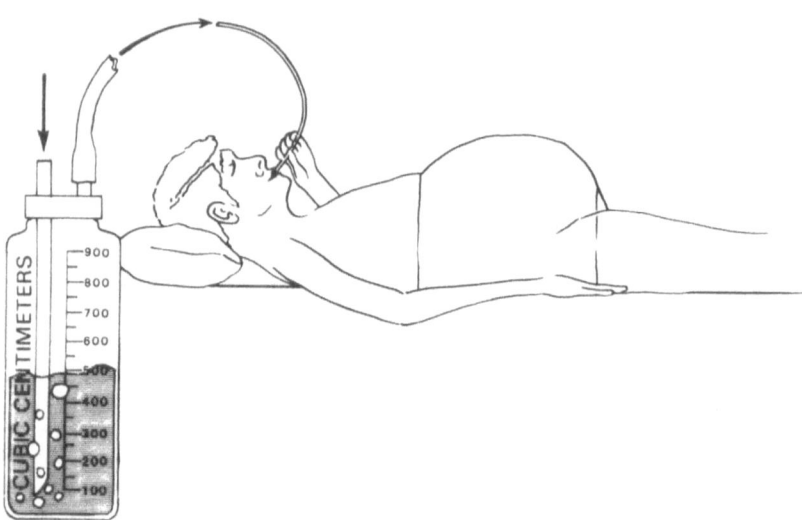

Figure 15   A tube is extended beneath the water level in a bottle and this patient inspires
against this resistance

Shunt misplacements are more likely to occur if lesser veins are chosen as the pathway for the venous tubing to enter the superior vena cava. The internal jugular vein is the straightest path to the superior vena cava. Nevertheless, some patients have no other access vein and the use of smaller veins is necessary. One such route is to pass the venous tube up from below. The saphenofemoral junction on the right is exposed and the saphenous vein ligated. As advised by Traverson and DenBesten[44], the venous tubing is detached from the valve and one end is attached to a water manometer via a three-way valve. The opened tip is advanced up the femoral vein while observing the pressure. It will be about 30 cm of water in the inferior vena cava and rise further on inspiration. As soon as the superior vena cava is reached, there is an abrupt fall in pressure with a further fall on inspiration. The tubing is pushed up 3–4 cm further. At this point, contrast agent is injected into the tubing and an X-ray is taken. If position is satisfactory, the tubing is secured at the saphenofemoral junction. The tubing is then reattached to the valve and implanted in the right lower quadrant. In the author's experience this route is often followed by slight swelling of the leg. Clots are also sometimes visible on a cavogram. Therefore the author does not advise this approach when there is other access via the large veins of the upper body. If the patient is in need of a shunt and no other access is available, the situation has required the insertion of venous tubing directly into the right atrium with complete success in an isolated case.

Postoperative management

Immediately after surgery, 40–48 mg furosemide is administered intravenously four to six times daily to ensure a maximal diuretic response and it is continued until the ascites has disappeared. Most of these patients have severe secondary hyperaldosteronism with marked elevations of plasma renin and aldosterone levels, and might not otherwise clear sufficient sodium chloride. Congestive heart failure may therefore be precipitated if furosemide is omitted. Cardiac patients will require, in addition, digitalis and bed-rest.

On the first or second day after the operation the patient puts on a firm, elastic abdominal binder, which augments intra-abdominal pressure. While the patient is lying supine he breathes vigorously against inspiratory resistance to increase the pressure differential between the peritoneal cavity and the superior vena cava (Figure 15). Any device that increases the resistance to respiration can be used; however, most incentive respirometers are totally unsatisfactory because they are only incentives for deep breathing and do not appreciably increase inspiratory resistance. Inspiration through a bottle with an underwater inlet tube is simple, as is inspiring through firmly woven cloth.

Because ascitic fluid is introduced into the circulation, the haematocrit may fall with haemodilution. If the ascitic fluid is emptied from the abdomen during surgery, haemodilution will be slight. Haemodilution is beneficial since it lowers blood viscosity. On rare occasions, the plasma volume expansion can be so extensive as to cause the haematocrit to fall below 20%, despite adequate diuretic treatment. If there is a large drop in the haematocrit, the patient should assume a sitting position, the abdominal binder should be removed, and intermittent positive-pressure breathing instituted. The haematocrit is easy to monitor and does not carry a danger of infection as does measurement of venous pressure.

During the postoperative period, body girth, urinary output, and body weight should be measured daily and serum electrolytes should be checked frequently (Figure 16). Hypokalaemia and tissue depletion of potassium may be present preoperatively because of the excessive use of diuretics. They can also occur postoperatively secondary to the marked diuresis that characterizes the early postoperative period. Because hypokalaemia and tissue depletion of potassium occur when the patient is still in state of secondary hyperaldosteronism (carried over from the preoperative period), potassium excretion is further enhanced. Therefore, potassium supplements are required until the serum potassium level has reached 4.0 mEq/l. In addition, spironolactone is of value in conserving the body's potassium because it counteracts the effect of aldosterone.

Later on, the hypokalaemia persists because as the patient puts on cellular mass a positive potassium phosphate and magnesium balance is associated with a positive nitrogen balance. This is related to the fact that intracellular electrolytes, potassium, magnesium, and phosphate are stored with the increase in cellular mass. Patients with hypokalaemia are often protein-depleted and should receive a full protein diet. If this causes symptoms of ammonia intoxication, then ion-exchange resins, lactulose, or both can be used to prevent absorption of ammonia from the gastrointestinal tract, allow a full protein diet and avert symptoms of ammonia intoxication.

A progressive, salt-restricted diet can be offered to the patient on the day after surgery. A diet containing 1–2 g salt/day can begin once the ascites has been absorbed and excreted. Diuretics and salt restriction should be discontinued when the ascites has disappeared. In Levy and co-workers' study[45], cirrhotic dogs with ascites were treated with a PV shunt and then placed on a high-salt diet. More salt was retained than excreted, leading to peripheral oedema; but in spite of the positive sodium balance, ascites did not reaccumulate. Thus, a late indication for diuretics in patients who have received a PV shunt is peripheral oedema which is unrelated to previous ascites. Diuretics are not to be used prophylactically to avoid the recurrence of ascites. Although more ascitic fluid may form with the normal use of salt, it may be beneficial to keep flow through the shunt reasonably high.

In the event of bleeding tendencies during surgery, a complete coagulation profile should be obtained immediately postoperatively. Patients with bleeding tendencies often have hypersplenism, resulting in thrombocytopenia and an unrelated tendency to thrombolysis. Disseminated intravascular coagulation was first described in a cirrhotic patient, and cirrhotics are prone to this disorder. Coagulation problems that appear preoperatively will be intensified operatively and postoperatively but have not been a problem if ascitic fluid is emptied from the abdomen and discarded. Bleeding from the wounds should alert the surgeon to the possibility of a consumptive coagulopathy (see the section on complications, below).

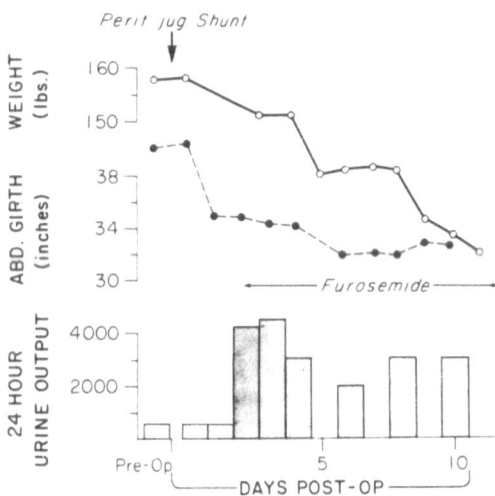

Figure 16   Body weight falls with loss of body girth and enhanced urinary output

RESULTS

Immediate results of shunt insertion

The successful response to the shunt operation is reflected by marked diuresis, weight loss, decrease in abdominal girth, improved urinary secretion, and reduction in plasma creatinine and blood urea nitrogen in patients with hepatorenal syndrome.

Physiological changes brought about by haemodilution with ascitic fluid

Heart

The haemodynamic effects caused by expansion of the plasma volume after a PV shunt were studied in nine patients. The ascitic fluid was not completely removed at the time of surgery in these patients. The cardiac output rose from an average value of 4.7 l/min to 7.1 l/min, an increase of 51%. In this time, the amount of ascitic fluid which had gained entrance to the circulation was sufficient to drop the haematocrit from an average of 39 to 30. This is equivalent to a haemodilution of 24%. If one assumes that the blood volume was really less than 51 in these patients, it means that at least 1250 cc had expanded the plasma volume and perhaps double that amount had expanded the interstitial fluid space (assuming the plasma protein concentration of ascitic fluid was approximately 2.5 g/dl).

Peripheral circulation

Patients with portal hypertension and ascites often sequester a good portion of their plasma volume in the ascitic fluid. The blood volume, although often normal when measured by the indicator dilution method, is really functionally reduced because of sequestration in the dilated venous bed of the splanchnic circulation. Such patients have a compensated functional hypovolaemia, as evidenced by peripheral vasoconstriction producing marked skin pallor. The peripheral veins are often collapsed and venous pressure is low. This situation is rectified by a PV shunt: the enhanced circulatory volume gives colour to the skin and the peripheral veins are filled.

Liver

Would the increased cardiac output raise portal vein pressure sufficiently to pose a threat of variceal rupture in patients with oesophageal varices? This problem was investigated in both dogs and humans.

The portal system of dogs was embolized with silicone oil to raise the portal vein pressure. At this point, plasma or dextran was infused to expand the plasma volume. Cardiac output rose but portal vein pressure dropped 1 cm for every 3.7-point drop in the haematocrit. The hepatic wedge pressure dropped a similar amount in patients after a PV shunt. The hepatic wedge pressure dropped from 25 to 16 (56%) in nine patients with PV shunts while cardiac output increased 51%.

Why should a fall in the haematocrit reduce portal vein pressure? The formula, blood pressure = resistance × flow is well known. Most physicians assume that resistance can only be lowered by vasodilatation and rarely take into account the possibility of decreasing the viscosity of blood[77]. Blood viscosity is primarily related to the concentration of erythrocytes. Compared to distilled water, the viscosity of plasma is about double. However, the viscosity of whole blood increases proportionally to the increase in red blood cell content and rises to 16 times that of distilled water at a haematocrit of 45 with low flow rates. Blood is less viscid at rapid flow rates, but in the obstructed venous system of portal hypertension the flow of blood is sluggish, contributing further to its viscosity. Aggregation of red blood cells produced by high plasma fibrinogen concentrations further increases blood viscosity.

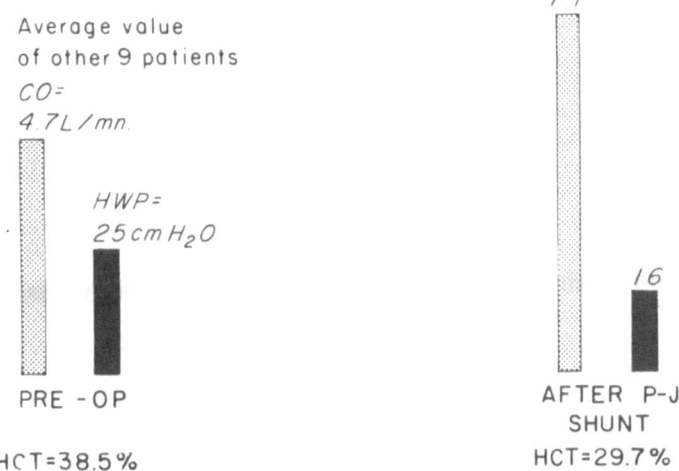

Figure 17   The effect of haemodilution on cardiac output, haematocrit, and hepatic wedge pressure is shown. In spite of the increase in cardiac output, wedge pressure fell after PV shunting

Haemodilution, even though accompanied by an increase in cardiac output beyond that which might occur with isovolemic haemodilution, does not elevate portal hypertension in cirrhosis during the acute haemodilution (Figure 17). Nonetheless, cardiac output remains elevated, the red cell mass is replenished with time, and the patient eventually does have an increased blood pressure, cardiac output and haematocrit in the later course of his recovery. This will cause an increase in portal hypertension, and rupture of oesophageal varices becomes a possibility.

In patients who have never bled, the incidence of bleeding from an oesophageal varix has not been significantly increased by a PV shunt as compared to patients with portal hypertension without a PV shunt. However, if the patient has had a previous bleeding episode, the chances that he will rebleed after a PV shunt are exceedingly high (about 85%). Our preference is for non-shunt surgery to obliterate varices at the time of a PV shunt[39].

Kidney

The measured renal blood flow in patients with hepatorenal syndrome (HRS) can also increase as much as 20 times after a PV shunt. Glomerular filtration rate increases significantly, as does urinary output. These changes are initiated by haemodilution which can increase perfusion even in the very vasospastic kidneys of HRS. The vasospasm, induced in experimental animals by injection of norepinephrine into the renal artery, is followed by fatal renal shutdown. Nonetheless, the majority of animals can be saved by haemodilution. The kidney possesses internal autoregulatory mechanisms for blood flow, controlled by the composition of the tubular urine. The initiation of urinary flow by haemodilution may, therefore, have effects other than those due solely to blood viscosity. Angiotensin concentration in peripheral blood has been shown by Laragh to be influenced by renal perfusion[20].

Although haemodilution by volume expansion does lower blood viscosity, the effect on volume receptors is also contributory to the changes in renal function. Total immersion of the body (except the head) in a bath tub of water rapidly expands the blood volume by compression of veins. This leads to natriuresis and increased renal blood flow in normal persons. It does the same in cirrhotics with ascites and tends to counteract sodium retention and hyperaldosteronism. Plasma renin levels are also lowered by immersion. This strong control of physiological mechanisms in normal persons elucidates some of the responses that were observed in cirrhotic ascites[19]. Since volume expansion by simple immersion can correct the pathophysiology observed in ascites, it is logical to assume that a reduction in effective blood volume is the cause for the abnormal renal function so long considered the renal basis for ascites. It also shows that diuretic therapy for ascites, by reducing the effective volume, further promotes the pathophysiology leading to salt retention. One can thus understand the dramatic improvement that takes place in renal physiology once volume has been expanded by a PV shunt.

The severe renal vasospasm which raised renal vascular resistance in HRS is partly overcome by lowering blood viscosity. Reduction of the haematocrit under such circumstances will lead to increased oxygen delivery to the tissue. HRS progresses to acute tubular necrosis, which many consider secondary to renal anoxia.

PV shunts, by lowering the haematocrit, will increase cardiac output. Volume expansion will reduce the concentration of vasopressors. This increase in cardiac output with lower resistance is responsible for greater oxygen delivery to the tissues even though the oxygen-carrying capacity of the blood may fall with the reduction in the blood haemoglobin concentration[39].

Long-term results of shunt insertion

Consideration of the results of shunt insertion has to be placed in context: patients who receive shunts that cure their ascites still have serious underlying disease that is going to affect their survival even though ascites is relieved. In most cases, the underlying disease is of the liver, such as alcoholic cirrhosis. In cases of malignant ascites, it is cancer.

Results from many groups have confirmed the usefulness of the shunt, at least for short-term benefit. Our colleagues, Wapnick et al.[38], demonstrated the superiority of the use of the PV shunt for ascites over conventional medical therapy in a randomized, prospective matched-pair study. Indeed, the study was terminated and attempts to provide medical therapy were abandoned as shunt insertion showed its superiority. Prospective studies from Toronto[42,46], and by Berkowitz et al.[47] and Ansley et al.[48] also demonstrated the value of shunt insertion. Our group[49] and another group[50] demonstrated the value of inserting the shunt when patients had HRS. Various groups[35,51-54] found the shunt helpful in improving the quality of life in patients with malignant ascites.

COMPLICATIONS: SHUNT FAILURE

Shunt failure is the most common postoperative complication. It becomes evident when the shunt fails to fully relieve ascites or ascites returns after a brief interval. Shunt failure can be immediate (no relief of ascites) or early (recurrence of ascites after a few days of relief). The time sequence is of some importance since the causes of early failures are usually different from the causes of late failures. An understanding of the basis of shunt failure helps provide an understanding of the basis of shunt patency tests, discussed later.

Immediate shunt failure

Initial shunt failures occur because of technical errors, because of inadequate postoperative care and because some patients have concealed cardiac disease and expansion of the extracellular fluid volume brings on heart failure.

Technical failures

Malplacement is a common cause of early and immediate failure, but the surgeon is usually unaware this has occurred or may not admit this possibility. One common malplacement occurs during introduction of the venous tube into the subclavian vein rather than into the vena cava. This may be caused by bending the patient's neck in such a fashion that the left side of the face is in apposition with the left shoulder. This straightens out the angle between the subclavian vein and the internal jugular vein, making it easier for the tube to go into the subclavian vein than the vena cava (Figure 18). When the cervical incision is made on the right side (the usual procedure), the head should be *rotated* slightly to the *left*, so that the right side of the face is uppermost but the neck must remain straight and the head must not be flexed laterally. Because the tube contains a radiopaque stripe, such malplacement can be diagnosed from an X-ray of the chest.

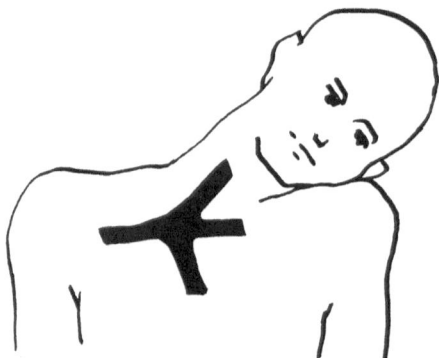

Figure 18   Lateral flexion of the head can open the angle between the internal jugular vein and the subclavian vein so that it is almost a straight line, making it easy for the venous tube to enter the subclavian vein

Another very common malplacement occurs when too little tubing is introduced into the jugular vein. The tip does not reach the superior vena cava and the flow of blood around the tube in the jugular vein is insufficient to prevent clotting. A clot often forms in the stump of the jugular vein, but this is of no consequence if the tip extends down to the superior vena cava. Too much tubing can be introduced and patients have been referred to the author with a non-functional shunt where the tube extended far into the inferior vena cava. Such a case has been reported by Holcroft et al.[55]. Also in certain instances the tubing has been found extending into the pulmonary artery or right ventricle.

Malplacements occur more frequently when the external jugular vein is chosen as the entry point for the venous tubing; the tube often goes out into the arm instead of into the chest (Figure 19). The external jugular vein often enters the subclavian vein at a very acute angle and it may be impossible to direct the venous tube in the proper direction. This is the main reason why this entry point should be avoided. Kinking in the vein has also occurred, with the passage of a loop into the chest.

In every instance of shunt insertion, the surgeon must avoid both kinking the tube and perforating it with a needle. Kinking may occur at the abdominal end near the valve but a functional test on the table rules out this possibility. If the tube is inadvertently perforated with, for example, a large needle during closure, it leaks ascitic fluid and allows blood to flow backwards toward the hole. Clotting then occurs in the tube tip (Figure 20).

Inadequate postoperative care

After surgery, patients must receive sufficient furosemide to produce maximal diuresis since patients have marked hyperaldosteronism and will otherwise retain salt. On the second or third postoperative day breathing exercises are started, with the patient lying flat on his back. A tight elastic binder is applied around the abdomen and the patient inhales against resistance. The binder increases the intra-abdominal pressure and raises the pressure gradient between the peritoneal cavity and the central venous system. Administration of furosemide and respiratory exercises are needed to empty the abdomen while the abdominal wall is flaccid and may or may not be required when abdominal tone returns. Many patients who have been referred for shunt failure were never instructed in the use of abdominal binders and breathing exercises, yet this is an essential aspect of early postoperative care.

Concealed cardiac disease

The patient with ascites can have a concealed cardiac problem. Cohn has pointed out that cirrhosis is commonly associated with cardiac disease[40]. Because the functional extracellular and intracellular fluid spaces become so depleted in the medically treated cardiac patient,

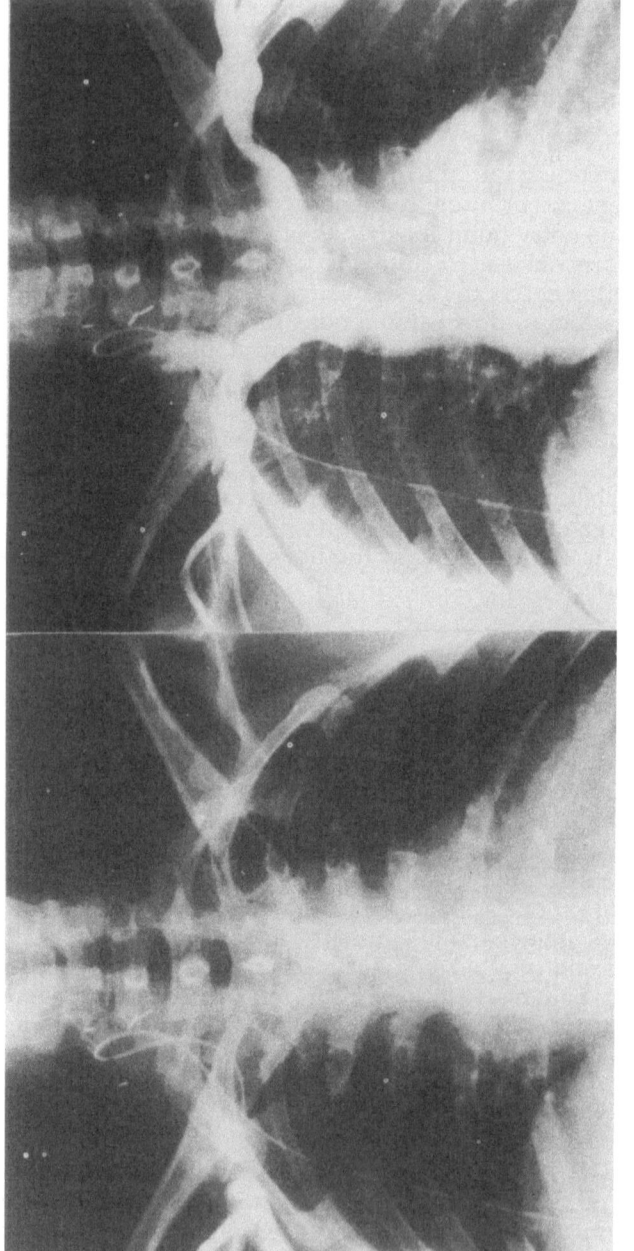

(A)

(B)

Figure 19 (A) The radiopaque stripe on the tubing makes it easy to recognize malplacement. The tube has entered the subclavian vein. (B) The position of the tubing is further demonstrated by angiography. The point of entry is the external jugular vein

cardiac decompensation may be unrecognized. As ascitic fluid expands the extracellular fluid space, cardiac insufficiency may become apparent. Such patients sometimes lose weight initially after shunt insertion, but the diuresis is inadequate, and haemodilution as evidenced by a fall in haematocrit does not occur. Surgeons have told us of cases in which the neck was re-explored a day or so after shunt insertion and in which the venous tube, when removed from the vein, dripped ascitic fluid. Yet haemodilution did not occur on insertion of the tube back into the vein. This is an important reason for testing the flow through the venous tubing at the table by the injection of dye into the venous tubing above the valve.

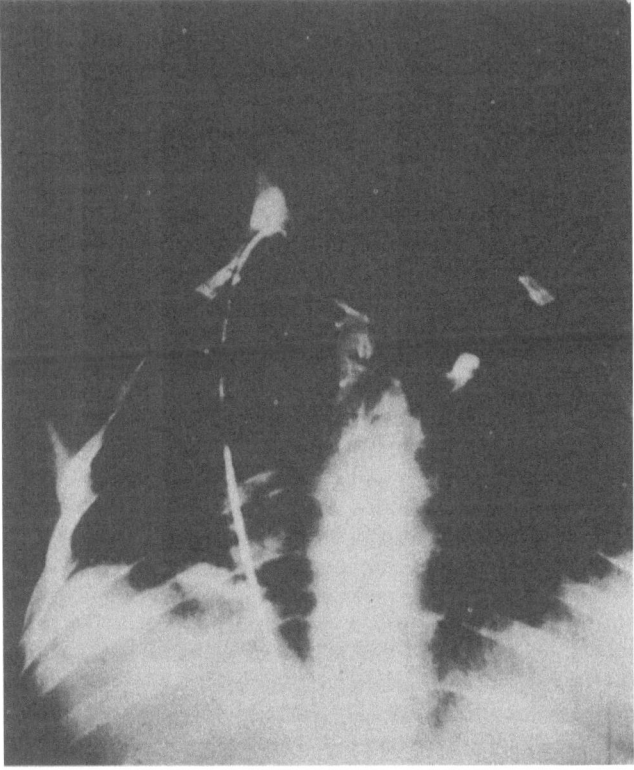

Figure 20 Shuntogram showing extravasation of dye from large puncture wound of venous tubing, allowing reflux of blood into tip of tubing

Patients with normal cardiac function do increase cardiac output in response to the infusion of ascitic fluid. Heart rate may not increase, but instead there is an increase in the stroke volume. Cardiac patients reach or exceed their maximal cardiac response with a small amount of volume expansion. Therefore, central venous pressure rises without a concomitant increase in cardiac output, demonstrating an abnormally high auricular pressure to cardiac output relationship (Starling curve). The cardiac response to a fluid load may be the only method to distinguish such patients preoperatively. In our experience an abnormal Starling curve has identified cardiac patients at risk, but this is difficult to institute as a routine test.

Infusion of ascitic fluid into cardiac patients will often decrease cardiac output, in contrast to infusion into normal persons. If the ensuing cardiac failure is predominantly right-sided, the central venous pressure will be raised. If the ensuing cardiac failure is left-sided, then pulmonary wedge pressure will rise and pulmonary oedema can occur. In our experience, central venous pressures in the range of 30 cm have been encountered in such patients without other significant evidence of cardiac failure. Schwartz and Miller[78] have also encountered such patients and advise a puncture of the venous tubing somewhere along its course to measure venous pressure. Pressure fluctuation during respiration is another indication of tube patency.

Cardiac insufficiency in patients with ascites can be diagnosed by recording central venous pressure with the patient in the reclining position, and can be suspected from observing pulsating neck veins. It is often apparent on chest films (Figure 21). Known cardiac patients can, nevertheless, be satisfactorily treated with a PV shunt. Removal of nearly all ascitic fluid at the beginning of the procedure (now recommended as a routine) can avoid cardiac overload and the problem of excreting large quantities of water and salt. During surgery, injection of a dye into the venous tubing will verify the flow of ascitic fluid into the vein. Treatment of heart failure after surgery for PV shunting must include bed-rest, digitalis, diuretics, and possibly paracentesis. These patients must perform respiratory exercises with suction bottles every 2 h for at least 5 or 10 min to avoid reaccumulation of ascites. Otherwise the differential pressure between the superior vena cava and the peritoneal cavity may not be adequate to empty fluid from the abdomen. Recall that shunt function depends on pressure differences between the peritoneal and intra-thoracic cavity; central venous pressures in cardiac patients, who may be asymptomatic, can be so elevated that the valve is prevented from opening.

Clotting in the vena cava is more prone to occur in cardiac patients with extremely high venous pressures because movement of fluids through the shunt is sluggish. Venous stasis can exist around the tube,

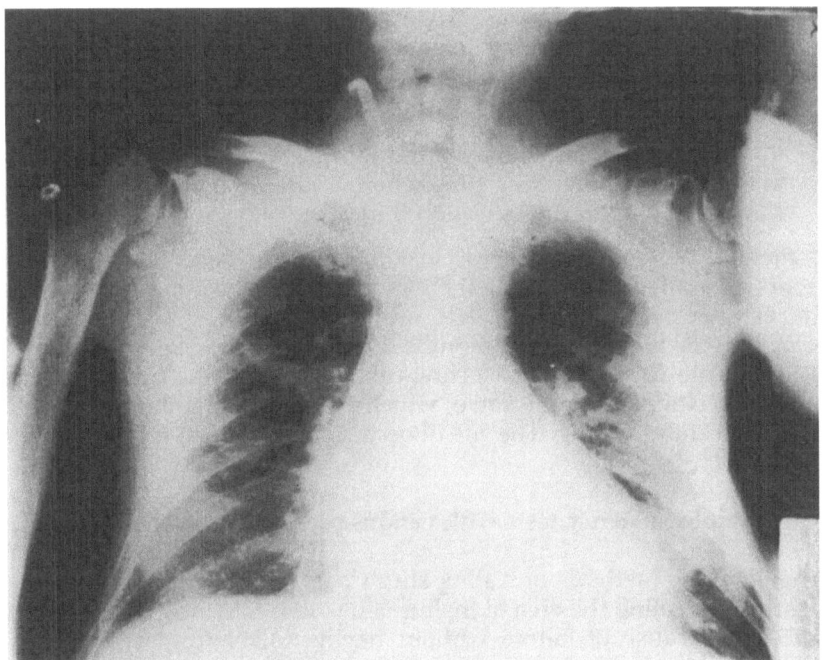

Figure 21 Shuntogram done on a patient who turned out to have concealed cardiac disease. The contrast agent took a long time to leave the tubing and some.is still present. The chest X-ray is characteristic of congestive heart failure

and stasis often initiates clotting[56-58]. If patients sit up continuously after surgery, stasis can initiate clotting.

Cardiac patients can be relieved of their ascites, but they require considerable attention and effort. Even with their co-operation, recovery is prolonged.

Postoperative test of shunt patency

Sometimes the patient fails to respond to the shunt immediately following its insertion and ascites is not relieved. This is the one situation where shunt patency might best be determined by injecting radionuclide into the peritoneal cavity and scanning the chest and abdomen 12 and 24 h later. This test has been described by many groups[59-63].

Clinical history usually makes the diagnosis of shunt occlusion quite obvious, and scanning results after intraperitoneal injection of radioactive nuclide do not add more information than is already known – i.e., the shunt is not functioning. Function must obviously be inadequate because the patient is not relieved of ascites.

Occlusion of the shunt can occur in two general areas:

(1) in the venous tube, with clot around the end, or
(2) at the valve or collecting tube where a foreign body or fat embolus can interfere with flow through the valve.

Immediate occlusion or early occlusion (that which occurs when ascites recurs after a few days of relief) are more likely to be due to occlusion at the venous outlet, whereas late occlusion (that which occurs when ascites recurs after weeks or months of relief) is more likely to be due to failure of the valve or the collecting tube. The collecting tube is less frequently occluded than the valve, which is itself less frequently occluded than the venous tubing. The site of occlusion must be determined radiographically.

Angiographic patency tests with venous pressure measurements

Angiographic methods of testing shunt patency have the advantage of clearly delineating the area of malfunction. This may make it possible to correct the cause of failure without having to remove or replace the entire shunt. Many workers, including Holcroft et al.[55], Stanley et al.[64], Ring and Rosato[65], and Freiman et al.[66] have successfully devised or applied angiographic methods of shunt patency testing. Our preference is for a two-step procedure.

The first step of our procedure is to visualize the superior vena cava by simultaneously injecting both cephalic veins with 60% contrast agent. This cavagram is necessary to ensure that no thrombi are present in the vena cava before the venous tube is injected (the second step). If only one arm vein is injected, a diagnosis of caval clot might erroneously be made from indentation of the dye column produced by blood flow from the opposite side. It is essential *not* to perform the second step of patency testing – injecting the shunt's venous tubing with contrast agent – if there is a vena caval clot. In one patient, injection of the venous tubing in the presence of vena caval clot precipitated a fatal pulmonary embolus. This possibility was the reason we decided not to place a pump in our valve system.

The second step of our procedure must be carried out with a fine-gauge needle, otherwise leakage will occur at the puncture site, permitting the back-flow of blood to obstruct the venous tubing. The puncture hole produced by a fine-gauge needle is of no significance. After the needle has been introduced into the tubing, it is connected to a water manometer (spinal manometer) and the pressure is measured. This will often reveal concealed cardicac dysfunction as venous pressures in excess of 30 cm of water have been encountered in the absence of obvious heart failure. Pressure fluctuations with respiration also denote shunt patency. After the conclusion of the pressure measurements, the tube is injected with contrast agent which should flow freely into the vena cava. If it enters the venous system without pooling, extravasation or accumulation, the venous end of the tube is patent and functional. The patient is then asked to take a forced inspiration with mouth and nose held shut. This manoeuvre should empty the contrast agent from the tubing. If contrast material enters the vena cava freely, but does not empty from the tubing with forced inspiration, the valve or peritoneal collecting tube is obstructed. It should be assumed that this procedure has delineated the problem in the situations described below.

Early shunt failure

In some cases, ascites recurs after a few days of relief. Assuming that the patient has had a rigorous trial of breathing exercises while wearing an abdominal binder, has received adequate bed-rest and has taken furosemide, and that shunt misplacement and cardiac failure have been ruled out, further investigation into the cause of early failure is mandatory. The two-step radiographic procedure is used to diagnose the cause of shunt failure in the same manner as it is used to diagnose the cause of immediate shunt failure.

Blood clots in vena cava causing early shunt failure

Superior vena cava syndrome due to caval thrombosis may occur shortly after shunt insertion because of clotting in the superior vena cava, especially in patients with cardiac disease and caval stasis. Caval thrombosis has occurred, however, as long as 1½ years after operation. Usually the tip of the venous tube is encased by thrombus (Figure 22). On occasion thrombosis in the superior vena cava has occurred with the tip of the tube extending below the clot, so that the ascites remains relieved and the superior vena caval syndrome appears without reappearance of ascites.

A question arises regarding the wisdom of removing the venous tube in patients with thrombosis of the superior vena cava. Two instances of caval thrombosis have been brought to our attention in which the clot dissolved during heparin therapy and ascites abated when shunt patency was restored by clot lysis. Thrombolytic therapy could have produced a similar result, and should be kept in mind.

In some cases the return of ascites is so tense and acute as to require paracentesis. In those cases where the entire superior vena cava is

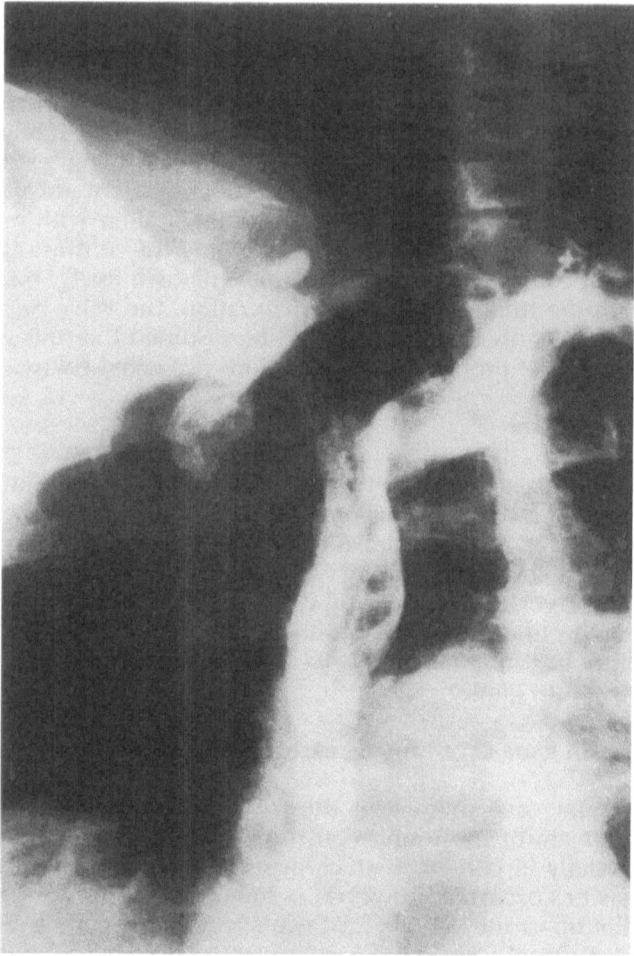

Figure 22 The right subclavian vein is obstructed with large collaterals visible in the shoulder area. The ascending vena cava is filled with clot. There is also some obstruction to the left side

obstructed by thrombosis no access veins are available and other entry to the superior vena cava must be sought. This has been encountered on seven occasions, and the author has threaded the venous tubing up the femoral vein into the superior vena cava. Although this technique proved successful in all seven cases, three patients developed swollen legs after placement of the valve, indicating that this may cause occlusion of the femoral vein, the iliac vein, or both.

Vaida and Laucius[67] reported an instance of early failure because of shunt dislodgement. They could not ascribe the dislodgement to surgical technique, to excessive patient movement during the early postoperative period, or to movement inside the body exerting traction on the shunt. Such cases are extremely rare.

Late shunt failure

Clotting

A clot can form at the tip of the venous tubing at any time. Late thrombosis is likely to be secondary to a bacterial thrombophlebitis originating from a bacteraemia. In such cases, a second venous tube should be inserted through the inferior vena cava to superior cava to relieve ascites. The patient must be placed on heparin and antibiotics. The superior vena caval syndrome should promptly resolve. Eckhauser *et al.*[57] described superior vena cava obstruction 8 months after shunt insertion, and Van Deventer *et al.*[58] described a case of superior vena cava syndrome occurring about 7 weeks after insertion.

If contrast enters the vena cava freely after injection into the tubing but does not empty on forced inspiration, the valve or peritoneal collecting tube is occluded. Similarly, an occluded valve often contains what appears to be fibrinoid material as the apparent cause of the occlusion. This fibrinoid material must be regarded as an inflammatory exudate and it should be irrigated from the valve into a sterile test tube and sent for culture and microscopic examination. Pus cells are frequently present confirm the inflammatory nature of the exudate. When such exudate is discovered in the valve, the patient should be placed on antibiotics and heparin for 2 weeks, even if no organism is identified and pus cells are not present. Since peritoneal fluid does not contain fibrin or fibrinogen but does contain split products, precipitate should not be assumed to be fibrin.

Late infection

Patients with ascites are prone to develop peritonitis, and insertion of a PV shunt does not prevent subsequent peritoneal infection. Such peritonitis invariably causes obstruction of the shunt and accounts for the presence of a white precipitate in the valve. In these cases, the valve should be discarded and replaced, not just disconnected, irrigated, and reconnected. The patients should always be treated with antibiotics and heparin as a precaution against subsequent infection and thrombosis.

The converse is also encountered. Septicaemia can occur in patients who have PV shunts and develop an infection. Patients who develop sepsis with bacteraemia and who have a shunt in place present a dilemma in management. Should the shunt be removed in such circumstances? In cases where the shunt was removed and cultured, no organisms were found and the shunt was not the cause of persistent bacteraemia. In our experience the shunt should not be removed; instead, the patient should be treated with massive doses of antibiotics similar to the treatment of subacute bacterial endocarditis. Several such cases have been encountered and the bacteraemia has responded to antibiotic therapy without removal of the shunt.

It seems reasonable to view patients with PV shunts as similar to those with prosthetic heart valves. Experience with shunted patients who develop bacteraemia after pneumonia or after acute upper respiratory tract infections has alerted us to the precaution that patients with a shunt must be treated with prophylactic antibiotics during any potentially infectious process, including teeth extractions.

Mechanical problems

Mechanical problems can also occur late in the convalescent or post-convalescent course. One patient was so exuberant at being relieved of ascites that he did a handstand. The exaggerated hyperextension of his neck withdrew the venous tube from the vein, and it had to be surgically replaced. Dieckmann *et al.*[68] reported an instance in which a shunted patient continued to do well until she fell at home and dislodged the venous tubing; the condition, confirmed by a dye study, was readily corrected.

OTHER COMPLICATIONS

Disseminated intravascular coagulation

Mild subcutaneous ecchymosis and purpura are frequently seen after shunt insertion. If such bleeding is severe and, in particular, is followed by impaired renal and cerebral function, the shunt should be ligated to avoid further deterioration. In these patients, the peritoneal cavity should be emptied of fluid and rinsed with saline before shunt function is restored. The ascitic fluid is toxic in these cases for reasons that are not adequately identified.

Among the postoperative complications arising from insertion of the PV shunt, disseminated intravascular coagulation (DIC, or consumptive coagulopathy) is among the most serious. This complication has been the subject of a number of reports[48, 69–76].

Although severe, life-threatening DIC is a rare occurrence, mild coagulopathies are frequent, especially with thrombolysis. Most of these occurrences can be handled satisfactorily without interruption of the shunt. Many cases are subclinical and self-limiting, recognized only from the results of laboratory tests without any apparent patient problems. On the other hand, patients who develop severe coagulopathy are recognized first by bleeding from their wounds; they may develop remote ecchymoses with blood in the urine or bleeding from other organ sites (Figure 23).

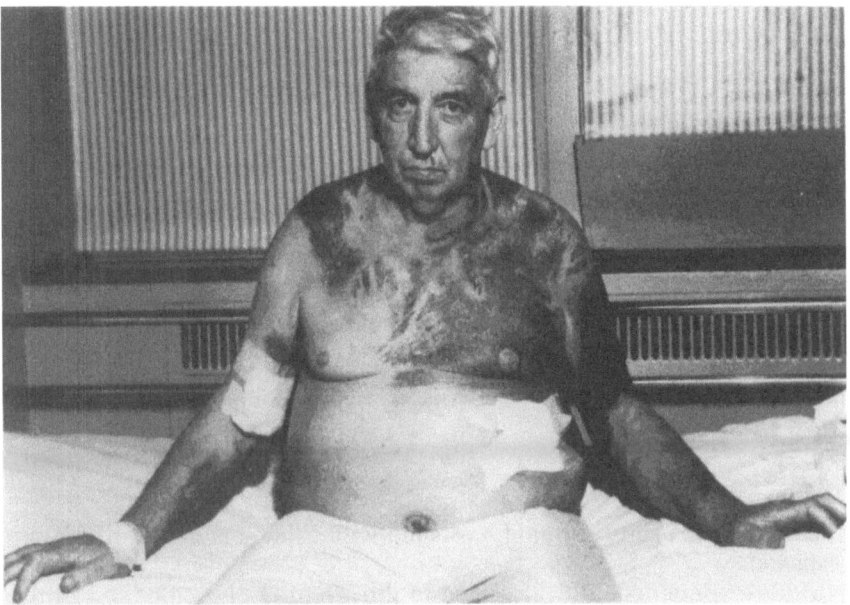

Figure 23 A patient with DIC is shown. Bleeding was present from the wounds and there were ecchymoses over wide areas of skin

A mild coagulopathy can usually be brought under control by treatment with platelet transfusions, fibrinogen, fresh frozen plasma, and epsilon-aminocaproic acid. Heparin may be added to this regimen. Control of the DIC can be observed by following coagulation parameters. The thromboelastograph is extremely useful in following therapy (Figure 24).

If the patient develops proteinuria, anaemia, or shock, the shunt should be immediately interrupted by a small incision over the venous tubing with ligature occlusion until the patient's condition improves.

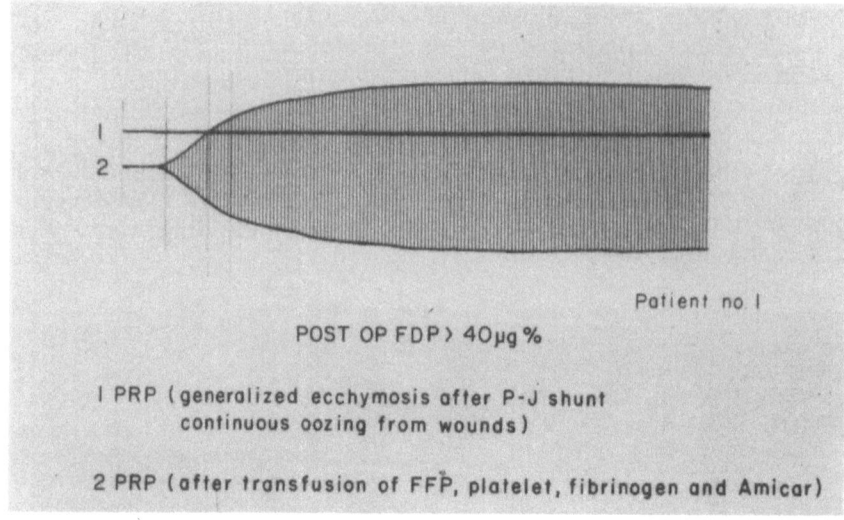

POST OP FDP ⟩ 40µg %

Patient no. I

I PRP (generalized ecchymosis after P-J shunt
continuous oozing from wounds)

2 PRP (after transfusion of FFP, platelet, fibrinogen and Amicar)

Figure 24 Two thromboelastograms are illustrated. These are tracings from an instrument that determines the tensile strength of a clot. The width of the band indicates the tensile strength of each specimen. Platelet rich plasma (PRP) is used to generate the clot. The tracing in specimen No. 1 is a straight line showing that no clot formed and that tensile strength is zero. In specimen No. 2, the same patient has been treated with fresh frozen plasma, fibrinogen and epsilon-aminocaproic acid (EACA) and the test reperformed. The thromboelastogram now appears quite normal with good tensile strength in the clot and no fibrinolysis

The peritoneal cavity should be washed with saline before shunt flow is restarted.

In our experience, DIC is related to the quantity of ascitic fluid introduced into the venous system. Our current technique for inserting the PV shunt calls for aspirating and discarding most of the ascitic fluid at operation, allowing very little ascitic fluid to enter the circulation. In our recent experience with more than 75 consecutive patients whose ascitic fluid was discarded before shunt insertion, DIC has not been encountered. Although the patient may need protein replacement, and although haemodilution is useful in correcting functional renal failure (HRS), it may be safer to perform haemodilution with infusions of plasma and serum albumin, rather than with ascitic fluid. The benefits derived from the reinfusion of a large quantity of ascitic fluid are not worth the risk of DIC.

Our previous description of the technique of inserting the PV shunt[79] did not call for disposal of the ascitic fluid. It is therefore unlikely that

ascitic fluid was discarded in most cited reports of DIC associated with
PV shunting.

The cause of DIC at first was thought to be an endotoxin known to be
present in the ascitic fluid of jaundiced patients. However, DIC has
been encountered after PV shunting for malignant ascites and it is difficult to explain such cases on the basis of endotoxin. If a piece of peritoneum is excised and placed on a fibrin plate, a large zone of lysis is
induced by activation of the plasminogen associated with the fibrin.
This unquestionably represents a secretion of the peritoneal endothelial
cell and accounts for the activation of plasminogen.

Small hernias and accumulations of fluid around the valve and tube
are possible if the closure of the peritoneum and muscle has been
incomplete. The endothelial cells in the peritoneal fluid can form a
closed sac which is not connected to the peritoneal cavity and which is
like a miniature coelomic cavity. These resemble hernias but are really
smooth walled sacs without outlets and their thin wall makes excision
difficult. A sac alongside the tubing can resemble an infant scrotal
hernia.

Fever

Slight fever is a mild postoperative complication which is unassociated
with a leukocytosis and blood cultures are always negative. This
responds to small doses of cortisone and does not last more than 2 or 3
days.

SUMMARY AND CONCLUSIONS

The technical requirements of PV shunt design have been outlined. The
indications for PV shunts, details of insertion and tests for patency have
been described. As surgeons gain experience with the procedure, the
risks to patients have declined. Most complications and shunt failures
are preventable.

The PV shunt is useful for relieving many, if not all, forms of ascites.
Its insertion enhances the quality of life and survival, with less risk and
greater benefit than conventional medical therapy.

Acknowledgment

The author would like to thank Michael S. Altus for editorial assistance
in the preparation of this chapter.

308   FRONTIERS IN GENERAL SURGERY

References

1 Atkinson, M. (1956). Ascites in liver disease. *Postgrad. Med. J.*, **32**, 482
2 Ratnoff, O. D. and Patek, A. J. (1942). The natural history of Laennec's cirrhosis of the liver. *Medicine*, **21**
3 Galambos, J. T. (1979). *Cirrhosis*, p. 96. (Philadelphia: Saunders)
4 Pequignot, G. (1974). Les problemes nutritionnels de la societe industrielle. *Vie Med. Can. Francais*, **3**, 216
5 Grossman, J. A and McDermott, W. V. (1974). Paroxysmal nocturnal hemoglobinuria associated with hepatic and portal venous thrombosis. *Am. J. Surg.*, **127**, 733
6 Retzlaff, K. and Monge J. H. (1973). Polcythemia vera with acute Budd–Chiari syndrome. *Minn. Med.*, **58**, 60
7 Hoyumpa, A. N., Schiff L. and Hefman, E. L. (1971). Budd–Chiari syndrome in women taking oral contraceptives. *Am. J. Med.*, **50**, 137
8 Lower, R. (1697). *Traite due Coeur*, p. 121. (French translation from the Latin), (Paris: Michallet)
9 Fortner, J. G., Kallum, B. O. and Kim, D. K. (1977). Surgical management of hepatic vein occlusion by tumor. *Arch. Surg.*, **112**, 727
10 Atkinson, M. and Losowsky, M. S. (1961). The mechanism of ascites formation in liver disease. *Q. J. Med.*, **30**, 153
11 Chalmers, T. C. (1960). Pathogenesis and treatment of hepatic failure. *N. Engl. J. Med.*, **163**, 23, 77
12 McKee, F. W., Schloerb, P. R., Schilling, J. A. *et al.* (1948). Protein metabolism and exchange as influenced by constriction of vena cava; experimental ascites and internal plasmapheresis; sodium chloride and protein intake, predominant factors. *J. Exp. Med.*, **87**, 457
13 Lieberman, F. L., Ito, S. and Reynolds, T. B. (1969). Effective plasma volume in cirrhosis with ascites. Evidence that a decreased value does not account for renal sodium retention, a spontaneous reduction in glomerular filtration rate (GFR), and of fall in GFR during drug-induced diuresis. *J. Clin. Invest.*, **48**, 975
14 Baldus, W. P., Summerskill, W. H., Hunt, J. C. *et al.* (1964). Renal circulation in cirrhosis: observations based on catheterization of the renal vein. *J. Clin. Invest.*, **43**, 1090
15 Summerskill, W. H. J., Barnado, D. E. and Baldus W. P. (1970). Disorders of water and electrolyte metabolism in liver disease. *Am. J. Clin. Nutr.*, **23**, 499
16 Daly, J. J., Roe, J. W. and Horrocks, P. (1967). A comparison of sodium excretion. *Clin. Sci.*, **33**, 481
17 Epstein, M., Berk, D. P., Hollenberg, N. K. *et al.* (1970). Renal failure in the patient with cirrhosis. *Am. J. Med.*, **49**, 175
18 Schroeder, E. T., Shear, L. and Sancetta, S. M. (1967). Renal failure in patients with cirrhosis of the liver. *Am. J. Med.*, **43**, 887
19 Epstein, M. (1979). Renal sodium handling in cirrhosis: a reappraisal. *Nephron*, **23**, 211
20 Laragh, J. H., Cannon, P. J. and Ames, R. P. (1964). Interaction between aldosterene secretion, sodium and potassium balance, and angiotensin activity in man: studies in hypertension and cirrhosis. *Can. Med. Assoc. J.*, **90**, 248
21 Garceau, A. J., Chalmers, T. C. *et al.* (1963). The natural history of cirrhosis. *N. Engl. J. Med.*, **268**, 469
22 Lieberman, F. L., Hudemura, R., Peters, R. L. and Reynolds, T. B. (1966). Pathogenesis treatment of hydrothorax complicating cirrhosis with ascites. *Ann. Intern. Med.*, **64**, 341
23 Lieberman, F. L. and Peters, R. L. (1970). Cirrhotic hydrothorax, *Arch. Intern. Med.*, **125**,114
24 Conn, H. (1964). Spontaneous peritonitis and bacteremia in Laennec's cirrhosis caused by enteric organisms, a relatively common but rarely recognized syndrome.

Ann. Intern. Med., **60**, 568

25 Wilkinson, P. and Sherlock, S. (1962). The effect of repeated albumin infusions in patients with cirrhosis. *Lancet*, **2**, 1125

26 Levy, V. G., Hecht, Y., Georgacopoulos H. *et al.* (1971). Assechement des cirrhotiques par reinjection veineuse continue du liquide d'ascite concentre. *Ann. Med. Interne*, **122**, 1075

27 Drummond, D. and Morison, R. (1896). A case of ascites due to cirrhosis of the liver. *Br. Med. J.*, **2**, 728

28 Neumann, C. G., Aldie, G. C. and Hinton, J. W. (1957). The absorption of ascitic fluid by means of ileo-entectropy in patients with advanced cirrhosis. *Ann. Surg.*, **146**, 700

29 Bollman, J. L. (1961). The animal with an Eck fistula. *Phys. Rev.*, **41**, 607

30 Warren, W. D. (1980). Reflections on the early development of the porto-caval shunt. *Ann. Surg.*, **191**, 519

31 Welch, H. F., Welch, C. H. and Carter, J. H. (1964). Prognosis after surgical treatment of ascites: results of side-to-side portacaval shunt in 40 patients. *Surgery*, **56**, 75

32 Voorhees, A. B., Caitman, E., Schneider, S., Nicholson, J., Kornfield, D. S. and Prices, J. B. (1973). Portal-systemic encephalopathy in the non-cirrhotic patient–effect of portal-systemic shunting. *Arch. Surg.*, **107**, 659

33 Smith, A. N., Preshaw, R. M. and Bisset, W. H. (1962). The drainage of resistant ascites by modification of the Spitz–Holter valve technique. *J. R. Coll. Surg. Edinburgh*, **7**, 289

34 LeVeen, H. H., Christoudias, G., Ip, M., Luft, R., Falk, G. and Grosberg, S. (1974). Peritoneovenous shunting for ascites. *Ann. Surg.*, **180**, 580

35 LeVeen, H. H., Wapnick, S., Grosberg, S. and Kinney, M. J. (1976). Further experiences with peritoneovenous shunt for ascites. *Ann. Surg.*, **184**, 574

36 Arroyo, V. and Rodes, J. (1975). A rational approach to the treatment of ascites. *Postgrad. Med. J.*, **51**, 5538

37 LeVeen, H. H., Wapnick, S., Guinto, R. and Kinney, M. (1978). Indications for peritoneo-jugular shunt for ascites. *World J. Surg.*, **2**, 367

38 Wapnick, S., Grosberg, S. J. and Evans, M. I. (1979). Randomized prospective matched pair study comparing peritoneovenous shunt and conventional therapy in massive ascites. *Br. J. Surg.*, **66**, 667

39 LeVeen, H. H. and Ip, M. (1980). Alternative methods for the control of variceal bleeding. In Narjarian, J. S. and Delaney, J. P. (eds), *Hepatic, Biliary, and Pancreatic Surgery*, pp. 635–648. (Chicago: Year Book Medical Publishers)

40 Cohn, J. L. (1975). Hepatocirculatory failure. *Med. Clin. N. Am.*, **59**, 955

41 LeVeen, H. H., Wapnick, S., Diaz, C., Grosberg, S. and Kinney, M. (1979). Ascites: its correction by peritoneovenous shunting. *Curr. Prob. Surg.*, **16**, 1

42 Greig, P. D., Langer, B., Blendis, L. M., Taylor, B. R. and Glynn, M. F. X. (1980). Complications after peritoneovenous shunting for ascites. *Am. J. Surg.*, **139**, 125

43 Garcia-Rinaldi, R., Gallagher, M. W. and Crumb, C. (1980). A simplified method for insertion of the LeVeen shunt. *Surg. Gynecol. Obstet.*, **150**, 894

44 Traverson, L. W. and DenBesten, L. (1979). The importance of venous manometry during placement of trans-saphenous peritoneovenous shunts. *Surgery*, **85**, 355

45 Levy, M., Wexler, M. J. and McCaffrey, C. (1979). Sodium retention in dogs with experimental cirrhosis following removal of ascites by continuous peritoneovenous shunting. *J. Lab. Clin. Med.*, **94**, 933

46 Blendis, L. M., Greig, P. D., Langer, B., Baigrie, R. S., Ruse, J. and Taylor J. R. (1979). The renal and hemodynamic effects of the peritoneovenous shunt for intractable hepatic ascites. *Gastroenterology*, **77**, 250

47 Berkowitz, H. D., Mullen, J. L., Miller, L. D. and Rosato, E. F. (1978). Improved renal function and inhibition of renin and aldosterone secretion following peritoneovenous (LeVeen) shunt. *Surgery*, **84**, 120

48 Ansley, J. D., Bethel, R. A., Bowen II, P. A. and Warren, W. D. (1978). Effect of peritoneovenous shunting with the LeVeen valve on ascites, renal function, and coagulation in six patients with intractable ascites. *Surgery*, **83**, 181

49 Kinney, M. J., Schneider, A., Wapnick, S. and LeVeen, H. (1979). The 'hepatorenal' syndrome and refractory ascites. *Nephron*, **23**, 228

50 Schwartz, M. L. and Vogel, S. B. (1980). Treatment of hepatorenal syndrome. *Am. J. Surg.*, **139**, 370

51 Straus, A. K., Roseman, D. L. and Shapiro, T. M. (1979). Peritoneovenous shunting in the management of malignant ascites. *Arch. Surg.*, **114**, 489

52 Raaf, J. H. and Stroehlein, J. R. (1980). Palliation of malignant ascites by the LeVeen peritoneovenous shunt. *Cancer*, **45**, 1019

53 Lokich, J., Reinhold, R., Silverman, M. and Tullis, J. (1981). Complications of peritoneovenous shunt for malignant ascites. *Cancer Treat. Rep.* (In press)

54 Sugarman, H. J., Prager, D., Post, R. M. and Hartzell, Jr. G. W. (1981). LeVeen peritoneovenous shunt for malignant ascites: a preliminary report. (Submitted for publication)

55 Holcroft, J., Kressel, H. Y., Prager, R., Trunkey, D. and Jacobs. R. P. (1976). An experience with a LeVeen ascites shunt. *Arch. Surg.*, **111**, 302

56 Dupas, J. L., Remond, A., Vermynck, J.-P., Capron, J.-P. and Lorriaux, A. (1978). Superior vena cava thrombosis as a complication of peritoneovenous shunt. *Gastroenterology*, **75**, 899

57 Eckhauser, F. E., Strodel, W. E., Knol, J. A. and Turcotte, J. G. (1979). Superior vena caval obstruction associated with long-term peritoneovenous shunting. *Ann. Surg.*, **190**, 758

58 Van Deventer, G. M., Snyder, N., III, and Patterson, M. (1979). The superior vena cava syndrome: a complication of the LeVeen shunt. *J. Am. Med. Assoc.*, **242**, 1655

59 Abdel-Dayem, H. M. (1979). False ascites in a patient with LeVeen shunt detected by intraperitoneal injection of ^{99m}Tc-sulfur colloid. *Clin. Nucl. Med.*, **4**, 1

60 Gorten, R. J. (1977). A test for evaluation of peritoneovenous shunt function: concise communication. *J. Nucl. Med.*, **18**, 29

61 Kirchmer, N., and Hart, U. (1977). Radionuclide assessment of LeVeen shunt patency. *Ann. Surg.*, **185**, 145

62 Rikkers, L. F., Fajman, W. A., Ansley, J. D. and Tarcan, Y. A. (1977). Patency of the peritoneovenous shunt. *Surg. Gynecol. Obstet.*, **145**, 745

63 Williamson, B. R. J., Lambert, M. J., III, Teates, C. D., Bray, S. T. and Wakefield, J. A. (1978). Patency evaluation of a LeVeen shunt using ^{99m}Tc-sulfur colloid. *Clin. Nucl. Med.*, **3**, 343

64 Stanley, M. M., Supan, W. A. P., Greenlee, H. B. and Reinhard, G. F. (1977). Radiographic visualization of outflow tube of LeVeen shunt for ascites: an aid in assessment of portion and function. *Gastroenterology*, **73**, A-50/1248 (abstr)

65 Ring, E. J. and Rosato, E. F. (1979). Assessment of peritoneojugular shunts by direct roentgenographic examination. *Surg. Gynecol. Obstet.*, **148**, 93

66 Freiman, D. B., Ring, E..J., Oleaga, J. A. and Rosato, E. F. (1978). Radiography of LeVeen type peritoneovenous shunts. *Am. J. Roentgenol.*, **131**, 916

67 Vaida, G. A. and Laucius, J. F. (1980). LeVeen shunt dislodgement. *J. Am. Med. Assoc.*, **243**, 149

68 Dieckmann, R. S., Rubinstein, M., Steinbaum, L. S. and Gregory, P. B. (1978). The peritoneovenous shunt in a patient with ascites and renal failure. *Dig. Dis.*, **23**, 62S (suppl.)

69 Harmon, D. C., Dermirjian, Z., Ellman, L. and Fischer, J. E. (1979). Disseminated intravascular coagulation with the peritoneovenous shunt. *Ann. Intern. Med.*, **90**, 774

70 Lerner, R. G., Nelson, J. C., Corines, P. and del Guerico, L. R. M. (1978). Disseminated intravascular coagulation. *J. Am. Med. Assoc.*, **249**, 2064

71 Lewis, R. T. (1979). Severe coagulopathy following insertion of the LeVeen shunt. A potentially fatal complication. *Can. J. Surg.*, **22**, 361

72 Mateshe, J. W., Beart, R. W., Bartholomew, L. G. and Baldus, W. P. (1978). Fatal disseminated intravascular coagulation after peritoneovenous shunt for intractable ascites. *Mayo Clin. Proc.*, **53**, 526

73 Samanta, A., Thakkar, V., Najem, A., Poskit, T. and Kiernan, T. (1978). Fibrin degradation products in ascites responsible for disseminated intravascular coagulopathy following peritoneojugular shunt. *Clin. Res.*, **26**, 324A

74 Schwartz, M. L., Swain, W. R. and Vogel, S. B. (1979). Coagulopathy following peritoneovenous shunting. *Surgery*, **85**, 671

75 Stein, S. F., Fulenwideer, J. T. and Ansley, J. D. (1978). Accelerated fibrinogen and platelet destruction after peritoneovenous shunting (LeVeen valve implantation) – abstract. *Gastroenterology*, **74**, 1161

76 Zarchy, T. M., Chan, C. H., DiBianco, R., Zeller, J., Banda, P. and Hoofnagle, J. H. (1978). Peritoneovenous shunt for intractable ascites: complications. *Gastroenterology*, **74**, 1169 (abstr.)

77 LeVeen, H. H., Ip, M., Ahmed, N., Mascardo, T., Guinto, R. B., Falk, G. and D'Ovidio, N. (1980). Lowering blood viscosity to overcome vascular resistance. *Surg. Gynecol. Obstet.*, **150**, 139

78 Schwartz, M. L. and Miller R. P. (1981). Angiographic assessment of LeVeen shunt malfunction. (Submitted for publication)

79 LeVeen, H. H. and Wapnick, S. (1975). Operative details of continuous peritoneovenous shunt for ascites. *Bull. Soc. Int. Chirurg.*, **6**, 579

10
The continent ileostomy

I. M. GELERNT, J. J. BAUER, B. A. SALKY AND I. KREEL

Total proctocolectomy will cure ulcerative volitis and familial polyposis. However large numbers of patients present late in the course of their illness, because of the reluctance of themselves, their families and their physicians to accept the required ileal stoma, with the need for a continuously worn appliance. The immediate maturation technique of Brooke[1], improved appliances, and the availability of trained stomal therapists have eliminated many of the complications of ileostomy. Nevertheless, the survey of ileostomy patients at the Mayo Clinic[2] points out that there are still considerable problems. Although most patients consider themselves in good health, 26% of these patients complained of significant peristomal problems and 16% felt that the time required for stomal care was excessive.

Therefore a continuing search has been made to safely preserve or restore faecal continence so that an appliance would no longer be necessary following total proctocolectomy.

In 1962 Nils Kock[3], working on a substitute for the urinary bladder, was able to construct a reservoir in which peristaltic waves would counteract each other. It was the extension of the principles learned in this experience that made possible the development of a continent ileostomy. It has been appreciated for some time that an obstructed stoma would produce rather severe ileostomy diarrhoea. Warren and McKitrick[4] described a syndrome which was termed ileostomy dysfunction in just this situation.

For proper reservoir function, a pouch for collecting stool in which no pressure waves would develop was necessary. Kock's contribution of constructing a reservoir in which motor activity would essentially counteract itself was a signal contribution in preparing a proper intestinal reservoir. The reservoir construction was such that although there would be a slow increase in basal pressure there would be no peristaltic waves traversing the pouch[5,6]. This was achieved by splitting an intestinal segment at its antimesenteric border and folding the segment twice. Having achieved a proper storage facility, Kock performed a number of these procedures in patients. It soon became obvious that for the desired result a valve mechanism was necessary. The first attempt by Kock at constructing a valve was the use of an antiperistaltic intestinal segment obliquely drawn through the rectus muscle. This attempt, though successful in a number of patients, had a significant failure rate. Of the 31 patients with this valve mechanism, eight had revisions to a new type of valve and 15 of the 21 remaining patients were incontinent. The next attempt utilized the concept of a nipple valve formed by the retrograde intussusception of the outflow tract. The construction of the nipple valve has gone through a number of definite advances so that now a reliable nipple valve is possible and can be achieved with a high degree of success[7-9].

SURGICAL TECHNIQUE

The procedure is the same when performed as a secondary manoeuvre or in conjunction with a total proctocolectomy; the procedure is performed with the surgeon on the patient's left. A total of 40 cm of terminal ileum is used to create the reservoir, nipple valve, and ouflow tract; 10 cm of the most terminal ileum (slightly more if there is a thick panniculus) are left untouched, to be used to form the valve and outflow tract. The remaining 30 cm of ileum are folded in a U-shaped pattern, with the outflow tract facing cephalad. The two 15 cm limbs are joined with a running absorbable suture along the antimesenteric borders (Figure 1A). The approximated limbs of the ileum are then incised along the suture line, extending the incision 2–3 cm more proximal than the suture line on the afferent limb. This facilitates separation of the afferent (inflow) and efferent (outflow) limbs when the reservoir is closed. A second continuous absorbable suture is then used to approximate the two cut edges of the limbs to constitute an inner layer (Figure 1B). The most terminal portion of the ileum is then intussuscepted in a retrograde fashion to form a 4–5 cm nipple (Figure 1C): satisfied that the nipple intussuscepts easily, it is reduced, and the serosa of that portion of the ileum is abraded with a fine orthopaedic rasp and then scored with cautery (Figure 1D).

Two rows of four number 2-O seromuscular sutures are placed to plicate both mesenteric edges of the ileum (Figure 2A). When tied, the mesenteric edges of the ileum will have been fixed in a retrograde

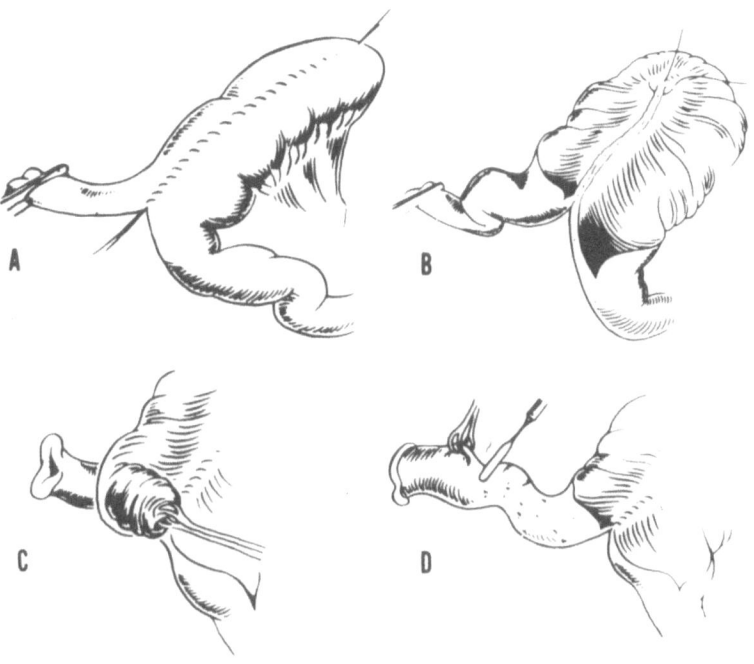

Figure 1   Construction of the continent ileostomy (see text)

intussuscepted fashion (Figure 2B). The remainder of the intussusception is then performed and a series of 12–16 number 2-O silk sutures are
placed circumferentially, perpendicular to the long axis of the nipple,
through both intestinal walls. A large-bore catheter or obturator should
be placed in the nipple valve during suture placement to prevent inadvertent occlusion of the lumen by suturing the bowel of the opposite
side. The sutures spare only the mesenteric aspect. The intestinal plate
is closed apex to apex, as demonstrated (Figure 2C), with two layers of a
running absorbable suture material (Figure 2D). The reservoir is folded
into the leaves of the mesentery, so that only the original suture line is
visible. Valvular function is tested by occluding the inflow portion of the
ileum, introducing a catheter into the reservoir, filling the reservoir with
air, and removing the catheter. No air should escape when the catheter
is removed. The catheter is again introduced and the air released.

A button of skin is excised in the right lower quadrant. The site is determined by choosing the site where the reservoir will fit best while
resting on the pelvic peritoneum. The stoma will usually exist best just
above the pubic hair line and will be concealed by undergarments. A

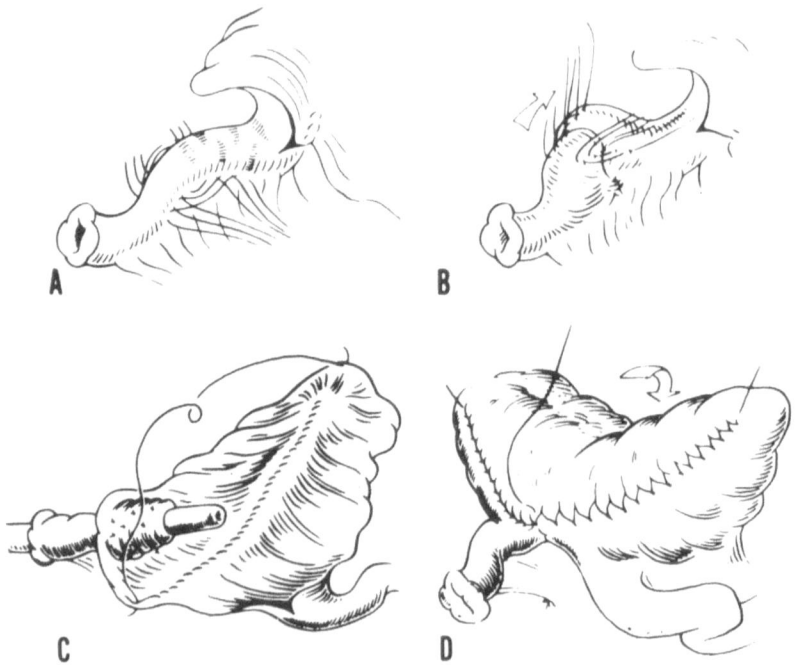

Figure 2 Construction of the continent ileostomy: formation of the nipple valve and closure of the reservoir (see text)

cruciate incision is made in the rectus fascia, and the muscle is divided bluntly in the direction of its fibres. An incision is made in the posterior fascia and peritoneum. To facilitate proper fixation of the pouch, the posterior aspect of the reservoir immediately behind the outflow tract is sutured to the inferior aspect of the peritoneal defect before the outflow tract is brought through the abdominal wall (Figure 3A). Silk sutures are used. After the pouch has been securely fastened to the lateral parieties (Figure 3B), the outflow tract is brought through the abdominal wall, and the remainder of the pouch about the outflow tract is securely sutured to the abdominal wall with interrupted 2-O silk. The entire outflow tract must lie within the body wall. The outflow tract is amputated at skin level and the ileostomy catheter (A. B. Medina, Kungsbacka, Sweden, number 28 Charriere) inserted into the pouch. It must traverse the canal easily and should be tested several times. The stoma is matured flush at skin level, and the catheter is placed in the reservoir. It is important to confirm that the catheter is in a dependent position and that all of its openings lie within the pouch. The catheter is sutured securely to the skin (Figure 3C). Soft rubber drains are placed in a lateral stab wound. The space lateral to the pouch is closed by suturing the mesentery of the ileum to the lateral parietal peritoneum. The ileostomy catheter is connected to a bedside bag via a wide-bore tube, and the wound is closed.

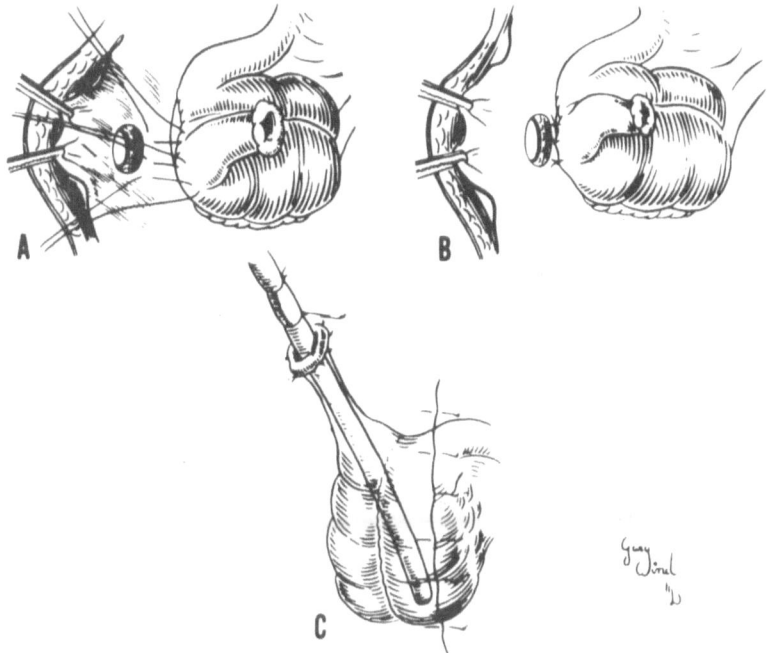

Figure 3 Construction of the continent ileostomy: formation and fixation of outflow tract and reservoir with intubation of the reservoir (see text)

POSTOPERATIVE MANAGEMENT

The catheter is left to gravity drainage for 14 days. It is irrigated frequently to ensure patency. On the fourteenth day the catheter is corked for 1 h intervals and left to gravity drainage at night. The duration of corking of the catheter is gradually increased and by the twentieth postoperative day the catheter is removed and the patient trained in its use. For several weeks the patient will be emptying the reservoir frequently, slowly increasing the time between emptying. Each patient is taught how to irrigate the reservoir in the event that it is ever needed.

Immediately following construction, the reservoir volume is approximately 75 cc. Postoperative management is designed to allow the reservoir to increase slowly in volume, preventing a sudden build-up of pressure within the pouch which might cause a de-intussusception of the nipple valve. Upon discharge the patient intubates the reservoir every 2 h, bimonthly increasing the period between intubation by 30 min until the reservoir is emptied four times each day. At this point the volume of the reservoir is approximately 500 cc. The patient will finally reach a regimen where intubation is necessary two to four times per day. Each patient must realize that he cannot go without intubation for too long a period. In our experience with patients who have had their surgery at other institutions, nipple valve slippage often follows a history of infrequent intubations in the early postoperative period. The diet following surgery is similar to that given patients after other types of bowel surgery, in that they are initially started on a liquid diet and gradually progress until a regular diet is reached. We suggest that our patients have no fruits or vegetables for the first month following surgery so that cellulose residue will not obstruct the catheter until there has been adequate healing of the nipple valve.

The patient with a continent ileostomy rapidly learns that thick stools will prolong the emptying period to the point of annoyance. Patients learn which liquids will keep their effluent thin so that emptying can be rapid. It has been our experience that grape or apple juice is quite effective in thinning stools; occasionaly patients will require periodic prune juice. On the average, patients will spend approximately 5 min from start to finish in emptying the reservoir. A small dressing is required to prevent mucus produced distal to the nipple valve from staining undergarments.

INDICATIONS FOR CONSTRUCTION OF A CONTINENT ILEOSTOMY

A continent ileostomy may be fashioned primarily whenever a patient undergoes a total proctocolectomy for ulcerative colitis or the familial polyposis syndrome. A standard ileostomy may be converted to a continent stoma where there are significant mechanical problems in stomal care (i.e. prolapse, retraction, skin erosion, stenosis) or when the stoma presents psychosocial problems to the patient.

There are now a number of studies[10-12] demonstrating improved psychosocial adjustments for reservoir-continent ileostomy patients. This is particularly obvious in a young patient who might otherwise find an ileostomy appliance extremely inhibitory in usual daily activities. One has only to see the improved adjustment in patients who have had conversions from standard to reservoir ileostomies to be impressed. All of the physicians, nurses and enterostomal therapists who have had a chance to observe these patients have noted a significant reduction in postoperative depression as compared to patients with a standard ileostomy.

CONTRAINDICATIONS TO RESERVOIR ILEOSTOMY

There are a number of contraindications to this procedure that must be strictly adhered to. There is no place for this procedure in patients undergoing emergency proctocolectomy, whether for toxic dilatation or haemorrhage. The additional time spent in constructing the continent ileostomy is not justified in this situation. It is much safer to construct the reservoir ileostomy at a second stage. A review of the series described in the literature indicates that mortalities have frequently occurred in this setting.

We feel that this procedure is not justified at the present time in patients with Crohn's colitis. The incidence of complications in patients with Crohn's disease was extremely high in Kock's series[6]. It is well known that the recurrence rate of the transmural inflammatory process is considerable and the risk of having to sacrifice 40–45 cm of terminal ileum is too great to justify the procedure in such patients. It is interesting to note that some of these patients have recurrences not only within the reservoir itself but also proximal to the reservoir, much the same as has been seen with procedures for Crohn's disease in which any anastomosis is performed (Figure 4).

The malnourished debilitated patient is a poor candidate for a procedure requiring long suture lines and increased operative time. Though 60% of our patients were receiving steroids at the time of surgery, we have not performed this procedure in the group showing severe cushingoid effects.

Patients undergoing a subtotal colectomy should have a standard ileostomy. The presence of a reservoir in the pelvis would make it extremely difficult to remove the rectum when it becomes necessary in the future. One is wiser in this instance to perform a standard ileostomy and, if the patient wishes, to convert the ileostomy to a reservoir ileostomy at the time of removal of the rectum.

The need for a co-operative, reliable patient is paramount for a successful result with this operation. The patient must be relied on to perform intubations in the proper manner, to adhere to the rather rigid schedule that we have outlined previously, and must be capable of inserting a catheter into a new orifice located on the abdomen. There

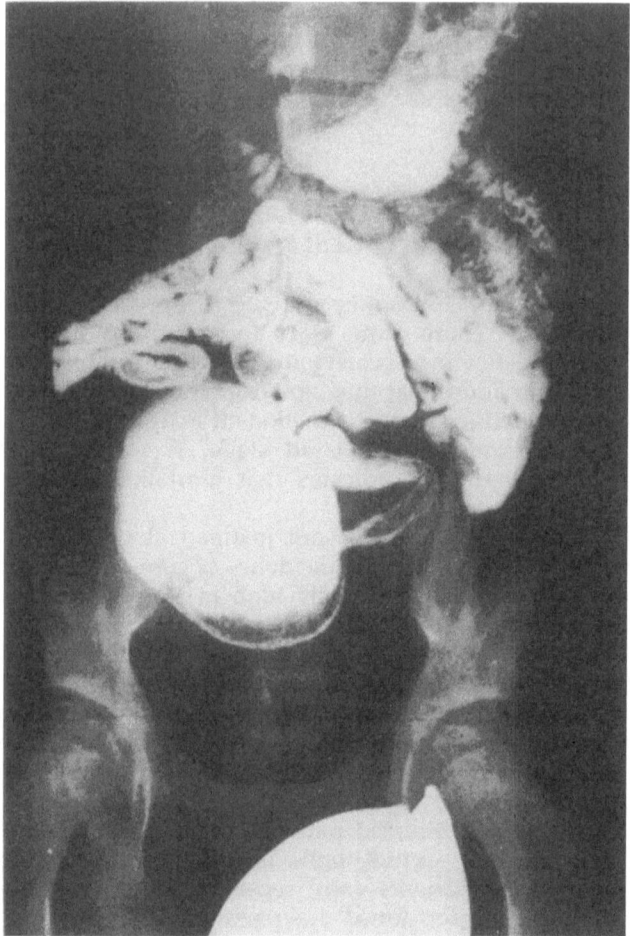

Figure 4 Small bowel barium series in a patient with a continent ileostomy and Crohn's disease involving both the reservoir and proximal intestine.

has been a rather frightening description of the psychiatric complications of the Kock reservoir in patients who were not psychologically suitable for this type of operative procedure[13]. We feel that the operation has no place in a very young child because of the unreliability of these patients. It has been our practice prior to accepting patients for the continent ileostomy, to spend considerable time in the initial preoperative interviews, explaining very vividly the method in which patients will have to empty the reservoir, and have the patient spend some time in discussing the operative procedure and the postoperative management of their ileostomy with patients who have had similar operations.

Finally, we feel that the procedure has a significantly higher failure rate in the markedly obese patient. In having had the opportunity to see many patients with poorly functioning reservoir ileostomies, we feel that there is a considerably higher valve failure rate in the obese patient. This is undoubtedly due to the inability to maintain a proper retrograde intussusception when one is dealing with a very fat, thickened mesentery.

MORPHOLOGY, PHYSIOLOGY, AND BACTERIOLOGY OF THE RESERVOIR ILEOSTOMY

The size and volume of the reservoir ileostomy increases considerably following surgery[5]. At the time of construction, the volume of the reservoir is approximately 75 cc. It is important that further increase in volume be permitted at a slow and gradual rate, otherwise pressure build-up in the reservoir will promote reduction of the intussusception which creates the nipple valve. The final volume and size of the reservoir is variable, depending on the patient's frequency of intubation. In our experience most patients reach a volume of 500–700 cc. Those patients in whom the reservoir reaches a capacity of more than 1 litre have no doubt been emptying the reservoir too infrequently and this may be associated with other problems described later in this chapter.

Conventional and continent ileostomies undergo changes in bacterial flora[14,15]. The increased number of aerobic intestinal bacteria are similar in both, but the prolonged periods of stool storage in the reservoir is no doubt responsible for the increased number of anaerobic organisms which have been demonstrated in the pouch. *Bacteroides* concentration is significantly higher in reservoirs than in normal ileum or conventional ileostomies. However, the available studies have made no attempt to correlate these findings with frequency of intubation and duration of time following surgery.

The postoperative changes which occur in the structure of the ileostomy reservoir are interesting. There is a gradual disappearance of the usual pattern of ileal rugal folds; on gross inspection the mucosa appears normal, however one can see some abrasive effect of the catheter along the outflow tract. These changes in the outflow tract disappear several weeks following construction of the reservoir and they are in part related to inexperience with catheterization, and the initial prolonged period of intubation. The silk sutures which have been placed in the nipple valve are usually extruded by the tenth postoperative month; occasionally, patients are aware of the sutures in the reservoir effluent.

Microscopically one sees a reduction in the height of the villi and crypts become somewhat more elongated[15,16]. Early biopsies reveal a non-specific inflammatory reaction which has usually disappeared by the first 100 postoperative days. The microvilli appear quite normal and areas of significant fibrosis are limited to the suture lines. There is an increase in the number of mitoses which begins soon after construction of the reservoir but stabilization occurs by the end of the first year. Philipson's studies[15,16] have revealed no difference in enterochromaffin or goblet cells between reservoir and standard ileostomies.

The microscopic changes in the ileal reservoir biopsies of the first year are not progressive and much of the early concern of continued morphological changes with possible serious consequences do not take place[17]. Animal studies suggest these changes are in good part reversible and that the ileal reservoir mucosa does not undergo continued harmful changes. This has been further documented in studies performed in patients 10 years following construction of continent ileostomies.

The motor function of the ileal reservoir in spite of significant attempts at alteration has many similarities to normal ileum[18]. The basal motor patterns in the resting reservoir are unchanged from normal ileum; however, one does not see true peristaltic waves traversing the reservoir.

Absorption from the ileal reservoir has been studied in a number of centres[16-19]. Electrolyte absorption is similar to that in normal ileum. There continues to be active mucosal absorption of sodium chloride with excretion of bicarbonate. The absorption of D-xylose and phenylalanine is unchanged from that of patients with standard ileostomies. The increased numbers of anaerobic bacteria as described above have caused considerable concern because of the possible consumption of vitamin B_{12} and bile salt deconjugation. Several studies have demonstrated there is in fact absorption of B_{12} from the reservoir. When reservoirs were studied using the instillation of vitamin B_{12} and intrinsic factor there was active absorption; however, the Schilling test was abnormal in a number of patients in the early postoperative period. Later studies revealed that only one patient in a study group of fourteen had an abnormal Schilling test. There were, however, a small number of patients with minimally subnormal Schilling tests and increased bile-acid excretion, but levels were similar to those of patients with standard ileostomies. A few investigators report significant increases in bile-salt excretion; however, these findings are not substantiated in other studies.

Vitamin B_{12} absorption and bile-salt excretion[20,21] are not only influenced by the status of the mucosa but also by bacteria. *Bacteroides,* the organism that shows the most significant increase when an ileal reservoir is constructed, can deconjugate bile salts and consume a great deal of vitamin B_{12}.

None of the studies to date demonstrate whether the slight change in B_{12} and cholic acid excretion is due to mucosal alteration or the presence of increased numbers of *Bacteroides* in the reservoir. Nilson and co-workers[22] have stated that the minimal alterations seen in the absorption of vitamin B_{12} and increased cholic acid excretion are of approximately the same magnitude as seen in conventional ileostomies and that significant metabolic consequences are no more likely to develop than in patients with conventional ileostomies.

EARLY COMPLICATIONS OF RESERVOIR ILEOSTOMIES AND THEIR MANAGEMENT

The early complications of this procedure are similar to that of any gastrointestinal operation. There are, however, a number which occur with some frequency and are related to the construction of the reservoir rather than proctocolectomy[22,24-26].

Suture line leak

The incidence of this complication can be reduced and almost eliminated by proper patient selection. Early suture line leaks are rare and will almost certainly need diversion of the faecal stream to control sepsis and achieve healing. Late suture line leaks occurring from the eighth to the twentieth day have responded quite well to sump tube drainage. Temporary diverting ileostomy has been necessary only on rare occasions. This complication is better prevented than treated. It can be avoided by choosing patients who are not severely debilitated or cushingoid and by making certain the ileal reservoir catheter is always patent.

Bleeding

This complication is similar to that seen with other gastrointestinal suture lines. It occurs at the end of the first postoperative week and will occasionally require blood transfusion. It is imperative that the catheter be continuously irrigated so that it is not occluded by clots. Bleeding suture lines have responded well to instillation of vasoconstrictors in the irrigating fluid or to intravenous pitressin.

Ischaemic loss of outflow tract

This complication can occur if the nipple valve is too long, especially in patients with a thick, fat-laden mesentery, or may occur with the combination of an oversized nipple valve and too small an opening in the abdominal wall. The patient will have a large volume of faecal leakage around the ileostomy catheter. This problem is best managed by keeping the reservoir empty with a sump-type drainage system. The outflow tract will rapidly shrink to the size of the catheter and can then be dealt with in an elective fashion. We have used an ordinary baby-pacifier to keep the tract in the abdominal wall open between intubations. Some have managed their reservoir so successfully in this fashion that they have been reluctant to have revisional surgery.

Other complications

Other complications occasionally described in the literature are volvulus of the reservoir because of improper fixation to the abdominal wall or perforation of the reservoir by a catheter. This latter complication has been described in patients with significant psychological disturbances[13].

LATE COMPLICATIONS

Slippage of nipple valve

This usually occurs at the mesenteric surface, and one can often obtain a history of the patient having gone for prolonged periods between intubations in the early postoperative period. The presentation is that of episodes of difficulty in intubation, followed by the patient noticing leakage of gas and stool. At the first episode of difficult intubation it is best to place a catheter in the reservoir and tape it securely in place for several weeks. If the slippage at this point has been minimal it will often fix in its new position and the patient will have no further difficulty. If the physician finds it difficult to insert the standard reservoir catheter into the pouch, it is best to use a small flexible catheter and then thread the large catheter over it. We have found it quite easy to intubate any reservoir using a flexible endoscope and guidewire. There are a number of patients in whom revision can be avoided if the nipple valve can be intussuscepted for its entire length using the flexible endoscope. If proper nipple valve configuration can be achieved with an endoscope, injections of the nipple with sclerosing solution through the endoscope can achieve permanent fixation[27,28]. As a rule, however, once slippage of the nipple valve has begun, revisional surgery will be necessary.

Fistula of nipple valve

Fistula can develop in the nipple valve when a full-thickness suture has been tied to occlude too much tissue. Occasionally it can be due to excessive cauterization of the bowel wall or too vigorous abrasion with a rasp. The manifestations of a fistula can occur early in the postoperative period with leakage about the ileostomy catheter or later, as manifest by incontinence without difficulty in intubation. The patient will not present with a history of prolonged intervals between intubation. Endoscopy will reveal a fistula which is usually rather small and near the base of the nipple valve. When fistulas are found at the distal end of the nipple valve, they are usually noted during routine endoscopic examination as they do not produce incontinence. Patients with nipple valve fistulas near the base of the valve (Figure 5) will require revisional surgery unless the opening is sufficiently small to be associated with minimal incontinence.

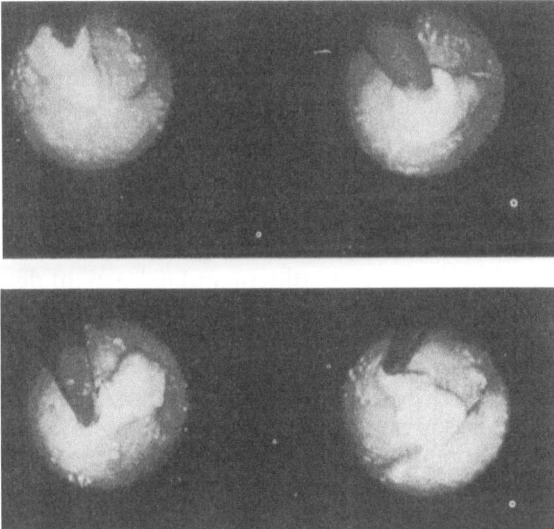

Figure 5   Upper: flexible endoscope traversing full length of nipple valve; lower: flexible endoscope exiting through fistula at base of nipple valve

Skin stricture

There are a group of patients who develop hypertrophic scars about the stoma. A skin stricture will also develop in patients in whom there has been slough of the most distal portion of the stoma. This problem can be managed in a number of patients with a baby-pacifier without further surgery. Most patients are somewhat reluctant to use a pacifier permanently and a Z-plasty will be necessary. This can be done using local anaesthesia and requires a minimal hospital stay.

Prolapse of nipple valve

Prolapse of an intact nipple valve occurs most often in patients who have had a number of operative revisions. The patient remains continent except during the period of prolapse. The nipple valve is easily reduced and catheterization can be achieved without difficulty. This problem has also occurred in patients doing strenuous exercise and occasionally in the last trimester of pregnancy. Patients having developed prolapse during pregnancy usually have no further difficulty once delivery has occurred. If prolapse continues as a problem because of repeated episodes revisional surgery will be necessary.

There have been isolated reports of late perforations by the ileostomy catheter. Several of these have been managed conservatively by keeping the pouch empty with sump tube drainage, providing there are no general peritoneal findings.

Pouchitis (diarrhoea)

The incidence of this complication and its intensity varies from series to series. In the full syndrome there is considerable diarrhoea, occasionally blood in the ileostomy reservoir effluent and the patient develops a low-grade temperature, feels poorly and loses weight. One must rule out recurrence of Crohn's disease, a major diagnostic error at the time of the initial procedure. More often it is related to prolonged periods between intubations in the early postoperative period. It has been our experience that there is a necessary period of mucosal adaptation before prolonged periods of intubation can be tolerated. Most patients with this syndrome respond rapidly to broad-spectrum antibiotics, frequent intubation and reservoir irrigation. The rapid response to broad-spectrum antibiotics suggests that there is a significant overgrowth of bacteria causing this inflammatory response. The endoscopic appearance of the reservoir during an episode of pouchitis reveals inflamed mucosa; there can be irregular, shallow ulcers covered by exudate and biopsies reveal a non-specific type of inflammation. In our experience we have seen patients who have been ascribed the diagnosis of pouchitis who in fact had low-grade adrenal insufficiency due to rapid lowering of steroids following surgery, and in one patient the underlying problem proved to be hyperthyroidism.

Crohn's disease

This complication occurs in patients having had a reservoir ileostomy constructed with an error in diagnosis. It can be avoided in most situations by strict criteria for patient selection, i.e., if there is any suggestion of Crohn's disease, do not construct a reservoir and never fashion a continent ileostomy from a standard ileostomy unless the colon pathology has been reviewed by a pathologist familiar with the diagnosis of ulcerative colitis and Crohn's disease. Occasionally when Crohn's disease occurs in the reservoir or the afferent loop an excellent response can be achieved with medical therapy. The reservoir provides a unique treatment situation because of the ease with which one can instil medications. We have found unusually good responses to steroid instillation and reservoir irrigation with non-absorbable antibiotics. If the recurrence is proximal to the reservoir it is often possible to resect the involved segment, leaving the reservoir intact. The best therapy, of course, is proper patient selection so the problem does not arise.

REVISIONAL SURGERY

There are three major problems requiring nipple valve revision: de-intussusception, nipple valve fistula, and prolapse of the nipple valve. The basic approach is the same for all three. A circumstomal incision with a medial extension of 2–3 cm and a lateral extension of 1–2 cm is preferable to using the previous abdominal incision. The outflow tract is carefully followed until the pouch is identified. The pouch is mobilized from the abdominal wall and the pouch and afferent loop can be delivered out of the abdomen. The pouch is opened at a suitable site to expose the nipple valve.

The repair of fistulas can usually be accompanied without difficulty as symptomatic fistulas are at or near the base of the nipple valve. The plane of serosal adherence on either side of the nipple valve fistula is identified at the base of the nipple and the valve is de-intussuscepted for a short distance beyond the fistula. The fistula is then divided and each opening is closed, so that the suture lines are not in apposition. The pouch is then closed and returned to the abdomen. It is again fixed to the abdominal wall, and the outflow tract wound is snugly closed. The stoma is matured flush at skin level. The tube is left in the pouch for 6 weeks but corking can begin at the end of the first week. The tube is left in place for a long period of time to avoid the possibility of traumatic intubation with damage to the suture line.

The technique for the repair of nipple valve reduction, once the pouch has been delivered and opened, is similar to the primary construction of the valve. The serosa is abraded, scored, and several rows of sutures are placed full-thickness through the nipple valve. We have also used staples to further secure the valve in place. Difficulties can be encountered if the area of slippage is fibrotic and adequate length of intussusception cannot be achieved or if the nipple valve was quite short to begin with. Both of these problems are best managed by the creation of a new nipple valve and outflow tract from the afferent limb. An incision is made in the mesentery of the afferent limb some 15 cm from the reservoir. The bowel is then transected and the distal portion (i.e., the previous afferent limb) is used to form a new valve and outflow tract using the method described in the primary procedure. The proximal end of the transected afferent limb is then anastomosed to the reservoir at the enterotomy site, the old outflow tract or any other suitable place on the reservoir. The patient is discharged with the ileostomy tube in place since it is best to leave the reservoir intubated for 6–8 weeks to ensure firm serosal bonding. This method is also used if there has been necrosis of the nipple valve.

The repair of nipple prolapse is difficult. It most often occurs in patients with a weakened abdominal wall from previous nipple revision. The outflow tract and exit from the pouch has been stretched and the nipple valve everts through it. Repair involves narrowing the outlet from the pouch, either by purse-string or plication. It is usually best to resite the stoma in an unused area of the abdominal wall adjacent to the old stoma. The patient should avoid increased abdominal pressure until adequate healing has occurred.

The problem of skin stricture is a minor one and this is best repaired by Z-plasty as has been described for standard ileostomy stomas.

CONCLUSION

In conclusion, the continent ileostomy represents a major advance in abdominal surgery. The primary procedure has a success rate[9] of better than 90%, and if revision is necessary it can be done safely with a high degree of success.

The quality of these patients' lives is clearly enhanced compared to those with standard ileostomies who require a continuous appliance[10-12,29]. Patients are more confident, less restricted in activity and their sexual adjustment to the surgery is excellent.

It has been interesting to note that 'well-adjusted' patients with well-functioning standard ileostomies feel that conversion to a continent ileostomy has provided significantly better quality of life.

Ten years of close observation of patients with continent ileostomies has eliminated many earlier fears concerning stool storage in an ileal reservoir. The incidence of non-specific inflammation (pouchitis) has been low, and the condition easily treated.

The need for valve revision has been significantly reduced as surgeons gain more experience with this procedure and follow the principles outlined in this chapter. The procedure has passed beyond the experimental stage and should now be part of the armamentarium of centres involved in the surgical therapy of inflammatory bowel disease.

References

1 Brooke, B. N. (1952). Management of ileostomy including its complications. *Lancet*, **2**, 102

2 Roy, P. H., Sauer, W. G., Beahrs, O. H. and Farrow, G. M. (1970). Experience with ileostomies, evaluation of long-term rehabilitation in 497 patients. *Am. J. Surg.*, **119**, 77

3 Kock, N. G. (1969). Intra-abdominal reservoir in patient with permanent ileostomy. Preliminary observations on a procedure resulting in fecal continence in five ileostomy patients. *Arch. Surg.*, **99**, 223

4 Warren, R. and McKittrick, L. S. (1951). Ileostomy for ulcerative colitis. *Surg. Gynecol. Obstet.*, **93**, 555

5 Kock, N. G. (1973). Continent ileostomy. *Progr. Surg.*, **12**, 180

6 Kock, N. G., Darle, N., Hulten, L., Kewenter, J., Myrvold, H. and Philipson, B. (1977). Ileostomy. In *Current Problems in Surgery*, Vol. XIV. (Chicago: Year Book Medical Publishers)

7 Gelernt, I. M., Bauer, J. J. and Kreel, I. (1976). The continent ileostomy in the pediatric patient. *J. Pediat. Surg.*, **11**, 773

8 Gelernt, I. M., Bauer, J. J. and Kreel, I. (1977). The reservoir ileostomy: early experience with 54 patients. *Ann. Surg.*, **185**, 175

9 Gelernt, I. M., Bauer, J. J. and Kreel, I. (1977). The continent ileostomy. *Pract. Gastroenterol.*, **1**, 47

10 Kock, N. G., Darle, N. and Kewenter, J. (1974). The quality of life after proctocolectomy and ileostomy – a study of patients with conventional ileostomies converted to continent ileostomies. *Dis. Colon Rectum*, **17**, 287

11 Bone, J. and Sorenson, F. H. (1974). Life with a conventional ileostomy. *Dis. Colon Rectum*, **17**, 194

12 Nilson, L. O., Kock, N. G., Kylberg, F., Myrvold, H. and Palselius, I. (1981). Sexual adjustment in ileostomy patients before and after conversion to continent ileostomy. (Submitted for publication)

13 Golden, H. K. (1976). Psychiatric casualties following revision. The continent Kock ileostomy. *Am. J. Dig. Dis.*, **21**, 969.

14 Brandberg, A., Kock, N. G. and Philipson, B. (1972). Bacterial flora in intraabdominal ileostomy reservoir. *Gastroenterology*, **63**, 413

15 Philipson, B., Brandberg, A., Jagenberg, R., Kock, N. G., Lager, I. and Ahren, C. (1975). Mucosal morphology, bacteriology and absorption in intra-abdominal ileostomy reservoir. *Scand. J. Gastroenterol.*, **10**, 145

16 Philipson, B., Kock, N. G., Robinson, W. L., Menge, H. and Mirkovitch, V. (1975). Function and structure of the mucosa of continent ileostomy reservoir in dogs. *Gut*, **16**, 132

17 Nilson, L. O., Kock, N. G., Lindgren, I., Myrvold, H., Philipson, B. and Ahren, C. (1980). Morphological and histochemical changes in the mucosa of the continent ileostomy reservoir 6–10 years after construction. *Scand. J. Gastroenterol.*, **15**, 4

18 Gadacz, T. R., Kelly, K. A. and Phillips, S. F. (1977). The continent ileal pouch,

absorptive and motor features. *Gastroenterology*, **72**, 1287

19 Jagenberg, R., Dotevall, G., Keuenter, I., Kock, N. G. and Philipson, B. (1971). Absorption studies in patients with intraabdominal ileostomy reservoirs and in patients with conventional ileostomies. *Gut*, **12**, 437

20 Anderson, H., Fasth, S., Filipson, P., Hellberg, L., Hulten, L., Nilson, L. O., Nordgren, S. and Kock, N. G. (1979). Fecal excretion of intravenously injected ¹⁴C-cholic in patients with conventional ileostomy and in patients with continent ileostomy reservoir. *Scand. J. Gastroenterol.*, **14**, 551

21 Jagenberg, R., Kock, N. G. and Philipson, B. (1975). Vitamin B-12 absorption in patients with continent ileostomies. *Scand. J. Gastroenterol.*, **10**, 141

22 Nilson, L. O., Anderson, H., Hulten, L., Jagenberg, R., Kock, N. G., Myrvold, H. E. and Philipson, B. (1979). Absorption studies in patients six to ten years after construction of ileostomy reservoir. *Gut*, **20**, 499

23 Goldman, S. L. and Rombea, J. L. (1978). The continent ileostomy: a collective review. *Dis. Colon Rectum*, **21**, 594

24 Halvorsen, J. F. and Heiman, P. (1979). The continent ileostomy of Kock (ileal intra-abdominal reservoir). *Br. J. Surg.*, **62**, 52

25 Stephens, D. H., Mantell, B. E. and Kelly, K. A., (1979). Radiology of continent ileostomy. *Am. J. Radiol.*, **132**, 717

26 Bearhrs, O. H. (1976). Present status of the continent ileal reservoir with ileostomy rather than ileostomy alone. *Dis. Colon Rectum*, **19**, 192

27 Waye, J. D., Gelernt, I. M. and Kreel, I. (1974). Endoscopy of the continent ileostomy. *Gastroenterology*, **66**, 829 (abstr.)

28 Waye, J. D., Kreel, I., Bauer, J. J. and Gelernt, I. M. (1977). The continent ileostomy diagnosis and treatment of problems by means of operative fiberoptic endoscopy. *Gastrointest. Endosc.*, **23**, 196

29 King, S. A. (1975). Quality of life: the continent ileostomy. *Ann. Surg.*, **182**, 29

11
Surgical management of supra-ampullary biliary obstruction in adults

S. S. HANNA, S. WILSON and D. W. JIRSCH

INTRODUCTION

Biliary tract obstruction is a common cause of morbidity and mortality. Our aim in writing this chapter is to outline the aetiology of biliary tract obstruction in adults with a discussion of new and pertinent advances in both diagnosis and the palliative and definitive relief of such obstructions exclusive of pancreatic and duodenal malignancy. Since we are confining our discussion to adults, biliary atresia will not be discussed.

In 1878 Schuppel classified bile duct obstruction into obstruction from within and obstruction from without the duct[1]. Based on this classification, a long list of possible causes of biliary tract obstruction can be constructed (Table 1). Biliary tract obstruction in adults is commonly due to choledocholithiasis. Most cases of biliary tract obstruction secondary to choledocholithiasis are partial but some are complete. Tumours of the extrahepatic bile ducts and iatrogenic bile duct strictures are particularly important since recognition can permit surgical correction. Iatrogenic bile duct injuries occur with an estimated frequency of 1 in 300 cholecystectomies[2].

Table 1   Major causes of surgical jaundice

A. *Intraluminal disease*
   (1) stones
   (2) parasites (*Clonorchis sinensis*)
   (3) blood (haematobilia)

B. *Intramural disease*
   (1) congenital: biliary atresia, biliary hypoplasia or choledochal cyst
   (2) traumatic: iatrogenic trauma, abdominal trauma (blunt or penetrating)
   (3) inflammatory: sclerosing cholangitis
   (4) neoplastic: benign tumours of the bile ducts (very rare); malignant tumours of the
       bile ducts (usually adenocarcinomas)

C. *Extrinsic lesions*
   (1) pancreatic lesions (e.g. carcinoma of the pancreas and acute or chronic pancreatitis)
   (2) lesions of the sphincter of Oddi
   (3) peptic ulcer
   (4) enlarged lymph nodes (metastatic, at or below the porta hepatis)
   (5) carcinoma of the ampulla of Vater and peri-ampullary tumours of duodenum

DIAGNOSIS OF BILIARY TRACT OBSTRUCTION

The diagnosis of biliary tract obstruction can often be made on the basis of a thorough history and physical examination, while at other times further investigation is necessary both for diagnosis and to identify the anatomy and probable pathology of the obstructive lesion. Figure 1 shows an appropriate sequence of investigation for patients presenting with jaundice.

The usual liver function tests include serum glutamic oxaloacetic transaminase (SGOT), serum glutamic pyruvic transaminase (SGPT), alkaline phosphatase and bilirubin; these are usually non-specific determinations which suggest the nature of underlying hepatobiliary disease. Many recent reports have documented the accuracy of ultrasonography in the diagnosis of obstructive biliary tract disease.

Diagnostic ultrasonography is a safe, rapidly performed, non-invasive technique which is highly accurate for study of the gallbladder (Figures 2 and 3) and the biliary tract. The normal ultrasound appearance of the biliary tree is shown in Figures 4–6. As this study is unaffected by the level of serum bilirubin, it is frequently the procedure of choice as an initial screening method for the patient with jaundice or increased alkaline phosphatase. While a low percentage of cases will have unsatisfactory examinations, usually related to bowel gas interference, the accuracy of detection of dilated bile ducts is greater than 90%[3-8]. The site of obstruction as well as the aetiology may also be determined (Figures 7–10) although with a lower frequency. False-positive results are uncommon although false-negative results occur in 5–10% of cases[3-8].

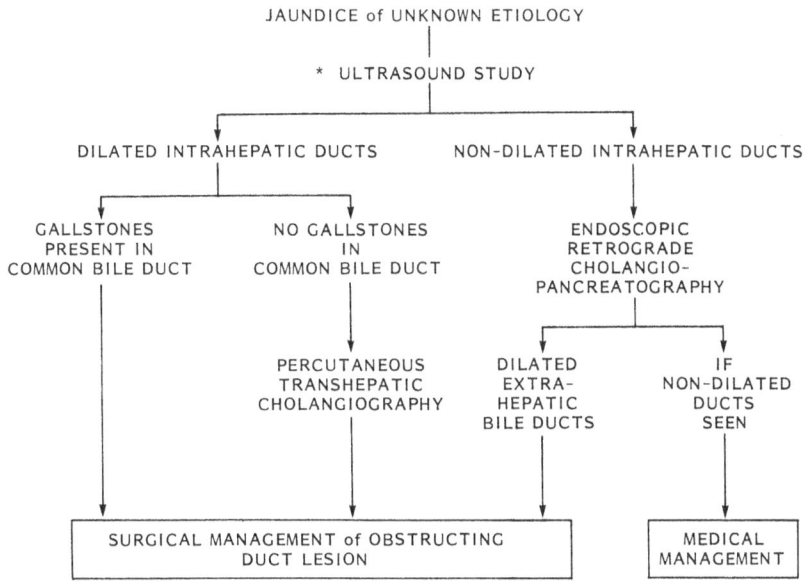

Figure 1 An approximate sequence of investigation in the jaundiced patient. Computerized axial tomograms (CAT scans) may be of value if the ultrasound study is non-specific, inconclusive or unavailable

In almost all cases then (97–98%), ultrasonography can differentiate medical from surgical jaundice, although it may not clearly indicate the cause or level of biliary tract obstruction. If the intrahepatic bile ducts are dilated on ultrasonography and if gallstones are visualized in the common bile duct (Figure 11), surgery is performed for presumed choledocholithiasis without any further diagnostic tests provided good operative cholangiography is available. If the intrahepatic bile ducts are dilated but no stones are seen in the biliary tree, percutaneous transhepatic cholangiography (PTC) is indicated (Figure 12). As currently employed, this procedure involves insertion under local anaesthesia of a fine-calibre or 'skinny needle', known as the Chiba needle, into the liver via the right 7th or 8th interspace in the mid or anterior axillary line with injection of contrast under fluoroscopy until a bile duct is located. The bile duct is then filled with contrast and cholangiograms are taken[9]. On the other hand, if the intrahepatic bile ducts are not dilated, then endoscopic retrograde cholangiopancreatography (ERCP) is indicated. If ultrasonography is not available or has proven inconclusive, computerized axial tomogram (CAT) scans can be used to determine whether

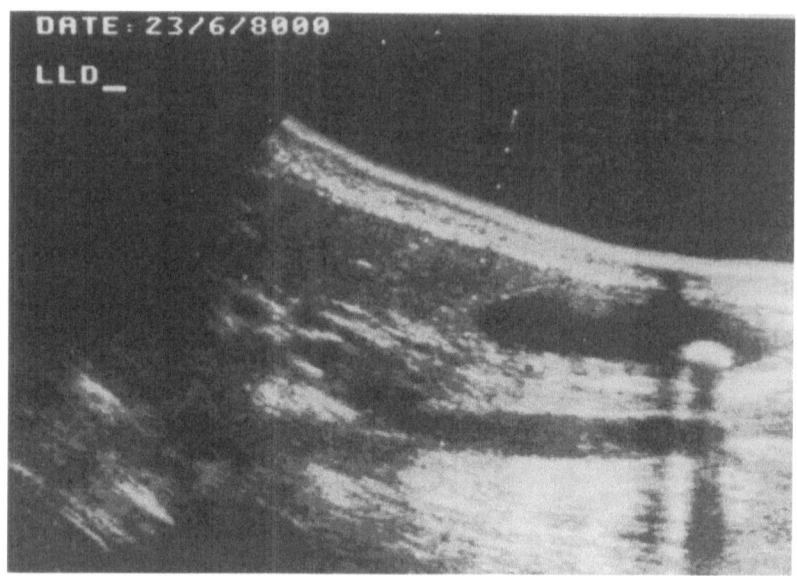

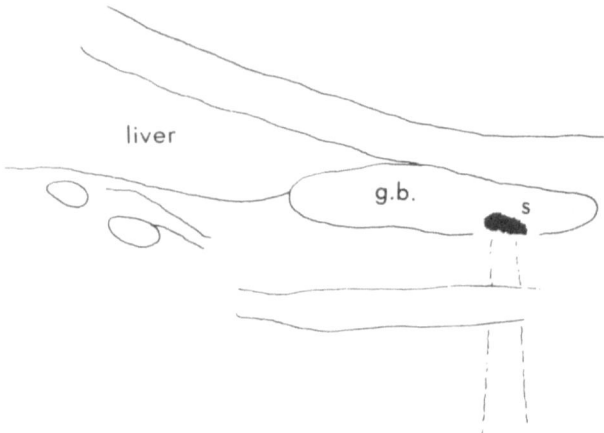

Figure 2 Cholelithiasis – a gallstone(s) is seen as an echogenic area within the gallbladder (g.b.). Distal to the stone there is an acoustic shadow related to attenuation of the sound beam

or not jaundice is due to a surgically correctable lesion (Figures 13–15). Once investigation is complete, the surgeon should know both the level and probable cause of biliary obstruction.

Preoperative preparation may involve administration of vitamin K

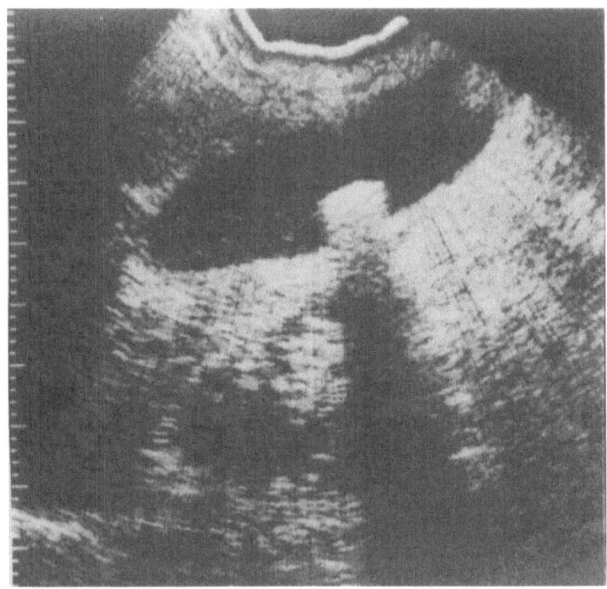

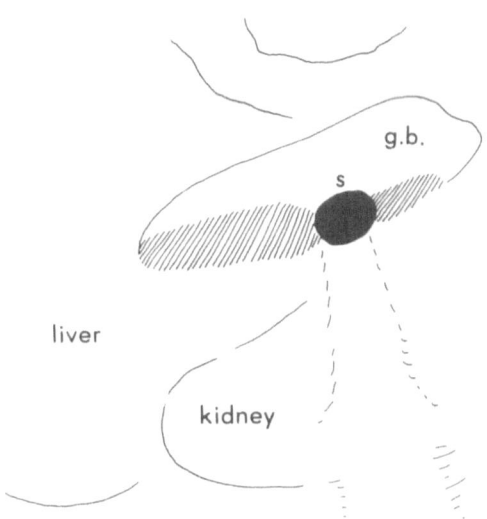

Figure 3 Acute cholecystitis – the gallbladder (g.b.) is large and contains a gallstone(s) and a dependent layer of sediment or debris

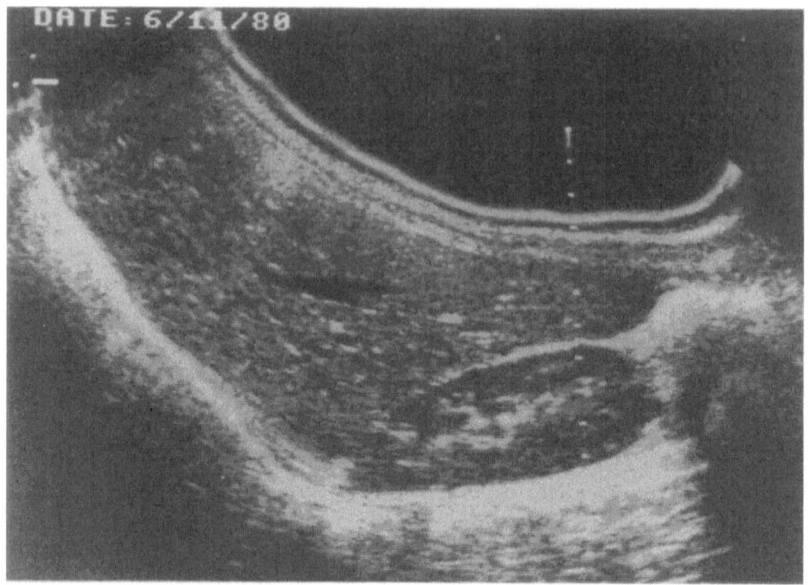

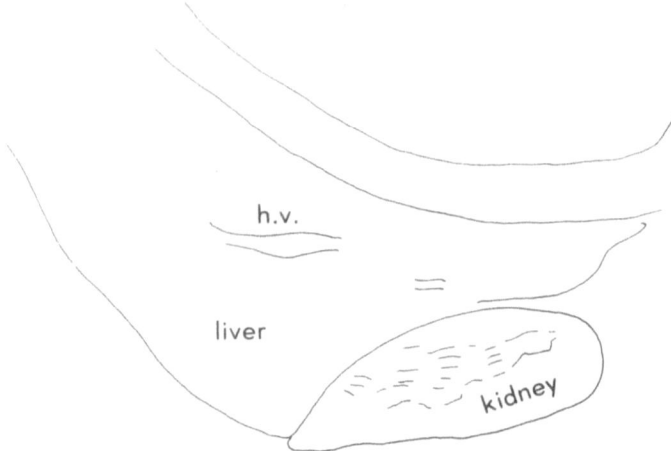

Figure 4 Sagittal section through the right lobe of the liver. The bile ducts are not identified. Portal veins and hepatic veins (h.v.) can be seen

and fresh frozen plasma to correct any coagulation defects. Prophylactic
antibiotics (cephalosporins) are administered transoperatively in an
attempt to prevent postoperative sepsis. In patients with significant and

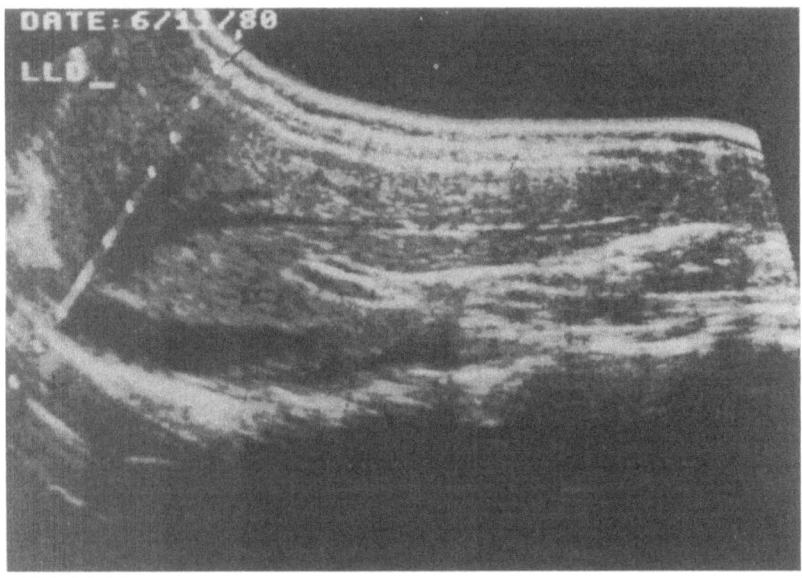

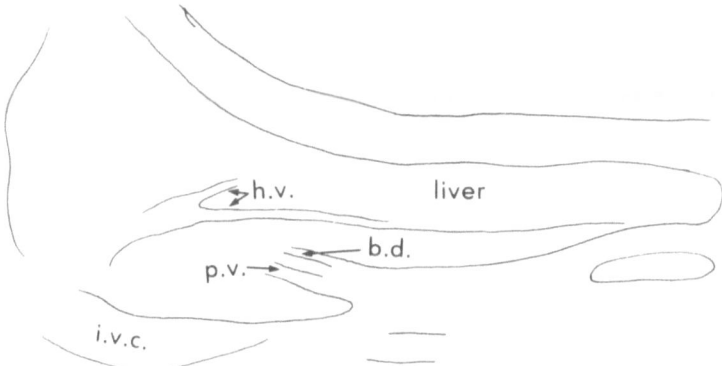

Figure 5 Sagittal section through the porta hepatis. The common hepatic duct (b.d.) lies anterior to the portal vein (p.v.) and the inferior vena cava (i.v.c.). The normal dimension of the common hepatic duct is 0.4 cm by ultrasonography

protracted hyperbilirubinaemia, preoperative drainage of the biliary tract after percutaneous transhepatic cholangiography should be considered (see below).

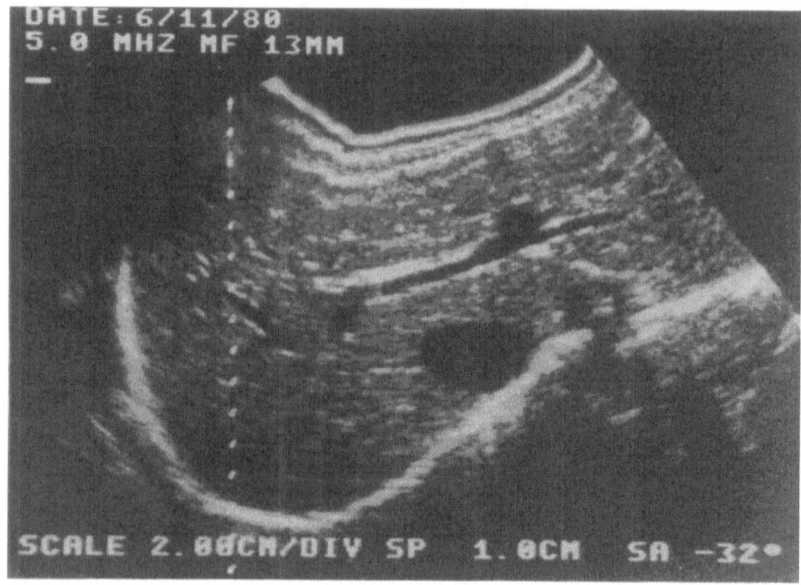

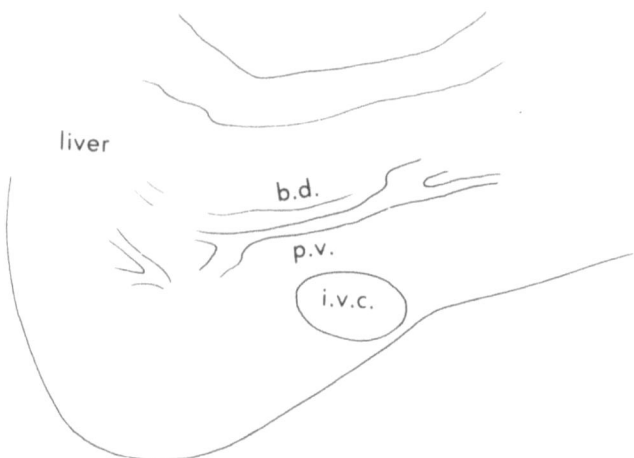

Figure 6 Subcostal oblique view of porta hepatis demonstrating the bifurcation of the portal vein (p.v.) into right and left branches. The normal-calibre right and left branches of the hepatic duct (b.d.) are seen

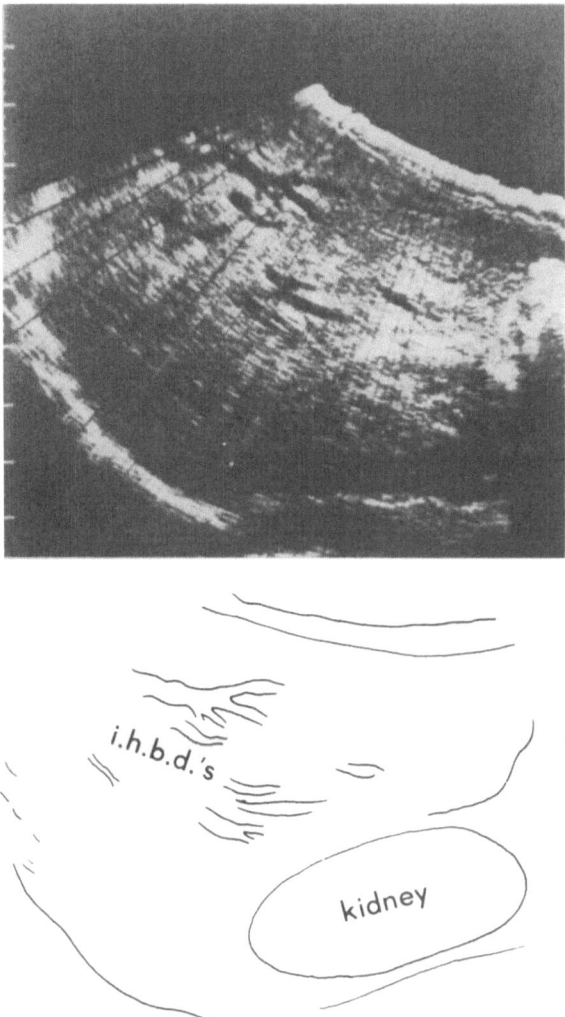

Figure 7 Sagittal section through the right lobe of the liver demonstrating multiple dilated intrahepatic ducts (i.h.b.d.)

CHOLEDOCHOLITHIASIS

Over 300 000 cholecystectomies are performed each year in the USA and the vast majority of these are performed for cholelithiasis[2]. Approximately 10% of patients undergoing cholecystectomy harbour common

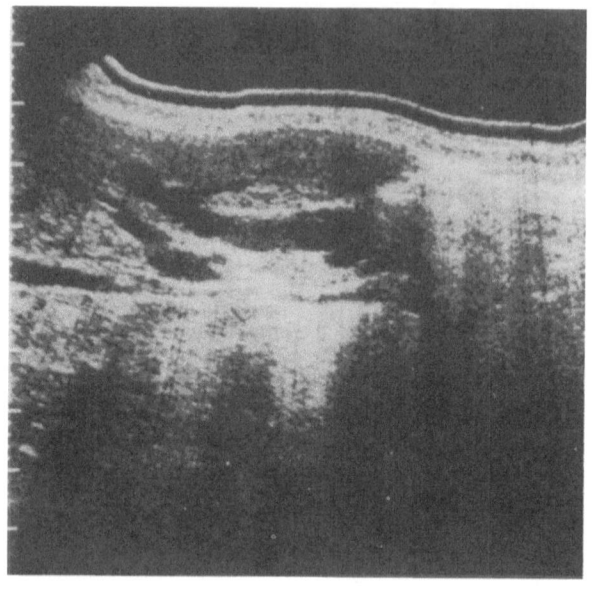

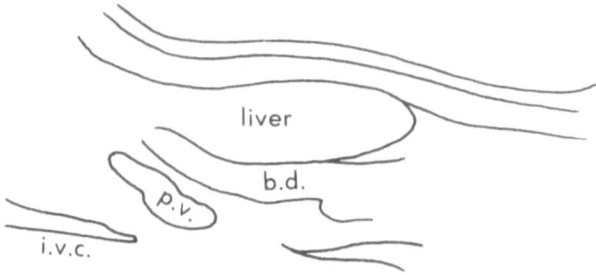

Figure 8 Sagittal section through the porta hepatis demonstrating a grossly dilated common bile duct (b.d.) lying anterior to the portal vein (p.v.) and the inferior vena cava (i.v.c.)

bile duct (CBD) stones, a coincidence which increases with age[10].

CBD stones may be primary or secondary. Primary CBD stones arise *de novo* in the CBD. Secondary CBD stones develop in the gallbladder and migrate into the CBD; these are thought to account for over 99% of all CBD stones in Europe and North America and primary CBD stones are rare. In the Far East, however, primary CBD stones are common, presumably because of bile duct contamination and infection with *E. coli* or enterococci and the prevalence of biliary tract colonization with the parasite *Clonorchis sinensis*.

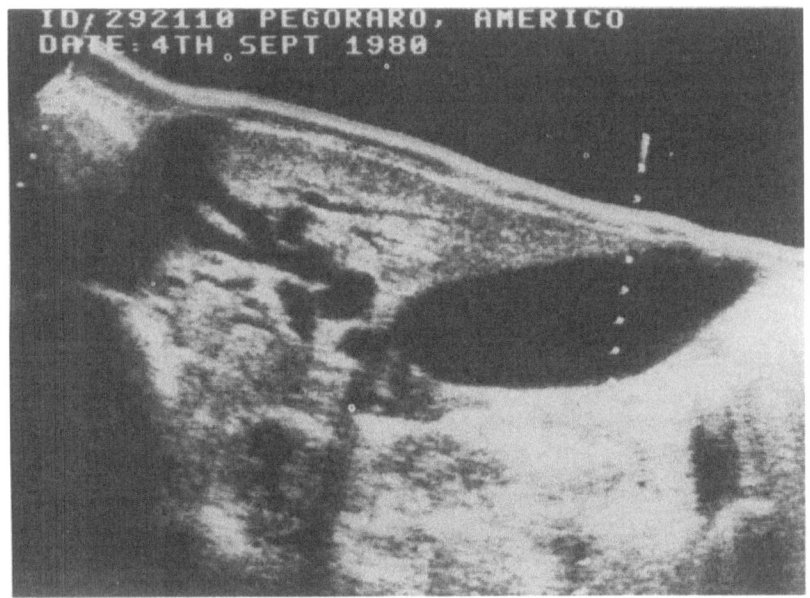

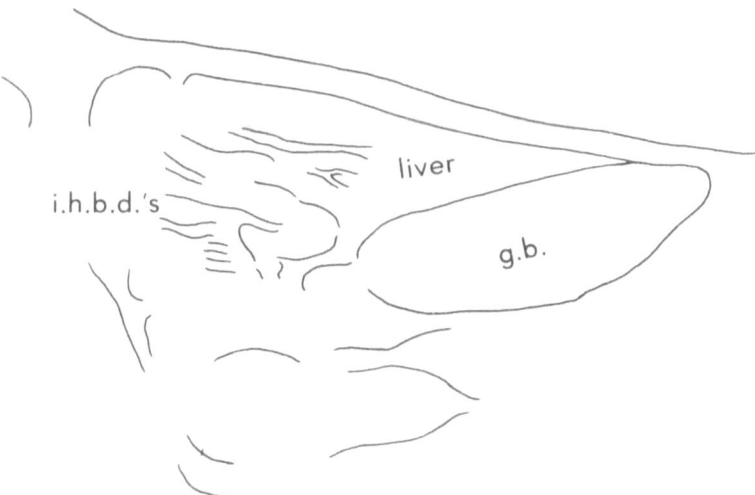

Figure 9 Sagittal section through the liver demonstrating a large and palpable 'Courvoisier' gallbladder (g.b.) and dilated intrahepatic bile ducts (i.h.b.d.)

Secondary CBD stones may be discovered and removed during cholecystectomy following operative cholangiography or they may be

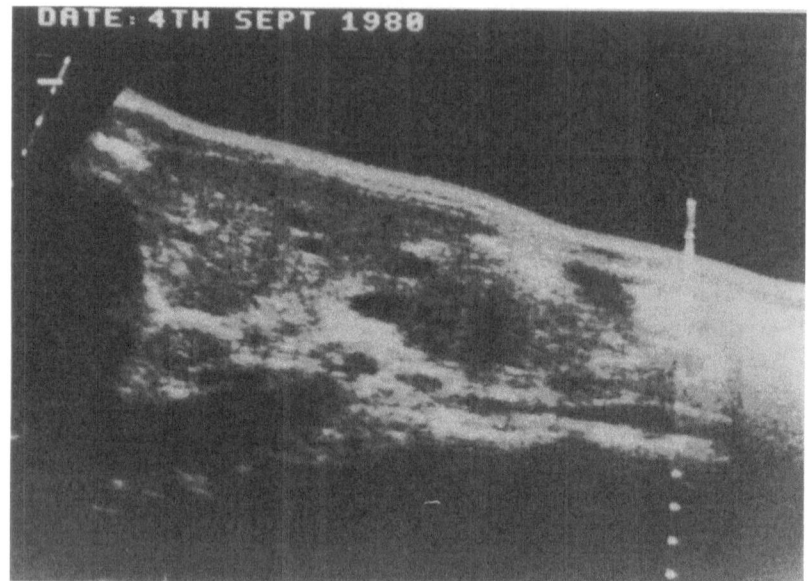

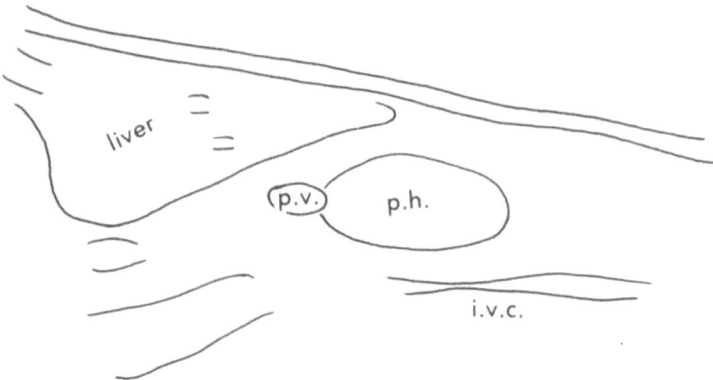

Figure 10 Sagittal section demonstrating a carcinoma in the pancreatic head (p.h.). The portal vein (p.v.) is seen in cross-section

missed during cholecystectomy and present days to years later. Hence, *the aim of surgery for calculous biliary tract disease is to identify and remove any and all stones at the time of initial cholecystectomy.*

The reported incidence of retained (residual) stones after CBD exploration ranges from 4 to 9%[10,11]. If stones are found in the CBD, however,

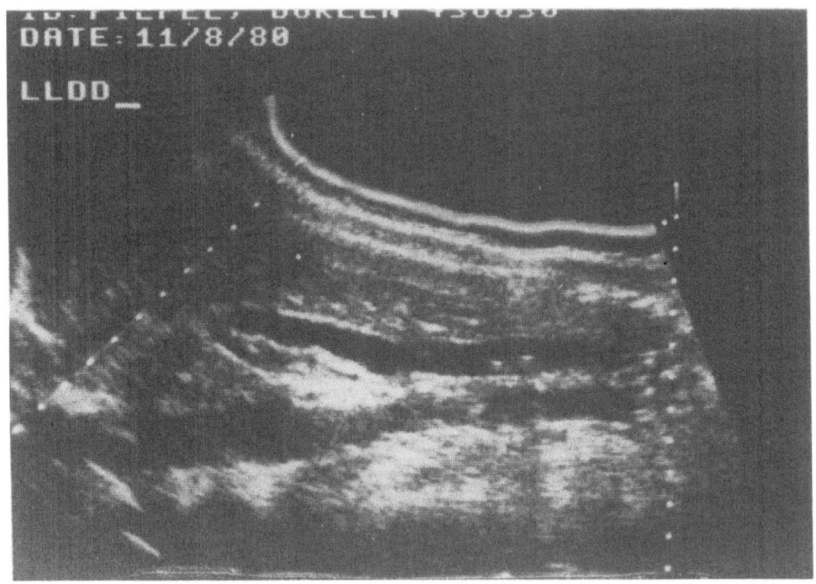

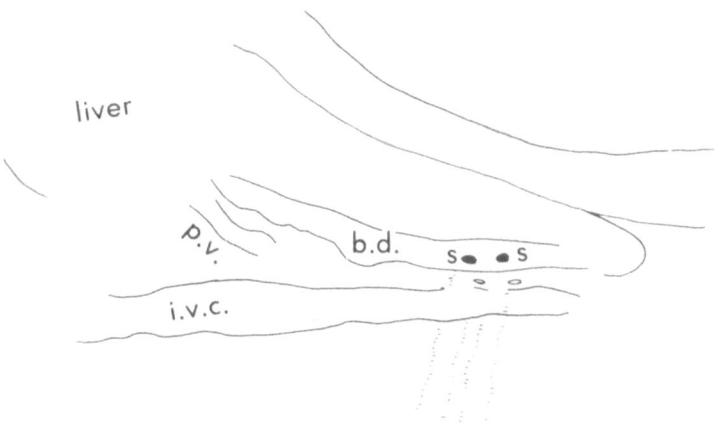

Figure 11 Choledocholithiasis – a dilated common bile duct (b.d.) is seen anterior to the portal vein (p.v.) and inferior vena cava (i.v.c.). Two stones (s) with distal acoustic shadows are noted within the duct

the incidence of retained stones is higher and varies from 14 to 22%[12–14]. Retained CBD stones can be prevented by identification at operation with a variety of procedures including routine operative cholangi-

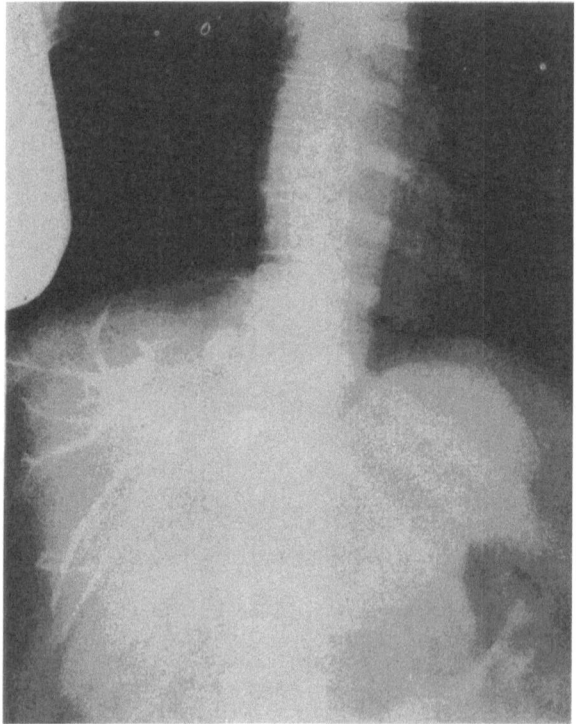

Figure 12 A percutaneous transhepatic cholangiogram (PTC) in a patient with obstructive jaundice showing a dilated right hepatic duct system. The left duct system barely fills with contrast. This indicates an obstructing lesion at the junction of right and left hepatic ducts with almost total occlusion of the left hepatic duct. This was secondary to metastatic lymph nodes at the porta hepatis

ography, operative manometry, pre- and post-CBD exploration cholangiograms and choledochoscopy.

Routine operative cholangiography

Two studies, each involving 400 or more operative cholangiograms, found that 4–11% of patients undergoing cholecystectomy will have unsuspected pathology, usually common duct stones, which would have been otherwise missed[15,16]. An additional 15–29% of patients undergoing cholecystectomy would have required a CBD exploration which would have been negative and, hence, unnecessary if operative cholangiography had not been performed[15,16]. Some surgeons argue

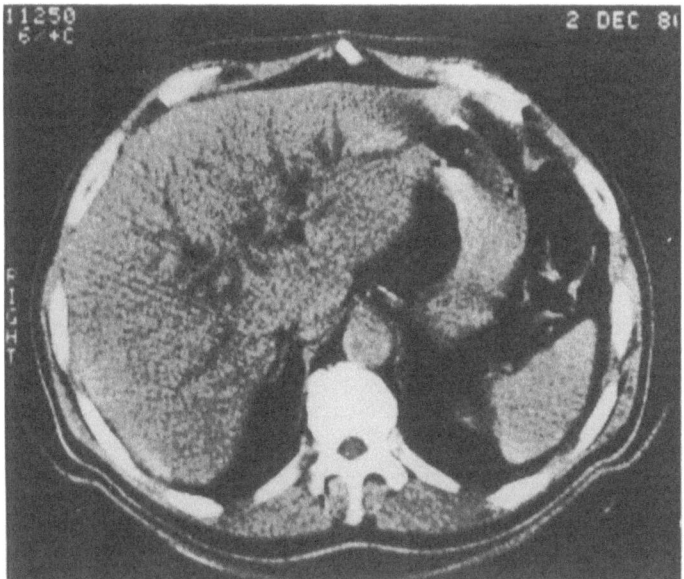

Figure 13 Computerized axial tomogram (CAT) scan through the liver demonstrating dilated intrahepatic bile ducts

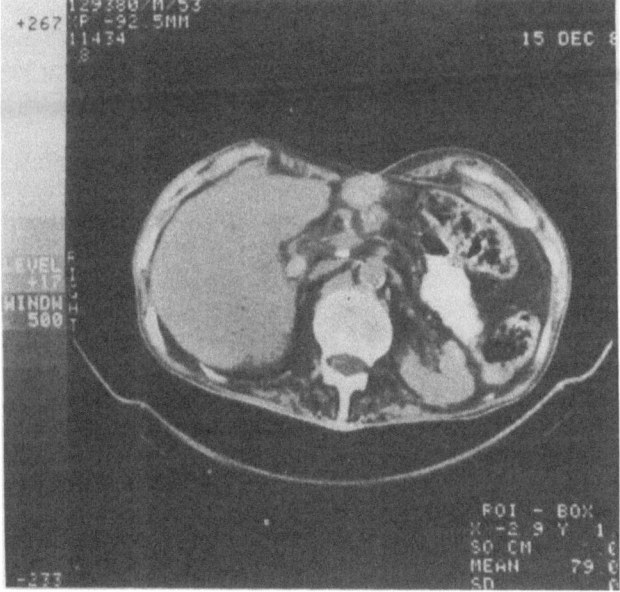

Figure 14 Choledocholithiasis on CAT scan of the abdomen

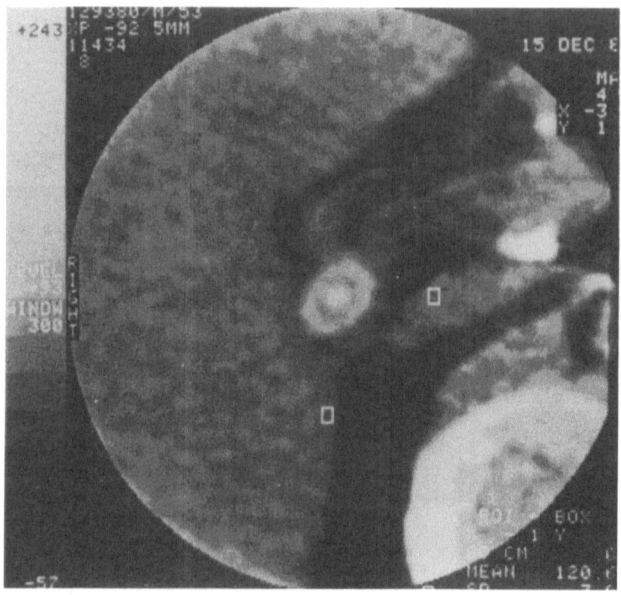

Figure 15   Magnified view of stone demonstrating laminations

that operative cholangiography is not required in patients with a single non-faceted stone in the gallbladder. This argument is not valid, as the authors have seen a number of such cases with associated choledocholithiasis. Operative cholangiography has proven clinical benefit in 15–16% of patients[15, 16] and in our view this is adequate justification for its routine use in association with cholecystectomy.

A negative cystic duct cholangiogram of acceptable quality more accurately excludes common duct stones than does duct exploration, with a reported 4.5% *versus* a 6% incidence of retained stones respectively[13]. On the other hand, a cystic duct cholangiogram which is positive, suggesting the presence of CBD stones, has been associated with a stone recovery rate of 78% compared with a 54% stone recovery rate when clinical criteria alone were used to dictate CBD exploration[13].

An adequate operative cholangiogram must show the entire extrahepatic biliary tree from the right and left hepatic ducts and their confluence to the ampulla of Vater, and it must demonstrate free flow of contrast into the duodenum. In order to obtain good-quality films, considerable attention to detail is mandatory. A scout film of the abdomen is recommended after induction of anaesthesia but before the abdomen is draped in order to determine the optimal radiographic exposure. An air bag placed under the patient's left lower chest is inflated prior to cholangiography in order to present superimposition of the spinal column and the lower end of the CBD on subsequent radiographs. A small plastic infant feeding tube (Bardic tube, C.R. Bard Canada, Ltd., Mississauga, Ontario) (No. 5 French) is introduced into the CBD via the cystic duct and is tied securely in place. The first radiograph is taken after injection of 5 cc of 20% Hypaque (Hypaque – M 60% (diatrizoate meglumine) Winthrop; diluted to 20% solution by addition of normal saline), the second following injection of 10 cc of contrast material, although larger volumes may be necessary if the biliary system is grossly dilated. Respiration must be temporarily suspended during X-ray exposure and radiographs of inadequate quality are repeated. If the ampulla of Vater appears to be in spasm, without flow of contrast into the duodenum, and if no stones are seen in the bile duct, 1 mg of gluca-gon is given intravenously. This relaxes the sphincter and allows con-trast to flow into the duodenum.

Operative manometry

In 1972 White from Seattle reported that manometric cholangiography using both flow and pressure measurements was 99% accurate in detecting biliary tract pathology. He also stated that operative chol-angiography had a 6% false negative rate and hence recommended routine manometric cholangiography as an adjunct to operative chol-angiography[17]. In 1978 White reported the 6–8-year follow-up after manometric cholangiography in 200 patients and these results contin-ued to show a 99% accuracy rate[18]. In this author's experience, mano-metry will demonstrate pathology missed by cholangiography in about 5% of patients[18].

White's technique is simple. The barrel of a 50 ml glass syringe is attached to gas-sterilized extension tubing by an intervening stopcock. The tubing is in turn connected to a plastic cannula. A rubber stopper with a glass tube is placed in the barrel of the syringe so that the glass tube is opposite the 10 ml mark (Figure 16). The cystic duct is cannulated so that the tip of the cannula lies in the CBD. The glass syringe is elev-ated so that the tip of the glass tube in the syringe lies 30 cm above the CBD. The stopcock is opened and saline is allowed to fill the duct until the rate of bubbling becomes constant. The quantity of saline flowing from the syringe in 1 min represents the flow rate and any flow greater than 10 ml/min at 30 cmH$_2$O pressure is considered normal. After flow measurements are taken, the syringe is disconnected and the fluid in the tubing is allowed to run into the CBD until it stops falling. The height of the fluid column above the CBD measures the resting pressure in the duct system, normally 15–16 cmH$_2$O; any pressure greater than

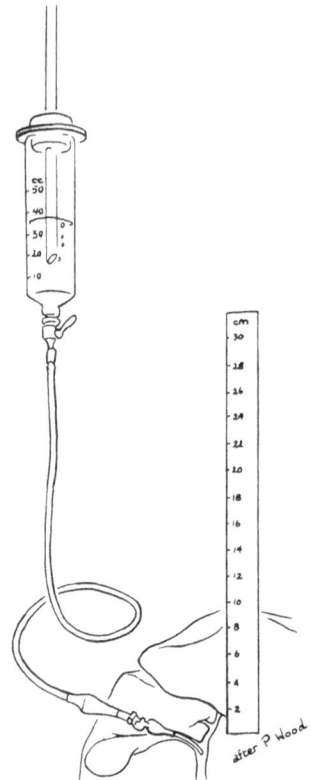

Figure 16   Technique of operative cholangiomanometry. See text

16 cmH$_2$O is considered abnormal.

Hopton[19] studied CBD perfusion with saline at a pressure of 30 cm in 204 patients and correlated the findings with operative cholangiography. He found that if the normal flow rate was regarded as 6 ml/ min or more there was a false-negative result in 3% of patients (i.e. the flow rate was normal but the operative cholangiogram was abnormal) and a false-positive result in 8% of patients (i.e. the flow rate was abnormal but the operative cholangiogram was normal). A mean flow of about 15 ml/min was found consistently in normal ducts. Hopton concluded that the results of flow studies are comparable with those of cholangiography in confirming the normality of the CBD but are less reliable in detecting stones. We have not had extensive experience with operative manometry since we insist on excellent operative cholangiography. Should excellent operative cholangiography not be available, however, the results of White and Hopton suggest that operative manometry can be of particular value.

Cholangiograms before and after CBD exploration

Pre-exploratory cholangiograms are useful to determine the number of stones in the duct before exploration and to outline the anatomy of the biliary tree. Two radiographs are usually obtained after injecting 5 and 10 ml of 20% Hypaque respectively.

Post-exploratory cholangiograms are routine to check the efficacy of CBD exploration. It must be emphasized that unless post-exploration cholangiograms are of good quality, stones can be overlooked in up to 22% of cases[12] and poor-quality films must be repeated. Close cooperation and communication between surgeon and radiologist are essential if missed stones are to be avoided.

Choledochoscopy

In a prospective multicentre study of 208 patients subjected to primary choledocholithotomy and choledochoscopy followed by intra-operative, post-exploratory T-tube cholangiograms, Nora et al.[20] reported an incidence of 2% unsuspected residual stones. This is lower than the 4–9% incidence of retained stones reported when choledochoscopy is not used[2, 11]. The rigid choledochoscope was used in this study.

In another study Kappas et al.[21] performed 121 duct explorations with the rigid choledochoscope. Pre-exploratory choledochoscopy was performed in 48 patients with a diagnostic accuracy of 94%. Post-exploratory choledochoscopy was used in 73 patients to define whether the CBD had been adequately cleared of stones. The accuracy of post-exploratory choledochoscopy alone was 87% and the accuracy of post-exploratory cholangiography was 82%, but when both were combined, there were no errors. The authors concluded that the addition of choledochoscopy to conventional radiological techniques should reduce the incidence of residual calculi after choledochotomy. In the context of these studies, we recommend rigid or flexible choledochoscopy after manual exploration of the CBD.

Management of retained CBD stones

To the dismay of the biliary tract surgeon, retained or residual CBD stones are not uncommonly found on a postoperative T-tube cholangiogram. Occasionally, however, they are discovered in a patient with symptomatic biliary tract disease long after previous cholecystectomy.

As mentioned 4–9%[2, 11] of all patients undergoing CBD exploration will have a residual stone or stones but this percentage rises to 14–22% if stones were found on initial duct exploration[12–14]. If a convalescent T-tube cholangiogram reveals a stone, it should be repeated 3–5 days later to rule out a radiographic artifact caused by an air bubble. If the presence of a stone is confirmed, management options include mechanical extraction, endoscopic papillotomy or sphincterotomy, chemical dissolution, operative removal or expectant treatment in the hope that the stone will pass.

Mechanical extraction – This is an ideal method for the removal of stones left in the biliary tree following surgery, provided access to the biliary tract is available through a T-tube or cholecystostomy tube. Mechanical extraction was first described by Mondet in 1962[22] and subsequently used in large numbers of patients by Mazzariello[23, 24] and Burhenne[25]. Recently, Mazzariello reported his 14-year experience with 1086 patients and documented a success rate of 96%[24]. He recommends waiting 1–2 months after operation before attempting extraction, to allow a fibrous tract to develop at the T-tube or cholecystostomy tube site. If the T-tube is a size 16 French or larger, the necessary instruments can be introduced through the fistulous tract; if the T-tube is smaller, the fistulous tract may require dilatation[24]. The technique of mechanical extraction involves introduction of a steerable basket under fluoroscopic control. The stone(s) are usually extracted but may alternately be pushed into the duodenum or crushed and removed piecemeal.

Mechanical extraction allows rapid removal of stones with minimal morbidity and mortality. This is usually performed on an out-patient basis with intravenous diazepam and meperidine analgesia and sedation. False passages in the fistulous tracks were created in 14 of the 1086 patients described by Mazzariello but in only two cases was the bile leak significant enough to require surgical correction[24]. Three patients developed pancreatitis: one responded to medical treatment, another required operation to extract a stone impacted at the ampulla of Vater and a third patient died. This death is the only mortality in Mazzariello's series and paradoxically, it occurred in an instance in which stone extraction was rapid and simple and no cause could be found for the pancreatitis[24].

While other series do not report results as excellent as those of Mazzariello[24] and Burhenne[25], the technique represents a major advance in the treatment of retained CBD stones. The technique requires, however, an experienced radiologist and appropriate equipment.

Endoscopic sphincterotomy (papillotomy) – This modality, first described by Classen and Demling in 1974[26], met with rapid acceptance resulting in several large series of cases[27-29]. It entails oral insertion of a side-viewing flexible duodenoscope, cannulation of the papilla of Vater and division of the latter with electrocautery.

An international study from 15 gastroenterology centres reported by Safrany showed that 3618 of 3853 attempted procedures (93%) were successful[27]. After endoscopic sphincterotomy, stones passed spontaneously (58.5%) or were removed (32%), thus rendering the procedure successful in 90.5% of cases; 9.5% of patients had residual stones and required surgery after failure of endoscopic sphincterotomy. The main complications associated with endoscopic sphincterotomy were bleeding, cholangitis, pancreatitis, perforation and stone impaction; these occurred in a total of 7% of cases. The mortality rate was 1.4%, and 2.3% of cases required emergency surgery for haemorrhage, cholangitis, perforation, stone impaction or pancreatitis. In Safrany's personal series of 562 patients subjected to endoscopic papillotomy, equally good results were reported[28].

Recently, Seifert described 955 cases of endoscopic sphincterotomy performed in nine centres over a 3-year period[29]. Of these, 92% were successful. There was a 7.3% incidence of complications, usually evident within 24 h of the procedure, and the mortality rate was 1.3%.

Endoscopic sphincterotomy has become an increasingly attractive therapeutic alternative for poor-risk surgical patients with choledocholithiasis. Since long-term follow-up studies are not yet available, however, Zimmon's suggestion that 'caution and judgement must temper the application of these relatively new techniques to patients under 50 years of age without increased surgical risk'[30] warrants consideration. Until such data are available, standard surgical therapy is appropriate for this group of patients.

Chemical dissolution – This method can only be used if a tube is already present in the bile duct. Best has extensively described a biliary flush regimen for dislodging retained CBD stones which includes ether and chloroform instillations via the T-tube[31, 32], although this regimen is no longer used because of the toxicity inherent in the chemicals used for instillation. Way has used sodium cholate infusions[33, 34] and Gardner has described the use of heparin in removing retained stones[35], although the reported success with these techniques has varied greatly (50–92%). Way described 30 patients with retained stones who received sodium cholate infusions with a 66% stone dissolution rate, although[33] 2 weeks of treatment were required. Failure most often occurred in patients with multiple stones, stones greater than 1.5 cm diameter and in patients with residual gallbladder stones after cholecystostomy. Diarrhoea is the most common side-effect of sodium cholate infusion and abdominal pain suggests increased biliary pressure or developing pancreatitis. Fever denotes cholangitis and requires stopping the infusion. Gardner et al.[35] reported successful dissolution of retained stones with heparin infusion in 31 of 43 patients (72%) but other investigators have been unable to reproduce these results[34].

A new agent called Capmul (Capital City Products Company, Columbus, Ohio) (mono-octanoin), a solvent for organic compounds including steroids, has been infused either via a T-tube or a catheter introduced endoscopically into the common bile duct[36]. This agent appears promising as it has been successful in dissolving retained stones in 75–83% of patients[36, 37].

In the authors' view, attempted chemical dissolution of retained stones is indicated if mechanical extraction has failed and before operative removal is undertaken (Figure 17).

Operative removal – Surgical removal of retained CBD stones is now less commonly necessary because of the success of non-operative treatment modalities. When these fail, however, operation is usually advised. Residual stone(s) are removed and a biliary–enteric anastomosis is often performed, particularly in patients likely to harbour missed stones: patients with a very large CBD and numerous stones, patients with intrahepatic stones and patients with suspected or proven primary choledocholithiasis.

There is controversy as to which biliary–enteric anastomosis is superior. The two procedures most commonly employed are lateral choledochoduodenostomy and transduodenal sphincteroplasty.

The so-called lateral choledochoduodenostomy is an anastomosis between the supraduodenal CBD and the mobilized duodenum; this operation is indicated in patients with large CBDs containing many stones. Although technically simple, the procedure has been criticized because of the development of the so-called 'sump syndrome' in a few patients in whom debris or stones have accumulated between the choledochoduodenostomy stoma and the ampulla of Vater[38]. Such debris may apparently produce abdominal pain characteristic of biliary tract obstruction but the frequency of this complication is unknown. It was not observed by Madden in 110 patients with choledochoduodenostomies performed over a 23-year period with an average follow-up of 10 years[39]. Madden reported a 2.7% operative mortality associated with choledochoduodenostomy and the results were described as excellent in 98 of the 99 patients who were available for follow-up. On the other hand, Smith described 25 patients referred to him with the 'sump syndrome'; all were successfully treated by subsequent sphincteroplasty although the choledochoduodenostomy was left in place[38].

Transduodenal sphincteroplasty, on the other hand, involves division of all the muscular fibres surrounding the distal CBD and

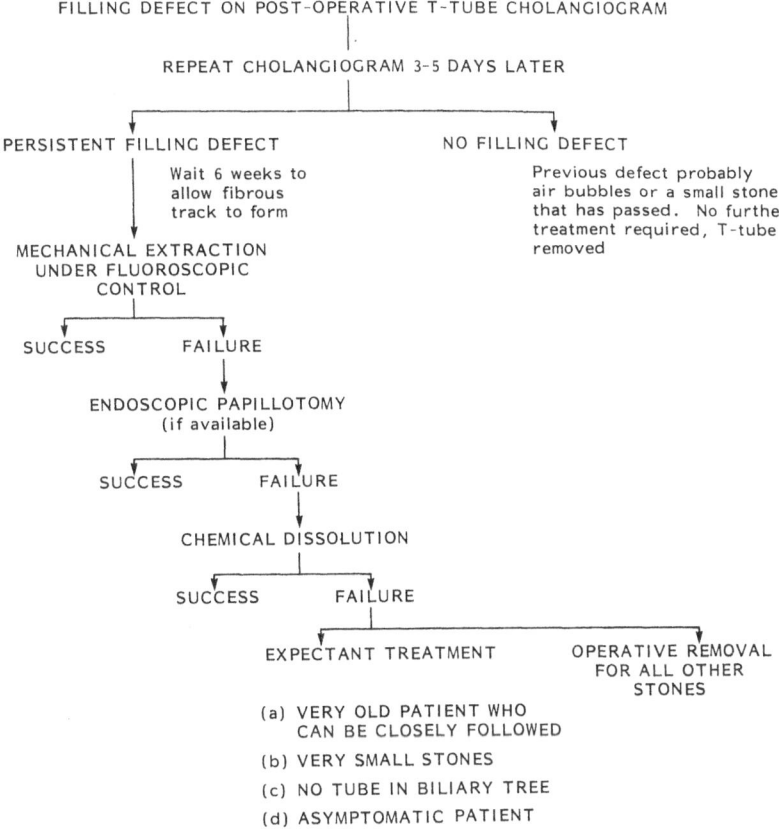

FILLING DEFECT ON POST-OPERATIVE T-TUBE CHOLANGIOGRAM

REPEAT CHOLANGIOGRAM 3-5 DAYS LATER

PERSISTENT FILLING DEFECT   NO FILLING DEFECT

Wait 6 weeks to   Previous defect probably
allow fibrous   air bubbles or a small stone
track to form   that has passed. No further
                                treatment required, T-tube
MECHANICAL EXTRACTION   removed
UNDER FLUOROSCOPIC
CONTROL

SUCCESS   FAILURE

ENDOSCOPIC PAPILLOTOMY
(if available)

SUCCESS   FAILURE

CHEMICAL DISSOLUTION

SUCCESS   FAILURE

EXPECTANT TREATMENT   OPERATIVE REMOVAL
                          FOR ALL OTHER
                          STONES

(a) VERY OLD PATIENT WHO
    CAN BE CLOSELY FOLLOWED
(b) VERY SMALL STONES
(c) NO TUBE IN BILIARY TREE
(d) ASYMPTOMATIC PATIENT

Figure 17   The management of retained common bile duct stone(s)

suture of the divided sphincter to the duodenum. The resulting stoma
has a diameter equal to that of the supraduodenal CBD. Sphincteroplasty has been championed by Austin Jones who has reported 189
sphincteroplasties for multiple stones with a follow-up of 2–7 years[40].
On postoperative T-tube cholangiograms, only five instances of duct
stones were seen and these passed after saline irrigation. The operative
mortality was about 1%. Sphincteroplasty is technically more difficult
than choledochoduodenostomy but has the advantage that it can be performed on normal-sized ducts. A lesser procedure, termed a sphincterotomy, divides only a portion of the sphincter mechanism and has been
used by many surgeons as an alternative to sphincteroplasty. In our

view, this does not matter unless there are known large residual calculi or the patient has primary choledocholithiasis.

In conclusion, lateral choledochoduodenostomy may be useful for retained stones in large common ducts (18 or more mm, in diameter)[40]. It is easily performed in aged or infirm patients, or in instances of common duct anatomical abnormality or pancreatic inflammation. Transduodenal sphincterotomy or sphincteroplasty is useful in normal-calibre ducts when a large number of stones have been removed or if there is doubt whether all stones have been removed. Many surgeons routinely fashion a sphincteroplasty or choledochoduodenostomy at the time of initial CBD exploration as a preventive measure if there are multiple stones, biliary sludge, or if there are irremovable hepatic calculi. We do not agree with this policy because there is a certain morbidity to these procedures and if further surgery is needed, it becomes more hazardous.

Expectant treatment – This may be prudent if there is no tube in the biliary tract, if the retained stones are very small and not associated with symptoms or if the patient is very old and can be followed closely. Generally, however, such patients remain amenable to endoscopic papillotomy and removal of retained stones is advised, as they will eventually cause symptoms.

IATROGENIC BILIARY STRICTURES

Non-malignant biliary strictures occur secondary to operative trauma or injury to the bile ducts. Elimination of these injuries would be a great advance in biliary tract surgery. Accurate statistics are not available but estimates place the incidence of iatrogenic biliary strictures at about 1 in 300 cholecystectomies[1, 41]. Although most injuries occur in association with cholecystectomy, bile duct injuries may occur after CBD exploration, gastric or pancreatic resection or in association with other intra-abdominal operation. The ultimate mortality from iatrogenic biliary strictures approximates 30%[41].

Aetiology

Poor surgical technique predisposes to biliary tract injury. In addition, the unusual anatomy so often present in the biliary tree makes injury more likely. For instance, a CBD of a narrow calibre may be confused with the cystic duct by the unwary surgeon; the right hepatic duct is absent in up to 25% of patients[41] and in some of these cases the right anterior duct is long, closely applied to the cystic duct and prone to

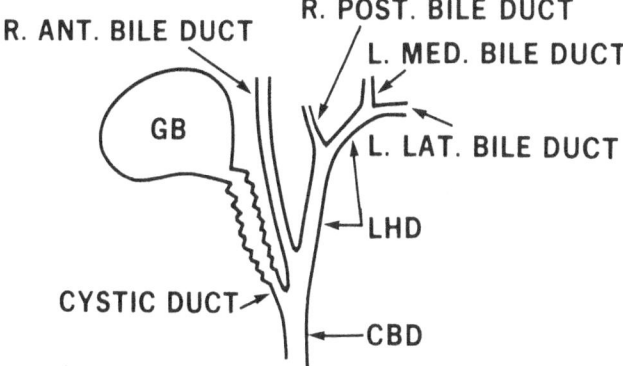

Figure 18 The right hepatic duct is absent. The right posterior bile duct joins the left hepatic duct (LHD). The right anterior bile duct is long and close to the cystic duct and thus prone to injury. It joins the LHD low to form a short common hepatic duct

injury (Figure 18). Other anomalies are also common: the right hepatic duct may pass close to the cystic duct (Figure 19); the cystic duct may join the right hepatic duct (Figure 20); the cystic duct may be short or absent (Figure 21) and the cystic duct may be adherent and parallel to the common hepatic duct (Figure 22). Excessive traction on the cystic duct is not a common cause of injury but may occur (Figure 23). Pathological factors can contribute to bile duct injury; for example, the oedema and friability of duct tissues in the presence of acute cholecystitis or extensive fibrosis in the porta hepatis following previous surgery may make dissection difficult and even hazardous.

Intra-operative haemorrhage can be a determining factor in the development of iatrogenic biliary strictures. Inadvertent haemorrhage can occur from the cystic artery or, less commonly, from the right hepatic artery. If clamps are applied blindly and impulsively, proximal bile duct injuries can occur. Should unexpected bleeding occur during cholecystectomy, a Pringle manoeuvre with pressure on the contents of the hepatoduodenal ligament will arrest haemorrhage and allow accurate localization and control of bleeding.

Bile duct injuries can occur during the course of a distal gastrectomy, especially in the context of a Billroth II anastomosis since division of the distal CBD can occur with mobilization or closure of the duodenal stump. Similarly, injury to the distal CBD can occur during excision of a duodenal diverticulum close to the ampulla of Vater or during pancreatic resection.

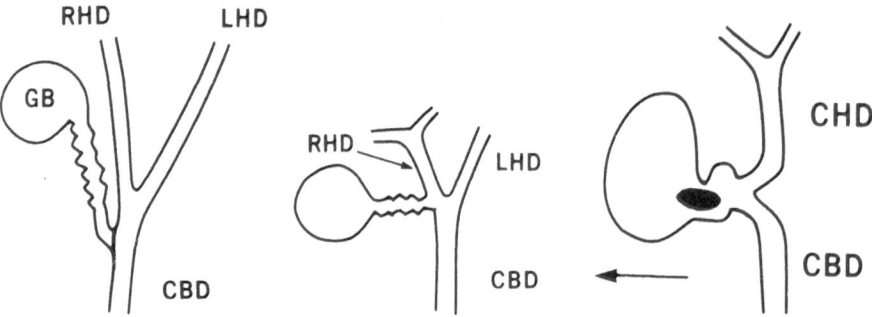

Figure 19 The right hepatic duct passes close to the cystic duct and is susceptible to injury

Figure 20 The cystic duct joins the right hepatic duct. If adhesions are present between these two, injury to the right hepatic duct is possible

Figure 21 The cystic duct is short or absent. Traction on the gallbladder tents the common hepatic duct (CHD) and the common bile duct (CBD) rendering them susceptible to injury

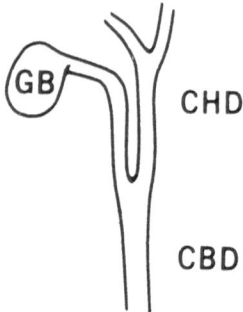

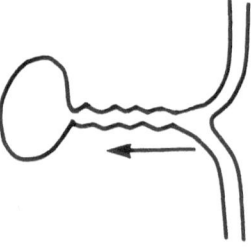

Figure 22 The cystic duct is long and adherent to the CHD making the latter susceptible to injury

Figure 23 Excessive traction on the gallbladder and cystic duct is a rare cause of common bile duct injury

Prevention

As Kune has noted, nearly all operative bile duct injuries are preventable[1,31]. Prevention is best accomplished with adequate demonstration of biliary tract anatomy. In this regard, an adequate incision facilitates proper exposure. The cystic artery should be identified to demonstrate that it enters the gallbladder and it should be ligated close to the gallbladder wall to avoid injury to the right hepatic duct, common hepatic duct or right hepatic artery.

Excessive traction on the gallbladder should be avoided. The critical triangle of Calot (Figure 24) formed by the common hepatic and right hepatic duct, the upper surface of the gallbladder and cystic duct and by the liver, is most important since it is in this area that large and unexpected bile ducts, such as the right anterior bile duct, may be present. The critical junction of cystic and common hepatic ducts must be clearly visible (Figure 25).

When dense fibrosis or oedema prevent precise dissection and identification of biliary anatomy, deliberate choledochotomy in the supraduodenal common bile duct with insertion of a probe to identify right and left hepatic ducts and the cystic duct is a very valuable technique. Deliberate choledochotomy may similarly be necessary in a difficult distal gastric resection when the CBD location is uncertain. A cholangiogram early in the course of cholecystectomy through the gallbladder, cystic duct or CBD, can be most useful in delineating biliary tract anatomy.

Pathology of bile duct injuries

At the site of bile duct transection, crush injury, ligature or other trauma, inflammation and fibrosis follow with a resultant biliary stricture. Bile ducts proximal to the stricture may dilate and are frequently thick-walled and fibrotic. Not only are epithelial changes present, but subepithelial fibrosis and inflammatory infiltrates are also seen. The bile ducts distal to the stricture undergo similar change and may become completely occluded by fibrous tissue. Bile in the ducts proximal to a stricture is almost always infected, usually with Gram-negative enteric organisms[41].

The iniquitous tendency of the injured bile duct to undergo fibrosis and stricture has been variously attributed to the necrotizing and desmoplastic effect of bile, to ischaemia, or a combination of factors. Recent resin-cast studies of the arterial blood supply of the human bile duct by Northover and Terblanche have shed light on the probable aetiology of many bile duct strictures[42]. The arterial supply of the supraduodenal bile duct is axial, with the main vessels, termed the 3 and 9 o'clock arteries, coursing along the lateral borders. Another vessel, termed the

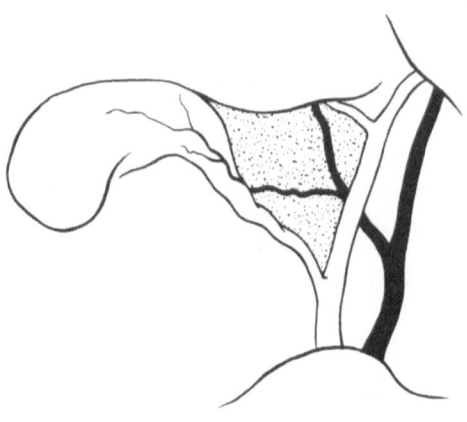

Figure 24 The triangle of Calot (dotted area) is very important since large and unexpected bile ducts, e.g. right anterior bile duct, may cross this area

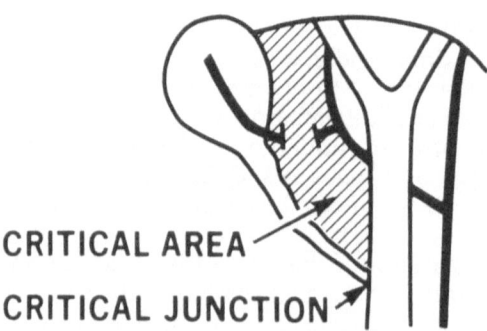

Figure 25 The critical junction of the cystic, common hepatic and common bile ducts should be clearly exposed at the time of cholecystectomy before any duct is ligated

retroportal artery and not previously described, was present in all of Terblanche's cast studies and was a major source of blood supply to the supraduodenal duct in 32% of instances. Damage to these vessels, which are 0.3 mm or less in diameter and which supply arterial blood to the CBD, may explain the long strictures sometimes seen after minimal surgical trauma in the area.

Surgical repair of traumatic biliary strictures is frequently followed by re-stenosis at the anastomotic area. Since biliary anastomoses heal by fibrosis, an internal splint is recommended in all established strictures. Rarely, a T-tube may be used as a splint for cases treated promptly at the time of initial injury. For established strictures, we use silastic splints (U-tubes) and leave them in place for 18 months so that anastomotic fibrosis and contraction will be complete at the time of removal.

If a biliary stricture is not corrected, the consequent stasis and superimposed infection will lead to periportal inflammation and fibrosis with eventual development of secondary biliary cirrhosis. As a further difficulty, 20% of patients with established biliary strictures develop portal hypertension which may induce bleeding from oesophageal varices[41].

Diagnosis

The diagnosis of biliary stricture is usually painfully obvious when the patient develops jaundice, excessive bile drainage or both, soon after cholecystectomy. In a few cases, the diagnosis is made at operation but in most cases it is made in the early postoperative period or less commonly, months or years later with the development of cholangitis or gradual jaundice. Laboratory investigations reveal a pattern of obstructive jaundice and ultrasonography or CAT demonstrates a dilated proximal biliary tree. A percutaneous transhepatic cholangiogram will reveal the anatomy of the proximal biliary tree and occasionally, an ERCP may be helpful to delineate biliary tract anatomy beyond the stricture.

Preoperative management

Since severe hyperbilirubinaemia predisposes to a higher operative mortality, it is often desirable to lower the serum bilirubin, release biliary pressure and assist hepatic function preoperatively[43]. In 1962 Glenn first suggested biliary catheterization for drainage as a prudent procedure following transhepatic cholangiography[44]. After diagnostic percutaneous transhepatic cholangiography gained popularity, percutaneous transhepatic drainage (PTD) has been used with therapeutic benefit as described in numerous recent publications[43-47]. In particular, the results of Nakayama's non-randomized study are impressive[43]: 105

patients with obstructive jaundice underwent attempted PTD with
success in 104 patients (84 had malignant and 21 had benign obstructive
lesions). In this series, 69 of 84 patients with malignant disease and 20 of
21 patients with benign disease underwent subsequent surgery and the
overall operative mortality was 8.2%. This group of 104 patients was
retrospectively compared to 148 patients on whom surgery was carried
out for malignant biliary tract obstruction without prior decompression
associated with an operative mortality of 28.3%. Operative mortality
was particularly high in patients with serum bilirubin levels greater than
10 mg/dl. We therefore advise PTD before radical or palliative surgery
whenever possible to reduce hyperbilirubinaemia, effect biliary decompression and assist hepatic function (Figure 26). According to Nakayama, this usually requires 1–2 weeks of drainage.

Recently, percutaneous insertion of a permanent endoprosthesis in
the biliary tree has been used in several centres for palliation of inoperable biliary tract malignancies[48-50]. We would not use this for benign
(iatrogenic) strictures but percutaneous drainage may have a place in
the management of inoperable malignancies.

Before biliary strictures are repaired, we recommend administration
of vitamin K and fresh frozen plasma as necessary to ensure normal coagulation. We also administer prophylactic cephalosporins, effective
against a narrow spectrum of Gram-negative organisms. Occasionally,
total parenteral nutrition may be advisable before surgical repair.

Operative treatment

The treatment of bile duct injuries is surgical. Unfortunately, bile duct
injury is not often recognized at cholecystectomy. If the surgeon recog-
nizes such injury but does not feel confident at repair, he should
provide adequate external bile duct drainage and prompt referral for definitive management. The experienced operator should assess the
extent of the injury in order to determine the most appropriate repair.
For example, for minimal bile duct injury when only a lateral defect is
present without other tissue loss, the defect can be closed transversely
after kocherizing the duodenum and mobilizing the head of pancreas to
avoid suture-line tension. The bile duct should be drained with a T-tube
thereafter, usually at a separate choledochotomy site. Circumferential
defects with loss of length are the most frequent type of injury, however,
and usually occur in ducts of normal or narrow calibre, making reconstruction difficult. In these, mucosa-to-mucosa apposition may be impossible and subsequent healing by fibrosis and stricture must be
anticipated. When loss of duct tissue has occurred, the type of reconstruction depends on whether or not the severed ends of duct can be re-
apposed without tension.

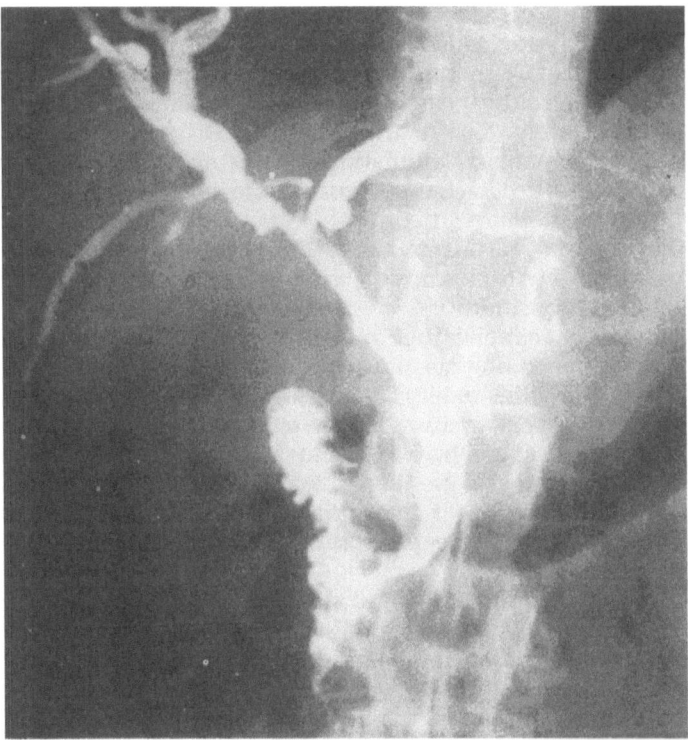

Figure 26 Cholangiogram obtained at the time of percutaneous transhepatic drainage (PTD). Since numerous liver metastases were seen on ultrasonography and documented by percutaneous liver biopsy, the patient was deemed incurable and palliation was accomplished with PTD

If the two ends of the bile duct can be apposed without tension and if bile duct injury is recognized at the time of operation, an end-to-end ductal anastomosis may be considered after the duodenum and head of pancreas are fully mobilized. We advocate such biliary anastomosis with a single layer of 4–O or 5–O interrupted sutures of polyglycolic acid. If possible, a T-tube should be inserted in the common duct below the anastomosis. One arm of the T-tube is used to splint and decompress the anastomosis for at least 3 months, after which the T-tube is removed if a cholangiogram performed at that time is satisfactory. If the two ends of the bile duct cannot be apposed without tension, however, a Roux-en-Y hepaticojejunostomy is required and the authors suggest that such an anastomosis is best splinted for a prolonged period after operation. T-tubes were formerly used to stent such anastomoses but are no longer advocated since they tend to fall out prematurely and this may permit recurrent stricture. Transhepatic tubes, as used by Smith, may allow more secure biliary intubation[51], but these also tend to be extruded prematurely. Saypol and Kurian[52] first used U-tubes to allow prolonged, secure biliary intubation in the management of benign biliary strictures. Terblanche and co-authors extended the use of U-tubes to malignant biliary strictures[53]. A major advantage of such tubes is that they do not fall out and they can be changed without further surgery, since a new tube can be joined to a previous tube and pulled ('railroaded') into position.

Unfortunately, most bile duct injuries are recognized after operation. In this context, one of the most important factors determining the fate of subsequent repair is the quality and accessibility of the *proximal bile duct*, the bile duct above the stricture. As the review of 900 cases of traumatic biliary stricture by Warren, McDonald and Kune[54] pointed out, the extent of the stricture and the quality and calibre of distal ducts are important in determining the choice of operation but the presence of other concurrent disease and the general condition of the patient can be equally significant.

Several types of operation are available. Staged repair can be performed in poor-risk patients including those with sepsis, subphrenic abscess or portal hypertension and bleeding varices. The first priority is to establish bile drainage and preserve hepatic function; this can be achieved without operation by percutaneous transhepatic drainage, permitting resolution of hyperbilirubinaemia and preparation for definitive bile duct repair. During this interval, other complicating factors such as sepsis or portal hypertension and bleeding varices can be controlled secondarily.

The Heineke–Mickulicz repair is indicated for a short or localized stricture, although this is rarely encountered (Figure 27). The stricture is divided longitudinally and sutured transversely to widen the duct lumen. The duodenum is mobilized to relieve tension and a T-tube is brought out as a splint below the anastomosis. Here the T-tube is usually removed after a cholangiogram, done 3 months postoperatively, reveals healing of the anastomosis.

Theoretically, duct-to-duct anastomosis after excision of a stricture is the best method of repair. In reality, however, the results of such repair are not better than those after a biliary–intestinal anastomosis[55] perhaps because of anastomotic tension or disturbed duct blood supply as mentioned above. In this regard, duct-to-duct anastomosis is recommended only if the two ends of the bile duct appear to have a good blood supply, are about the same diameter and can be anastomosed without tension (Figure 28). If these conditions cannot be met, a biliary–intestinal

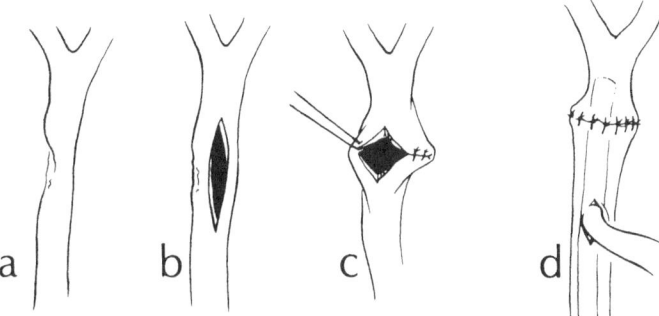

Figure 27 If a short stricture is encountered, a Heineke–Mickulicz repair may be possible. The stricture is divided longitudinally and sutured horizontally. A T-tube is inserted below the anastomosis

anastomosis is recommended, since it is more likely to be successful[54,55]. Biliary–intestinal anastomosis is consequently necessary for a large number of biliary strictures. For strictures of the distal CBD, a choledochoduodenostomy may be performed, or a Roux-en-Y choledochojejunostomy for strictures of the proximal CBD. For common hepatic duct strictures, a Roux-en-Y hepaticojejunostomy with a U-tube stent is advocated as the Roux loop minimizes or prevents intestinal reflux. The U-tube stent is required since such anastomoses are technically difficult and mucosa-to-mucosa apposition is poor; without prolonged stenting the incidence of re-stricture is extremely high[55].

Surgical technique

Exposure is usually facilitated by a generous right subcostal incision with extension to the left side if necessary. Adhesions from previous surgery are severed and the hepatic flexure of colon and the duodenum are mobilized to afford excellent exposure. The bile duct proximal to the stricture is usually found anteromedial to the hepatic artery at the hepatic hilum. The dilated, occluded proximal duct may be identified by needle aspiration of bile, by the preoperative insertion of a percutaneous transhepatic catheter, or by an intraoperative transhepatic cholangiogram. When the proximal bile duct is found, it is freed from surrounding scar or other tissues and trimmed until a rim of duct at least 6–8 mm long is obtained for anastomosis, although excessive mobilization may harm the duct's precarious blood supply. The proximal biliary tree is carefully explored and irrigated with saline. The most difficult cases involve the confluence of the right and left hepatic ducts

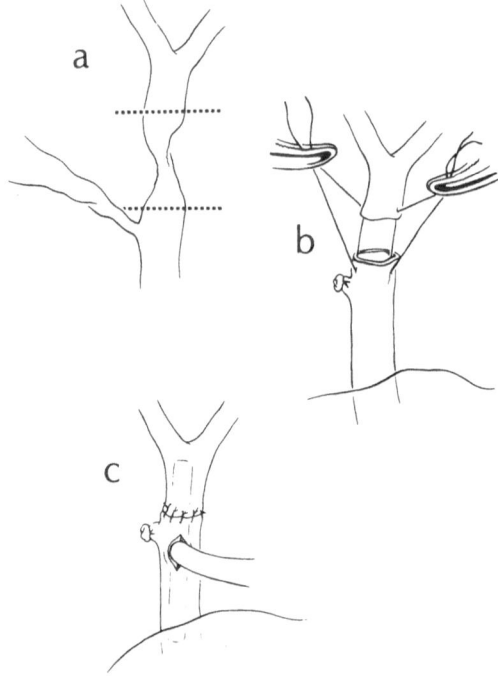

Figure 28   This short and favourable biliary stricture was excised and a duct-to-duct anastomosis was performed over a T-tube without tension

or strictures of individual hepatic ducts. If the proximal end of the stricture stops at the level of union of the two hepatic ducts, the 'carina' should be excised to permit hepaticojejunostomy with a wider stoma (Figure 29). The aim of subsequent surgical manoeuvres is to achieve duct mucosa-to-mucosa apposition with the widest possible stoma and without tension[51] and the operators' use of magnifying loops may be helpful. The principles of duct repair are difficult to meet in most established strictures and an internal splint is essential.

If preoperative PTC and/or ERCP indicate that the distal bile duct may be useful for anastomosis it is looked for, otherwise a Roux-en-Y hepaticojejunostomy is performed without any attempt at locating the distal duct. If it is decided to locate the distal bile duct, the lymph node that lies above the duodenum and lateral to the CBD, the so-called common duct gland may be a useful landmark in locating the CBD obscured by previous surgery. Alternately, if dissection in the supraduodenal area appears unrewarding, a duodenotomy and insertion of a probe through

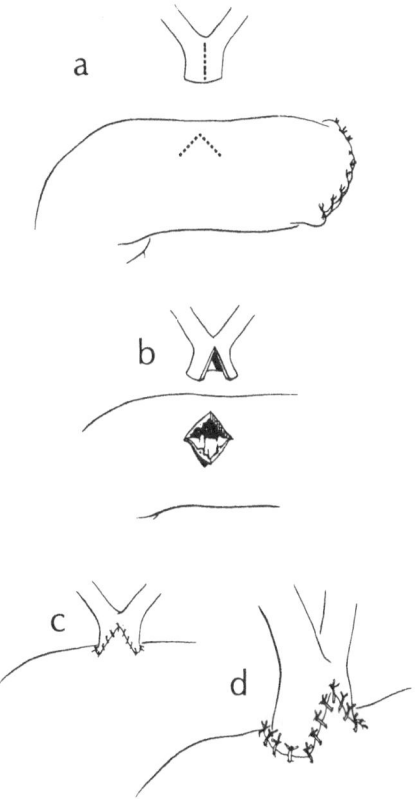

Figure 29   If the proximal end of a biliary stricture stops at the level of union of right and left hepatic ducts (a), the 'carina' should be excised (b) to allow a wider stoma for hepatico-jejunostomy (c) and (d)

the ampulla of Vater may be necessary. Once bile duct distal to the stric-ture is located, it is trimmed and examined to determine if it is suitable for anastomosis. As is commonly the case, if it is occluded with scar, of small calibre or so fibrotic that it will not distend to 10 mm diameter, it is considered unsuitable for anastomosis. The distal duct should be fully explored, of course, to ensure that no further obstruction exists.

The first step in a Roux-en-Y hepaticojejunostomy is to construct a defunctioned segment of jejunum approximately 40 cm long (Figure 30). The end of the jejunal segment is closed and an enterotomy is made in the side of the jejunum near the end. End-to-side anastomosis to proxi-mal duct is performed with a single row of through-and-through inter-

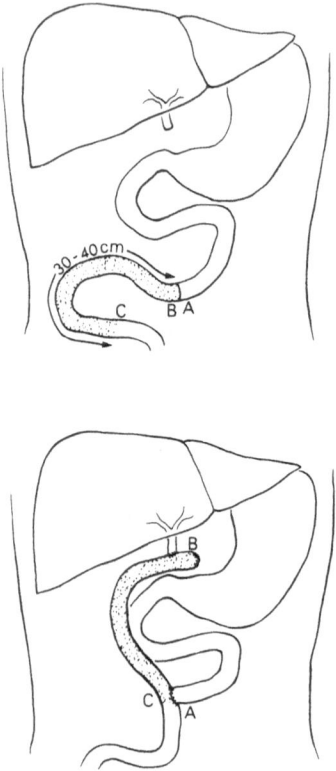

Figure 30 A Roux-en-Y limb of jejunum is constructed by division of the jejunum distal to the ligament of Treitz (top) with an end-to-side jejunojejunostomy. The end of the jejunal limb is closed and an end-to-side Roux-en-Y hepaticojejunostomy is formed (bottom)

rupted sutures of 4–O polyglycolic acid and the posterior row of sutures is placed first. The hepatojejunal anastomosis is splinted with a U-tube or tubes (Figure 31) inserted before the anterior row of polyglycolic acid sutures. A Randall's stone forcep is passed up the right or left hepatic duct as far as possible, bringing the forceps close to Glisson's capsule at the liver surface. Pushing the stone forceps through the intervening bridge of liver tissue enables the operator to grasp a silastic tube (Dow Corning, Mississauga, Ontario, Canada) of appropriate length and diameter which is pulled through the liver substance into the duct remnant, through the anastomosis and out the lateral wall of the jejunal segment. This tube is brought through the anterior abdominal wall at two sites, one close to its exit from the liver, the other close to its exit from the jejunal segment; it resembles a U lying sideways, and hence its name. One or two U-tubes can be inserted into the biliary tree depending on the location and extent of the lesion. After U-tube placement, the hepaticojejunal anastomosis is completed and the intestinal limb containing the hepaticojejunostomy is suspended to the undersurface of the liver by a few sutures to prevent any pull on the anastomosis.

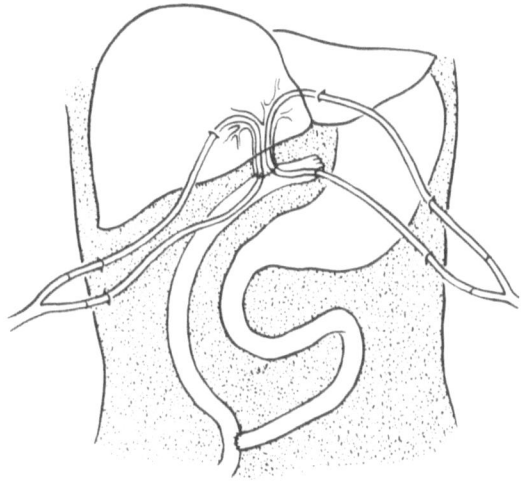

Figure 31   Two U-tubes have been inserted, one through the right and one through the left hepatic ducts

A modification of the Roux-en-Y hepaticojejunostomy was introduced by Rodney Smith in 1967 and reported in 1969[56]. In constructing the hepaticojejunal anastomosis, a circular seromuscular disc is excised from the jejunum and the mucosa is left intact. A small balloon-tipped transhepatic catheter is passed through the common hepatic duct into the jejunum through a small incision in the jejunal mucosa. The balloon is inflated and what has been termed a 'mucosal–jejunal graft' is pulled up to the hepatic ducts (Figure 32). No sutures are used in anastomosis although the jejunum is tethered to the undersurface of the liver with several sutures. The long-term results of this mucosal graft operation are largely unknown but the preliminary (6–18 months) results published in 1975 are encouraging [57]: 50 patients underwent 61 mucosal graft operations with a 65% success rate per operation and an 85% ultimate success rate. The operative mortality was 6%, the average hospitalization period was 19.6 days and the transhepatic catheter tube was removed after 3 months.

Much controversy surrounds the subject of splinting duct–intestinal anastomoses and there are two schools of thought. Proponents of the

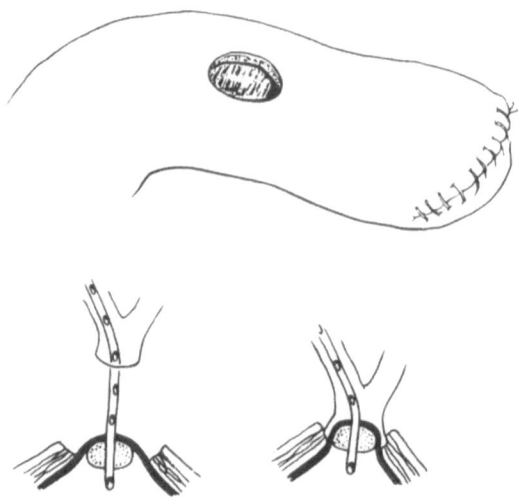

Figure 32 The Rodney Smith mucosal graft technique. A seromuscular disc is excised from the Roux-en-Y jejunal limb (top). A small balloon-tipped transhepatic catheter has been passed through the common hepatic duct and into the jejunum through a small incision in the jejunal mucosa (bottom left). The balloon is inflated and pulled up to effect a 'mucosal graft' of the bile duct (bottom right)

first advocate a short period of splinting of about 3 months[57,58] while others advocate prolonged internal splinting[54,55] since a number of investigators have considered their results optimal with splinting of such anastomoses for 12–18 months[55] (Figure 33). A recent Russian publication states that 2 years is the optimal time for a U-tube to be left in the biliary tree after benign strictures are repaired[59]. Our experience with prolonged splinting has been excellent and we advocate this whenever a duct-enteric anastomosis is under tension, has poor blood supply, does not have a wide stoma, or is performed for a recurrent biliary stricture, since the advantages of a secure anastomosis far outweigh the risks of recurrent stricture, sepsis and further operation. The use of the U-tube as an adjunct in the treatment of benign biliary strictures represents a major advance in abdominal surgery.

In spite of improved diagnosis and treatment of biliary strictures, an operative mortality of 5–8% attends operations directed at such repair[41]. Although figures for large series using prolonged U-tube stenting are not available, from previous studies there is a 10% incidence of major complications and a 35% incidence of re-stenosis, usually within 3 years. Ultimately, however, 60–70% of patients who have sustained an operative injury to the bile ducts are restored to normal health if their

BILIARY STRICTURES

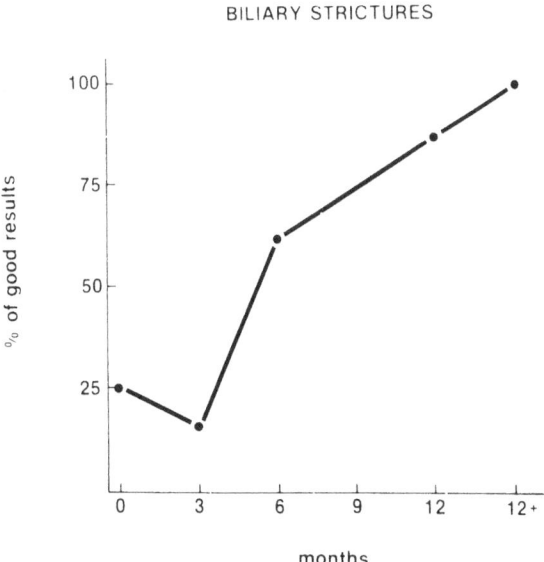

Figure 33 The percentage of good results after repair of biliary structures is plotted against the length of time biliary stents were left *in situ*. It is noted that the longer the stent is left in place, the better the results. Reprinted with permission from Kune *et al.*[55]

repair is performed by experienced surgeons. Those patients who die following the development or redevelopment of a biliary stricture usually do so secondary to hepatic failure or portal hypertension with bleeding gastro-oesophageal varices.

Portal hypertension has been noted in 20% of patients with established biliary stricture but once biliary strictures are effectively treated, significant complications of portal hypertension are uncommon. In one series of patients with failed repair of biliary strictures, portal hypertension developed 2–5 years after the diagnosis of a biliary stricture and bleeding varices were noted within 1–9 years of diagnosis, with an average delay of 5 years. Michie[60], however, noted that in a few cases cirrhosis developed within several months of bile duct injury, with established cirrhosis present at 1 year and death from bleeding varices within 32 months. Obviously, when portal hypertension coexists with a biliary stricture, preservation of hepatic function is paramount. This usually mandates prompt repair of the biliary stricture although later operation for portal hypertension may be necessary.

MALIGNANT BILIARY OBSTRUCTION

Bile duct cancer represents 2.9–4.6% of all malignant tumours found at autopsy.[61] A third to a half of bile duct cancers occur high in the hilum of the liver, involving the right or left hepatic duct or their confluence[11,62]. Accurate diagnosis was difficult before PTC, ERCP, ultrasonography and CAT, but localization and the probable diagnosis of tumour are now readily apparent, permitting successful resection or palliative intubation in a large number of patients. Patients with malignant biliary obstruction usually present with obstructive jaundice and pain is present in about half of cases[62,63]. The pattern of the obstructive jaundice caused by these tumours is not unique and requires the standard investigation referred to hitherto (Figure 1). Precise pathological diagnosis usually requires laparotomy.

Microscopically, the majority (95%) of bile duct tumours are adenocarcinomas[11,62] derived from bile duct epithelium and three gross types of duct malignancy are observed[62,64]. Local or nodular carcinomas are small, well-localized, firm to hard tumours, often located in the upper bile duct; they are less common but more amenable to resection than infiltrating carcinomas. In the diffuse or infiltrative growths, the wall of the bile duct over an extensive area is thickened with fibrous tissue and clinical and pathological differentiation from sclerosing cholangitis is difficult. Papillary carcinomas are the third type of tumour and grow within the lumen of bile ducts. Although intraoperative choledochoscopy may reveal multiple sites of tumour growth, some authors suggest that this tumour type has a better prognosis[65] than the nodular or infiltrative growths.

Although bile duct tumours are sometimes small and well localized, they usually involve the hepatic artery and/or portal vein early in their course and frequently extend into the hepatic parenchyma, making complete tumour excision impossible without either extensive liver resection or liver transplantation. In a series of 30 supraduodenal bile duct cancers, Takasan et al. reported that 20 were infiltrating carcinomas, and of these, only one was resectable[64]. Distant metastases from bile duct carcinoma are uncommon and occur late in the course of the disease[65]. Early mortality is thus commonly due to hepatic failure or cholangitis secondary to prolonged biliary obstruction. Recognition of this clinical course has led to a variety of procedures which afford excellent palliation by relieving biliary obstruction.

As has been mentioned, tumours of the hepatic ducts were difficult to diagnose until the recent widespread use of PTC, ERCP, ultrasonography and CAT. Hence, much of the literature before the advent of newer investigative modalities documents many cases in which diagnosis was delayed, as it was, for example, in 9 of Klatskin's 13 cases[65], 8 of Longmire's 25 cases[11], and 11 of our 80 cases[62]; all too often the diagnosis of a bile duct carcinoma was missed at laparotomy for obstructive jaundice. Such recognition now occurs early: obstruction of right, left or both hepatic ducts as visualized preoperatively by transhepatic cholangiography with uniformly dilated proximal intrahepatic ducts in a patient who has not had previous biliary tract surgery indicates a malignant obstruction.

Treatment

Since most patients with biliary tumours present with jaundice, preoperative percutaneous transhepatic drainage should be performed on patients with hyperbilirubinaemia (greater than 10 mg/dl) to minimize operative mortality[43]. The treatment and prognosis of bile duct cancers obviously depend on tumour location, histology and spread. For purposes of discussion, the extrahepatic biliary tract can be divided into three parts (Figure 34):

Tumours of the hepatic ducts (upper third tumours)

These are tumours involving the right or left hepatic duct, the common hepatic duct or the cystic duct (Figure 34). Tumours involving the junction of the right and left hepatic duct are known as Klatskin tumours after the author who first described these tumours in detail and reported 13 cases in 1965[65].

Radical excision of bile duct tumours is advised whenever possible as it offers the only hope of cure; unfortunately, however, only 7–18% of tumours are resectable[11,62–64]. A bile duct tumour involving the right hepatic duct and growing into the right lobe of the liver can be removed en bloc with the right lobe of the liver, provided the left hepatic duct, the left hepatic artery and the left portal vein are tumour-free. Because of the juxtaposition of vital anatomical structures in this area, the majority of proximal bile duct tumours are unresectable due to local spread to the hepatic parenchyma, involvement of the hepatic artery or portal vein. Radiotherapy should be routinely employed after radical resection to eradicate the residual microscopic foci of tumour cells that are almost always left behind, even after so-called 'radical resection'[62].

If complete resection is impossible, significant palliation can be achieved by removal of as much obstructing tumour as possible with a subsequent Roux-en-Y hepaticojejunostomy stented with a U-tube (see above), by dilatation of obstructing tumour and U-tube insertion or by a modified Longmire procedure (see below). Following any of these palliative procedures, radiotherapy is indicated[62,66–68], since it has been found to prolong survival. This is facilitated by delineating tumour at

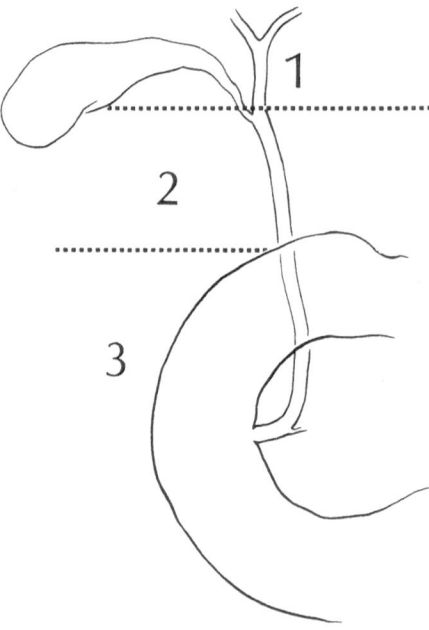

Figure 34   The biliary tract can be divided into three areas. The upper third (1) includes the right, left and common hepatic ducts down to the junction with the cystic duct. The middle third (2) of the biliary tract is the supraduodenal portion of the common bile duct. The lower third (3) of the biliary tract includes the retroduodenal, intrapancreatic and transduodenal portions of the common bile duct

operation with metal clips. Patients with biliary tumours and distant metastases, or patients who are very poor operative risks, can be palliated with percutaneous transhepatic drainage plus radiotherapy, although such drainage tubes tend to fall out or block and are clearly a poor alternative to more definitive management. Our experience with chemotherapy of bile duct cancers is limited and we have not observed real benefit.

If the bile duct malignancy is unresectable, dilatation with rigid dilators followed by insertion of a transhepatic U-tube coursing through tumour and out of the CBD below the tumour can afford useful palliation and this can be followed by radiotherapy with benefit. In some cases, where surgical access to the porta hepatis is impossible because of tumour invasion, a modified Longmire procedure may be useful. The Longmire procedure as originally described involves amputation of part or most of the left lateral segment of the liver with a Roux-en-Y hepaticojejunostomy, anastomosing the exposed left hepatic duct to a limb of jejunum. Since this procedure often proved unsuccessful, with stricture formation and occlusion of the hepaticojejunostomy, it has been modified by inserting a silastic tube through the exposed bile duct and through the Roux-en-Y limb to enhance biliary drainage. Such a procedure is of occasional use when the porta hepatis is inaccessible.

Tumours of the middle third

Tumours of the middle third of the bile ducts (Figure 34) are more often resectable (31–40%)[11,58] than tumours of the upper third and they are associated with a better survival. In Longmire's series, roughly half such patients survive 3 years, although only 8% survive 5 years or more[11]. As for upper third tumours, surgical resection is the best treatment but if not feasible, a palliative bypass or resection and stenting should be performed and adjunctive radiotherapy has been associated with benefit.

Tumours of the distal third

Tumours of the distal third or lower common bile duct (Figure 34) are generally grouped with periampullary tumours. They have a better prognosis than either carcinomas of the head of the pancreas or carcinomas of the upper bile duct. The better prognosis is related to a higher resectability rate (75–82%)[11,58] because of a more favourable location, although 5-year survival rates are poor (15%)[58]. The treatment of these tumours usually requires a pancreaticoduodenectomy (Whipple procedure) or a total pancreatectomy and duodenectomy. Reconstruction usually requires Roux-en-Y hepaticojejunostomy with a T-tube left in place for a short period thereafter. Here a short period of stenting is indicated, since the anastomosis is more secure because of a larger bile duct.

SCLEROSING CHOLANGITIS

Sclerosing cholangitis is a rare disease of unknown aetiology that was first described by Delbet in 1924[69]. Sclerosing cholangitis may be segmental or diffuse and can involve only segments of or the entire biliary tree[70,71]. The rarity of this disease is demonstrated by the fact that Glenn found but 20 patients with sclerosing cholangitis among 11 000 patients treated surgically for biliary tract disease over a 45-year review period[72]. Glenn further states that only 150–200 cases have been described worldwide[72].

In an effort to define sclerosing cholangitis more precisely, Holubitsky and McKenzie established the following diagnostic criteria[73]:

absence of previous operative trauma to the biliary tract, absence of calculi in the gallbladder and common bile duct, sclerosis and stenosis involving all or almost all of the extrahepatic ducts and exclusion of biliary tract malignancy. Others[74] have excluded patients with associated ulcerative colitis, Crohn's disease, biliary cirrhosis or retroperitoneal fibrosis. This exclusion does not seem justifiable, since the biliary tract disease in these cases follows the same clinical and pathological course as sclerosing cholangitis without such association.

The disease entity is characterized by a diffuse mural thickening of a segment of, or the entire, common bile duct, diminishing its lumen. The fibrosis and inflammation which involves the common duct can extend to the adjoining structures in the hepatoduodenal ligament and regional lymphadenopathy is usually present. Pruritus and jaundice are the most common symptoms and itching frequently precedes jaundice by weeks or months. Most patients complain of vague right upper abdominal distress and two-thirds of patients have hepatosplenomegaly[11] but fever is unusual. Serum bilirubin and alkaline phosphatase are generally elevated. The disease tends to exhibit remissions and exacerbations and an unpredictable course with usual slow progression and ultimate death with liver failure in 2–3 years, although other cases linger with chronic disease for many years.

The recurrent obstructive jaundice with which these patients present requires a percutaneous transhepatic cholangiogram (PTC) and/or an endoscopic retrograde cholangiopancreatogram (ERCP) as part of diagnostic work-up. The PTC will usually fail because of the small, thick-walled ducts but an ERCP may suggest the diagnosis preoperatively. A preoperative or operative cholangiogram of good quality with complete filling of the intra- and extrahepatic ductal system is very valuable in differentiating sclerosing cholangitis from a sclerosing bile duct carcinoma. In sclerosing cholangitis, there is diffuse narrowing of the biliary tree with alternating areas of constriction and dilatation, whereas with bile duct carcinoma, there is an obstruction with uniform dilatation above it.

The diagnosis of sclerosing cholangitis is usually established at operation and the most important objective of operation is to distinguish sclerosing cholangitis from sclerosing carcinoma by biopsy of the duct wall[11]. In some doubtful cases the final diagnosis must await the outcome of clinical follow-up over a period of years[11]. A T-tube is usually inserted following duct exploration. Longmire advises that this be removed within 2 weeks to avoid bacterial contamination of the biliary tree[11], an attitude we agree with, since prolonged T-tube drainage has not been shown to improve the disease. If one accepts that sclerosing cholangitis may be segmental and operative cholangiograms indicate a localized stenosis in the extrahepatic biliary tree with proximal dilatation, as described by Grodsinsky et al.[70] and Caroli et al.[71], then excision of the stricture with duct-enteric anastomosis may afford long-term benefit. The therapeutic administration of corticosteroids is controversial and, apart from imparting a general sense of well-being, is not clearly beneficial[72]. If bacterial cholangitis occurs, a cephalosporin and an aminoglycoside antibiotic should be administered until appropriate culture studies are available. Cholestyramine can be helpful in reducing pruritus.

FIBROSIS OF THE SPHINCTER OF ODDI

Longmire put the problem well when he stated that 'One of the most controversial problems of biliary tract surgery relates to correlation of clinical symptoms with dysfunction of the sphincter of Oddi. The problem is made even more complex by the fact that symptoms of sphincter dysfunction may be related to the biliary tract, to the pancreas or to both systems'[9,11].

Stenosis of the sphincter of Oddi was first described by Florshen in 1912[75]. Fourteen years later, Del Valle and Donovan[76] presented a clinicopathological analysis of patients with total or partial common bile duct obstruction resulting from chronic fibrosis of the papilla of Vater. The true incidence of this condition is unknown but Yvergneaux et al. from Belgium[77], in a series of 1150 biliary tract operations in which radiomanometry was performed and in which contrast was injected under known pressure, diagnosed 65 cases (5.7%) of 'benign Oddi stenosis'. In 50 of these 65 cases, associated pathology was found, usually on the basis of calculous disease, leaving only 15 cases in which 'benign Oddi stenosis' was an isolated circumstance: an incidence of 1.3% of biliary tract operations.

A variety of symptoms have been positively associated with this disease. Pain is said to be present in 90% of cases. This can be continuous or intermittent and noted in the right upper quadrant or epigastrium and it may radiate to the back or lower scapula. Jaundice or a history thereof is present in 50% of patients and more than 80% of patients have had one or more previous biliary tract operations without relief of symptoms. A preoperative ERCP that shows delayed emptying of the CBD is said to suggest fibrosis of the sphincter of Oddi but the definitive diagnosis is made at surgery, although definite diagnostic criteria have not been established. Some surgeons diagnose the condition on inability to pass a No. 3 Bakes dilator through the sphincter of Oddi but this manoeuvre is unreliable and possibly dangerous[11,78] since it can lead to perforation or a false passage.

The diagnosis has been noted pathologically with evidence of extensive fibrosis in tissues submitted at the time of sphincteroplasty[79], although again, there are no definite pathological criteria available for diagnosis. Fibrosis of the sphincter of Oddi remains a poorly defined entity. Transduodenal sphincteroplasty (rather than sphincterotomy) with submission of the tissue excised from the ampulla of Vater for pathological examination would seem to be the treatment of choice if other biliary tract and other intra-abdominal disease has been excluded by careful investigation.

SUMMARY

Significant advances have recently been made in the diagnosis and treatment of biliary tract obstruction. The newer diagnostic modalities include ultrasonography, computerized axial tomography, percutaneous transhepatic cholangiography and endoscopic retrograde cholangiopancreatography. These permit early localization and probable diagnosis prior to operation, which can be planned more carefully.

The biliary surgeon now has an expanded therapeutic armamentarium. There are a variety of techniques whereby retained common duct stones can be prevented and even if retained stones are apparent, mechanical extraction, chemical dissolution or endoscopic papillotomy make reoperation seldom necessary. Better delineation of the 'normal' biliary tract anatomy makes iatrogenic stricture formation less likely but the principles of repair with long-term stenting of biliary intestinal anastomoses make biliary strictures less formidable problems than they once were. The newer diagnostic modalities may permit early detection and excision of biliary tract malignancies. Even if these are unresectable, however, significant palliation can often be obtained by percutaneous hepatic drainage or easily replaceable U-tubes. Better care is available for patients with biliary tract obstruction of diverse aetiologies.

References

1 Schuppel, O. (1878). Die Krankheiten der Gallenwege und der Pfortader in von Ziemssen, H. (ed.): Handbuch der Speziellen Pathologie und Therapie, lief XXII, 4 (Leipzig: F. C. W. Vogen)
2 Thorbjarnarson, B. (1975). Surgery of the Biliary Tract (Toronto: W. B. Saunders)
3 Stoller, J. L., Copperberg P. L. and Simpson, W. M. (1979). Diagnostic ultrasonography in aucte cholecystitis. Can. J. Surg., 22, 374
4 McKay, A. J., Duncan, J. G., Lam, P. et al. (1979). The role of grey scale ultrasonography in acute cholecystitis. Can. J. Surg., 22, 374
5 McCluskey, P. L., Prinz, R. A., Guico, R. et al. (1979). Use of ultrasound to demonstrate gallstones in symptomatic patients with normal oral cholecystograms. Am. J. Surg., 138, 655
6 Prian, G. W., Norton, L. W., Eule, J, Jr et al. (1977). Clinical indications and accuracy

of grey scale ultrasonography in the patient with suspected biliary tract disease. *Am. J. Surg.*, **134,** 705

7   Taylor, K. J. W. and Rosenfield, A. T. (1977). Grey-scale ultrasonography in the differential diagnosis of jaundice. *Arch. Surg.*, **112,** 820

8   Cintora, I., Ben-Ora, A., MacNeil, R. *et al.* (1979). Cholecystosonography for the decision to operate when acute cholecystitis is suspected. *Am. J. Surg.*, **138,** 818

9   Okuda, K., Tanikawa, K., Emura, T. *et al.* (1974). Non-surgical, percutaneous transhepatic cholangiography – diagnostic significance in medical problems of the liver. *Dig. Dis.*, **19,** 21

10 Glenn, E. and McSherry, C. K. (1975). Calculous biliary tract disease. *Curr. Prob. Surg.*, June

11 Longmire, W. P. Jr. (1977). The diverse causes of biliary obstruction and their remedies. *Curr. Prob. Surg.*, **XIV** (7) 1–59, July 1977.

12 Corlette, M. B., Schatzki, S. and Ackroyd, F. (1978). Operative cholangiography and overlooked stones. *Arch. Surg.*, **113,** 729

13 Jolly, P. C., Baker, J. W., Schmidt, H. M. *et al.* (1968). Operative cholangiography: case for its routine use. *Ann. Surg.*, **168,** 551

14 Way, L. W., Admirand, W. H. and Dunphy, J. E. (1972). Management of choledocholithiasis. *Ann. Surg.*, **176,** 247

15 Faris, I., Thompson, J. P. S., Grundy, D. J. and LeQuesne L. P. (1975). Operative cholangiography: a reappraisal based upon a review of 400 cholangiograms. *Br. J. Surg.*, **62,** 966

16 Brendan Devlin, H., Sabay, A. K., Tiwari, P. N. *et al.* (1978). Cholecystectomy and a simple technique of operative cholangiography. *Br. J. Surg.*, **65,** 848

17 White, T. T., Waisman, H., Hopton, D. *et al.* (1972). Radiomanometry, flow rate and cholangiography in the evaluation of common bile duct disease. *Am. J. Surg.*, **123,** 73

18 White, T. T. and Bordley, J, IV (1978). One percent incidence of recurrent gallstones six to eight years after manometric cholangiography. *Ann. Surg.*, **188,** 562

19 Hopton, D. (1978). Common bile duct perfusion combined with operative cholangiography. *Br. J. Surg.*, **65,** 852

20 Nora, P. F., Berci, G., Dorazio, R. A. *et al.* (1977). Operative choledochoscopy: results of a prospective study in several institutions. *Am. J. Surg.*, **133,** 105

21 Kappas, A., Alexander-Williams, J., Keighley, M. R. B. *et al.* (1979). Operative choledochoscopy. *Br. J. Surg.*, **66,** 177

22 Mondet, A. (1962). Tecnica de la extraccion incruenta de los calculos en la litiasis residual del coledoco. *Bol. Soc. Cir. Buenos Aires*, **46,** 278

23 Mazzariello, R. M. (1976). Residual biliary tract stones: non-operative treatment of 570 patients. *Surg. Ann.*, **8,** 113

24 Mazzariello, R. M. (1980). Non-operative treatment of residual biliary tract stones. In Maingot, R. (ed.) *Abdominal Operations*, Vol. I, pp. 1166–1175. (New York: Appleton-Century-Crofts)

25 Burhenne, H. J. (1974). Non-operative roentgenologic instrumentation technics of the post-operative biliary tract. *Am. J. Surg.*, **128,** 111

26 Classen, M. and Demling, L. (1974). Endoskopische sphincterotomie der papilla Vateri und steinextraktion aus dem ductus choledochus. *Dtsch. Med. Wochenschr.*, **99,** 496

27 Safrany, L. (1978). Endoscopic treatment of biliary tract disease. An international study. *Lancet*, **2,** 983

28 Safrany, L. (1978). Transduodenal endoscopic sphincterotomy and extraction of bile duct stones. *World J. Surg.*, **2,** 457

29 Seifert, E. (1978). Endoscopic papillotomy and removal of gallstones. *Am. J. Gastroenterol.*, **69,** 154

30 Zimmon, D. S. (1978). Invited commentary. *World J. Surg.*, **2,** 463

31 Best, R. R. (1938). Cholangiographic demonstration of the remaining common duct stone and its non-operative management. *Surg. Gynecol. Obstet.*, **66**, 1040
32 Best, R. R. (1965). Editorial. *Rev. Surg.*, **22**, 405
33 Way, L. W. (1973). Retained common duct stones. *Surg. Clin. N. Am.*, **53**, 1139
34 Way, L. W. and Motson, R. W. (1976). Dissolution of retained common duct stones. *Adv. Surg.*, **10**, 99
35 Gardner, B., Dennis, C. R. and Patti, J. (1975). Current status of heparin dissolution of gallstones. *Am. J. Surg.*, **130**, 293
36 Witzel, L., Weiderholt, J. and Wolbergs, E. (1980). Dissolution of gallstones by perfusion with Capmul via a catheter introduced endoscopically into the bile duct. *N. Engl. J. Med.*, **303**, 465
37 Thistle, J. L., Carlson, G. L., Hofmann, A. F. *et al.* (1980). Monooctanoin, a dissolution agent for retained cholesterol bile duct stones: physical properties and clinical application. *Gastroenterology*, **78**, 1016
38 Smith, R. (1980). Personal communication as quoted by Austin Jones. In Maingot, R. (ed.). *Abdominal Operations*, Vol. I, Chap. 68, p. 1124. (New York: Appleton-Century-Crofts)
39 Madden, J. L. (1976). Choledochoduodenostomy. In Varco, R. L. and Delaney, J. P. (eds.). *Controversy in Surgery*, Chap. 11, pp. 235–240. (Toronto: W. B. Saunders)
40 Austin Jones, S. (1980). Transduodenal sphincteroplasty (not sphincterotomy) in the prophylaxis and treatment of residual common duct stones. In Maingot, R. (ed.). *Abdominal Operations*, pp. 1113–1127. (New York: Appleton-Century-Crofts)
41 Kune, G. (1972). *Current Practice of Biliary Surgery*. (New York: Little, Brown & Company)
42 Northover, J. M. A. and Terblanche, J. (1979). A new look at the arterial supply of the bile duct in man and its surgical implications. *Br. J. Surg.*, **66**, 379
43 Nakayama, T., Ikeda, A. and Okuda, K. (1978). Percutaneous transhepatic drainage of the biliary tract. Technique and results in 104 cases. *Gastroenterology*, **74**, 554
44 Glenn, F., Evans, J. A., Mujahed, Z. *et al.* (1962). Percutaneous transhepatic cholangiography. *Ann. Surg.*, **156**, 451
45 Mori, K., Misumi, A., Sugiyama, M. *et al.* (1977). Percutaneous transhepatic bile drainage. *Ann. Surg.*, **185**, 111
46 Hansson, J. A., Hoevels, J., Simert, G. *et al.* (1979). Clinical aspects of non-surgical percutaneous transhepatic bile drainage in obstructive lesions of the extrahepatic bile ducts. *Ann. Surg.*, **189**, 58
47 Ring, E. J., Husted, J. W., Oleaga, J. A. *et al.* (1979). A multihole catheter for maintaining long-term percutaneous antegrade biliary drainage. *Radiology*, **132**, 752
48 Pereiras, R. V. Jr., Rheingold, O. J., Hutson D. *et al.* (1978). Relief of malignant obstructive jaundice by percutaneous insertion of a permanent prosthesis in the biliary tree. *Ann. Intern. Med.*, **89**, 589
49 Hoevels, J. and Ihse, I. (1979). Percutaneous transhepatic insertion of a permanent endoprosthesis in obstructive lesions of the extrahepatic bile ducts. *Gastrointest. Radiol.*, **4**, 367
50 Burcharth, F., Jensen, L. I. and Olesen, K. (1979). Endoprosthesis for internal drainage of the biliary tract. Technique and results in 48 cases. *Gastroenterology*, **77**, 133
51 Smith, R. (1964). Hepaticojejunostomy with transhepatic intubation. A technique for very high strictures of the hepatic ducts. *Br. J. Surg.*, **51**, 186
52 Saypol, G. M. and Kurian, G. (1969). A technique of repair of stricture of the bile duct. *Surg. Gynecol. Obstet.*, **128**, 1071
53 Terblanche, J, Saunders, S. J. and Louw, J. H. (1972). Prolonged palliation in carcinoma of the main hepatic duct junction. *Surgery*, **71**, 720
54 Warren, K. W., McDonald, W. M. and Kune, G. A. (1966). Bile duct strictures. New concepts in the management of an old problem. In Irvine, W. T. (ed.). *Modern Trends*

in Surgery, (2nd edn) (London: Butterworth)
55 Kune, G. A., Hardy, K. J., Brown, G. *et al.* (1969). Operative injuries of the bile ducts. *Med. J. Aust.*, **2**, 233
56 Smith, R. (1969). Strictures of the bile ducts. *Proc. R. Soc. Med.*, **62**, 131
57 Wexler, M. J. and Smith, R. (1975). Jejunal mucosal graft. A sutureless technic for repair of high bile duct strictures. *Am. J. Surg.*, **129**, 204
58 Hertzer, N. R., Gray, H. W., Hoerr, S. O. *et al.* (1973). The use of T-tube splints in bile duct repairs. *Surg. Gynecol. Obstet.*, **137**, 413
59 Galperin, E. I. and Kuzovlev, N. F. (1980). Exchangeable transhepatic drainage in benign obstructions of the proximal hepatic duct. *Surg. Gynecol. Obstet.*, **151**, 325
60 Michie, W. and Gunn, A. (1964). Bile duct injuries. A new suggestion for their repair. *Br. J. Surg.*, **51**, 96
61 Sako, K., Seitzinger, G. L. and Garside, E. (1957). Carcinoma of the extrahepatic bile ducts; review of the literature and report of six cases. *Surgery*, **4**, 416
62 Black, K., Hanna, S. S., Langer, B., Jirsch, D. W. and Rider, W. D. (1978). Management of carcinoma of the extrahepatic bile ducts. *Can. J. Surg.*, **21**, 542
63 Ross, A. P., Braasch, J. W. and Warren, K. W. (1973). Carcinoma of the proximal bile ducts. *Surg. Gynecol. Obstet.*, **136**, 923
64 Takasan, H., Kim, C. I., Arii, S. *et al.* (1980). Clinicopathologic study of seventy patients with carcinoma of the biliary tract. *Surg. Gynecol. Obstet.*, **150**, 721
65 Klatskin, G. (1965). Adenocarcinoma of the hepatic duct at its bifurcation within the porta hepatis. *Am. J. Med.*, **38**, 241
66 Hanna, S. S. and Rider, W. D. (1978). Carcinoma of the gallbladder or extrahepatic bile ducts: the role of radiotherapy. *Can. Med. Assoc. J.*, **118**, 59
67 Green, N., Mikkelson, W. P. and Kernen, J. A. (1973). Cancer of the common hepatic bile ducts – palliative radiotherapy. *Radiology*, **109**, 687
68 Kopelson, G., Harisiadis, L., Tretter, P. *et al.* (1977). The role of radiation therapy in cancer of the extrahepatic biliary system. *Int. J. Radiat. Oncol. Biol. Phys.*, **2**, 883
69 Delbet, P. (1974). *Bull. Mem. Soc. Chir. Paris*, **50**, 1144
70 Grodsinsky, C., Block, H. A. and Brush, B. E. (1974). Varieties of sclerosing cholangitis, surgical significance. *Bull. Soc. Int. Chir.*, **33**, 487
71 Caroli, J. and Rosener, D. (1976). Cholangitis. In Backus, H. L. (ed.). *Gastroenterology*, Vol. 3, p. 865. (Philadelphia: W. B. Saunders Company)
72 Glenn, F. (1980). Idiopathic sclerosing choledochitis. In Maingot, R. (ed.). *Abdominal Operations*, pp. 1193–1197. (New York: Appleton-Century-Crofts)
73 Holubitsky, I. B. and McKenzie, A. D. (1964). Primary sclerosing cholangitis of the extrahepatic bile ducts. *Can. J. Surg.*, **7**, 277
74 Meyers, R. N., Cooper, J. H. and Padis, N. (1970). Primary sclerosing cholangitis. *Am. J. Gastroenterol.*, **53**, 327
75 Florcken, H. (1912), *Dtsch. Z. Chir.*, **123**, 604
76 Del Valle, D. and Donovan, R. (1926). *Arch. Argent. Enferm. Ap. Digest*, **4**, 1
77 Yvergneaux, J. P., Bouwens, E. and Yvergneaux E. (1974). Diagnostic de la sténose oddienne dans une série homogène de 1150 interventions biliaires sous radiomanometrie. *Ann. Chir.*, **28**, 545
78 Boyden, A. M. (1973). Discussion in paper by White, T. T. *et al.* Indications for sphincteroplasty as opposed to choledochoduodenostomy. *Am. J. Surg.*, **126**, 165
79 Acosta, J. M., Civantos, F., Nardi, G. L. *et al.* (1967). Fibrosis of the papilla of Vater. *Surg. Gynecol. Obstet.*, **124**, 787

Subject Index

abscesses
  CAT localization 67–9
    accuracy 69
  paracolic 70
  subdiaphragmatic 70, 71
    drainage 78
  see also subcutaneous drainage
accidents, trauma and embolism in 108, 111, 112
adjuvant therapy
  animal studies 165, 166
  BCG, methanol extraction residue 159
  breast cancer 163–77
  and cancer staging 148
  early stage breast cancer 174, 175
  endocrine effects 169, 170
  gastrointestinal cancer 143–60
  groups benefiting in breast cancer 167, 168
  irradiation 158
  principles in breast cancer 166
  risks 172–4
  see also 5-FU, Milan trial
adrenalectomy 175
adrenals 65–7, 75
adriamycin 171
alcoholism and ascites 258, 259
aldosterone tumours 66
amino acid mixtures
  and encephalopathy 211
  in intravenous hyperalimentation 196, 211
AMP, cyclic and gastric secretion 239
amylopectin sulphate 242
angiodysplasia 96, 99
  blood loss in elderly 100
  incidence 98

silicone injection 99
angiography
  angiodysplasia 96–9
  camera use 85, 86
  coeliac 90
  diagnosis and control of bleeding 85–116
  diverticular haemorrhage 97, 98, 100
  gastrointestinal tract bleeding 89–102
  gastro-oesophageal varices 95
  haemoptysis 114, 115
  hepatic haemorrhage 100, 101
  lower gastrointestinal tract haemorrhage 96–102
  mortality after trauma 111
  musculoskeletal haemorrhage 108
  obturator artery 111
  pancreatic haemorrhage 101, 102
  peritoneovenous shunt patency 300, 301
  prostate and embolization 108, 109
  and renal function in trauma 103
  small bowel, arteriovenous malformation 94
  splenic, haemorrhage 113, 114
  stomach, bleeding control 90–2
  trauma from accidents 108, 111–13
  ulcers 90, 93
  upper gastrointestinal tract haemorrhage 90–6
  urinogenital tract haemorrhage 103–8
  see also arteriography
antacids 240–2
antigens
  carcinoma-associated in culture 135
  cell mediated immune response 186, 187
  colonic mucoprotein 135
  gastric cancer 128–30
  glycoprotein 123

antigens *(continued)*
  non-cross reacting 126
  oncofetal in gastrointestinal cancer 123–
    37
  pancreas-associated oncofetal 124, 125
  pancreatic cancer 124–8
  tumour-associated 123
  see also α-fetoprotein, carcinoembryonic
    and individual antigens
antithrombin III deficiency 205
arteriography 96
  brachiocephalic 115, 116
  inferior mesenteric 98
  liver 100, 101
  superior mesenteric 97, 98
ascites
  Baldus' classification 263, 264
  cardiogenic 261, 262
  causes 258–62
  chylous, fat 260
  definition 257
  fluid accumulation rate 262, 263
  fluid diversion 269
  malignant, prognosis 261
  management, previous 268, 269
  nephrogenic 261
  nutritional 262
  peritoneovenous shunt 257, 266, 269–304
  portacaval shunt, hazards 269
  postoperative and shunts 261
  prognosis 264, 265
  renal pathophysiology 263, 264
  salt restriction 268
  sequelae 265–8
  surgical treatment 257–307
  see also Budd–Chiari syndrome, perito-
    venous shunt
aspiration
  biopsy results 76
  CAT use 75
  skinny needle in pancreatic carcinoma 72
azotaemia 264

balloons in haemorrhage control 116
barium enema in colorectal cancer 130
basal energy expenditure (BEE) 184–5
bile duct
  pathology of injuries 357, 359
  see also common bile duct
bile duct tumours 370–3
  localization and types 370
  Longmire procedure 371–3
  resectable, numbers 371

Roux-en-Y, hepaticojejunostomy 371–3
  treatment 371–3
bile salts and gastric mucosa 224, 225
biliary obstruction
  CAT 346
  diagnosis 332–9
  extrahepatic 15
  investigation sequence 332, 333
  malignant 370–3
  supra-ampullary, surgical management
    331–76
  surgery
    antibiotics 336
    preparation for 334, 336, 337
  ultrasonography 332–43
  see also common bile duct stones
biliary strictures, iatrogenic 354–70
  aetiology 354–6
  diagnostic methods 359
  ductal anastomosis 361, 364
  Heineke–Mickulicz repair 362, 363
  incidence 354
  poor surgical technique 354–6
  preoperative management 359, 360
  prevention 357, 358
  Roux-en-Y hepaticojejunostomy 363–7
  surgical technique 363–9
  type of operation 362
biopsy
  CAT use 69–78
  complications 72
  malignancy confirmation 74, 75
  Menghini needle biopsy 75, 76
  needle aspiration 15, 29
  needle, presacral and CAT 73
  needle size 71
  renal and arteriovenous fistula 103
bleeding, angiography and 85–116
BPF *see* serum basic ferroprotein
breast cancer
  adjuvant therapy 163–77
  aims of future trials 177
  anti-oestrogens 176
  combination chemotherapy 167, 168
  early stage management 174
  endocrine effects, drugs 169, 170
  hormonal therapy 176
  incidence 163
  metastases, incidence 164
  oestrogen receptors in 170
  recommendations for systemic therapy
    174–7
  systemic therapy 163

bronchial artery and haemoptysis control 115
Budd–Chiari syndrome 275
  and ascites 259, 260
  fatal 260
  fluid accumulation 262
  induced and malnutrition 265

cancer
  alimentary tract and endoscopy 3
  breast 163–77
  cervical, bleeding control 110
  chemotherapy and carcinoembryonic antigen 133
  classification 130, 131
  colorectal 21, 22, 26, 128, 130–6, 146–59
  duodenal, diagnosis 9, 10
  gastric, diagnosis 9, 128–30
  gastrointestinal 143–60
    antigens 123–37
  hepatocellular 46
  pancreatic 16, 54, 72, 124–9, 342
  renal 61, 62
  squamous cell 47
  see also individual organs
carbenoxolene
  in duodenal ulcer 244
  and gastrointestinal mucosa protection 243, 244
  mineralocorticoid side-effects 244
  mode of action 243
carbohydrates, daily requirements 193
carcinoembryonic antigen (CEA) 123
  and cancer staging 131
  during chemotherapy 133
  and chemotherapy assessment 134
  colorectal cancer 130–6
  false positives 126
  gastrointestinal malignancy 129, 130
  monitoring recurrence of colorectal cancer 132–4
  pancreatic cancer 126–8
  in pancreatitis 127
  stage of sampling 134
  tumour marker 123
  use in colorectal cancer 132
  usefulness 136, 155
carcinoembryonic antigen-S from colon 135
catheter
  balloon occlusion 88
  central venous in IVH 200–2
  infection 206, 207
  silastic for home use 205

sterilization 200
C3DNA-binding protein 129
CEA see carcinoembryonic antigen
chemotherapy
  cancer and carcinoembryonic antigen 133–5
  combination 157, 167–71; see also Milan trial
  combination and hormonal in breast cancer 176
  cytotoxicity 172, 173
  and second malignancies 173
  toxicities 173, 174
cholangiography
  bile duct exploration 349
  bile duct perfusion 348
  operative manometry 347–9
  percutaneous transhepatic 333, 344, 374
  routine operative 344, 346, 347
cholecystectomy 339
cholecystitis
  acute, ultrasonography 335
  gangrenous 101
choledochoduodenostomy 363
choledocholithiasis 343
choledochoscopy 349–54
choledoscopy and endoscopic types 17
cholelithiasis, ultrasonography 334
cimetidine
  actions 230
  duodenal ulcer healing 230–3
  gastric ulcer healing 233, 234
  gastrointestinal bleeding 235
  gastro-oesophageal reflux 234, 235
  intrinsic factor secretion 237
  maintenance therapy 232, 233
  and remission 233
  side-effects 237, 238
  surgery and recurrent ulceration 234
  therapeutic uses 230
  in Zollinger–Ellison syndrome 236
cirrhosis
  and ascites 258, 259
  causes 259
  diet 264
  and heart disease 277
  renal function 263, 264
Clonorchis sinensis, biliary tract colonization 340
colonic diverticular bleeding, control 97
colonoscopy 18–26
  analgesia 19
  biopsy safety 21

colonoscopy (continued)
  cancer screening 21, 22, 26
  diagnostic indications 20, 21
  fluoroscopy use 19, 20
  foreign bodies 25
  Hippocrates 18
  instruments available 18, 19
  origins 18
  special applications 25
  strictures 25
  technique 19
colorectal cancer
  antigens 130
  Dukes' staging 130
  TMN classification 131
combined modality see adjuvant therapy
common bile duct stones 333, 340–3
  chemical dissolution 351, 352
  endoscopic sphincterotomy, success 350,
    351
  management of retained 349, 353
  mechanical extraction, success 350
  operative removal 352–4
  retained, incidence 342, 343, 349, 350
computerized axial tomography (CAT, CT)
  adrenals 65–7
  bile ducts 345
  biliary system 50–2
  biopsy and aspiration 69–78
  contrast material 72, 74
  cystic disease, liver 44
  diagnostic accuracy 48, 69
  gallstone laminations 346
  haemangiomas 44, 45
  intra-abdominal abscess 67–9
  intra-abdominal disease, diagnosis 41–79
  and jaundice 333
  kidneys 59–63
  liver scan 42–50
  and laparoscopy 29
  needle biopsy 15
  non-Hodgkin's lymphomas 65
  pancreas 52–9
  pancreatic pseudocyst 57
  principles 41
  renal masses 103
  retroperitoneum 63–5
contrast enema 20
coronary vein, Gelfoam occlusion 95
corrosive chemicals 10
Crohn's disease 9, 27
  and ileostomy, contraindications 319, 327
  and malnutrition 191

cyanoacrylate and pancreatic surgery 101,
    102, 104
cyclophosphamide 167

diarrhoea
  in continent ileostomy 326
  and 5-FU 150, 156
diazepam, use in endoscopy 15, 19
disseminated intravascular coagulation
    (DIC)
  coagulopathy 305
  and endotoxin 307
  and peritovenous shunt 276, 304–7
  rarity 305
  remote ecchymoses 305
diverticula 7
doxorubicin, cardiotoxicity 173
drugs
  anticholinergic 229
  antigastrin 229, 230
  antihistamines 230
  peptic ulcers 227–46
  see also individual drugs
duodenal ulcers
  carbenoxolone 244
  and cimetidine 230–3
  control of bleeding 90, 93
  transcatheter embolization 93
duodenoscopy 5–11
duodenum
  mucosal barrier 226
  neoplasms 9, 10

Eastern Cooperative Oncology Group
    (ECOG) 127
eating and IVH 190
ECRP see endoscopic retrograde cholangio-
    pancreatography
EDC1 126
electrocautery
  and gastrointestinal bleeding 13
  polyps, colorectal 22–5
  and stone removal 16
embolization, transcatheter
  autologous clot 87, 105
  complications 89, 105
  contraindications 114
  detachable silicone balloons 88, 89
  isobutyl-2-cyanoacrylate 89
  kidney 105–7
  liver bleeding 101
  pancreatic haemorrhage 101, 102, 104
  polyvinyl alcohol 88

prostate 108, 109
steel coils 88
surgical gelatin 87, 88, 92, 93, 105
endoscopic retrograde cholangiopancreatography (ERCP) 374
  anaesthesia 14, 15
  calculi crushing 16
  therapeutic applications 16, 17
  use 15
endoscopy
  biliary 17
  gastrointestinal disease 1–30
  inflammatory bowel disease 27
  origins in sword swallowing 3
  reliability 1
  slow acceptance by surgeons 2
  understanding of gastric bleeding 12, 13
energy, daily requirements 193
enteral hyperalimentation 188, 189
epistaxis 115
essential fatty acids
  daily requirement 192, 194
  deficiency and symptoms 194, 195

familial polyposis 318
femoral artery, false aneurysm occlusion
113
fetal sulphoglycoprotein antigen (FSA)
127–9
α-fetoprotein (AFP) 123
  in pancreatic cancer 125
5-fluoro-2-deoxyuridine
  colorectal cancer 146
  loss of 147
  resurrection of 157
  stomach cancer 146
5-fluoro-2'-deoxyuridine-5'-
monophosphate 152
5-fluorouracil (5-FU)
  adjuvant courses 151
  assessment of usefulness 159, 160
  breast cancer 167
  circumstances for toxicity 149, 150
  colorectal cancer 146–8, 156, 157
  combination chemotherapy 157, 172
  compared with radiation 144
  compared with surgery 147
  dosing regimes 148, 152, 156
  drug-related death 149
  Dukes staging 153–5
  effect on CEA levels 135
  homeopathic doses 157
  intra-arterial 144

poor-risk patients 150
rectal cancer 158
recurrence 154, 155
resection adjuvant in colonic cancer 153
risk assessment 150, 151
stomach cancer 144, 145
and survival in cancer 144, 145
toxicity 147, 149, 151, 156
white blood cell counts 151
see also adjuvant therapy

gallbladder
  abnormalities 51
  CAT image 42, 50
  'Courvoisier' 341
  obstruction 51
  see also biliary obstruction
gallstones, numbers of operations 17
gastric acid 220–2
gastric cancer
  antigenic indicators 128–30
  chemotherapy 144
  Japan 144
  treatments 144, 145
gastric mucosa
  barrier components 222–4
  bile salt ultrastructural damage 224, 225
  cell loss 226
  damage to 224, 238, 245, 246
  damage and histamine release 235
  mucus 222
  resistance of 222–6, 228
gastric polyps, snare cautery 9
gastric resection and cancer risk 238
gastric ulcers 8, 90
  and cimetidine 233, 234
  see also peptic ulcers
gastrin and gastric acid secretion 221, 222
gastrointestinal bleeding 89–102
  angiography 89–109
  cimetidine 235, 236
  endoscopy 11–14
  H_2 receptor antagonists 236
  lower 13, 14, 96–109
  surgical measures 11
  upper 11–13, 90–6
gastrointestinal cancer
  adjuvant therapy 143–60
  antigens in 123–37
  dismal prognosis 143
gastrointestinal disease
  diagnostic methods 1, 2
  use of endoscopy 1–30

gastroscopy 5–11
Gelfoam
    phagocytosis of particles 87
    renal bleeding control 105–7
genitourinary tract see urinogenital tract
geranyl farnesyl acetate 245
Gianturco–Anderson coils 88
von Gierke's disease 49
α-2-glycoprotein 126
granulocytopenia and cimetidine 237

haematochezia and diagnosis 98
haemoptysis, angiography contraindica-
    tions 114
haemorrhage
    head and neck 115, 116
    neoplastic erosion of arteries 116
    trauma 111
    see also individual organs
Harris–Benedict equation 184
hepatectomy and trauma 100
hepatic artery ligation and embolization
    101, 102
hepatitis, viral and ascites 259
hepatocellular failure 150
hepatorenal syndrome
    in ascites 264
    renal blood flow 292
hernia
    and ascites 267, 268
    perforation 276
hiatus hernia 7
histamine and gastric acid secretion 220
human chorionic gonadotrophin 126
hydrothorax
    in ascites 265, 267, 275, 276
    and diaphragm defect 267
hyperammonaemia 197
hyperbilirubinaemia and operative morta-
    lity 359
hypertension 86, 87
    portal 101
    portal and biliary strictures 369
hypophosphataemia 197

ileostomy, continent 313–29
    absorption from reservoir 332
    bacteriology and morphology 321–3
    barium, small bowel 320
    catheter duration 317
    complications 323–8
    contraindications 319–21
    Crohn's disease 319, 327

indications 318, 319
nipple valve fistula 325
nipple valve formation 315, 316
nipple valve prolapse 326
nipple valve slippage 318, 324, 325
nipple valve surgery, revisional 327, 328
outflow tract formation and fixation 316,
    317
postoperative management 317, 318
pouchitis 326
psychological effects 318–21
reservoir 319
    peristaltic counteraction 313, 314
skin stricture 325, 326
success rate 328
surgical construction 314–17
ileostomy dysfunction 313
ileostomy, standard 319
iliolumbar artery, embolization after acci-
    dent 112
inflammatory bowel disease 27
intensive care, angiography suite 85
intra-abdominal abscess, percutaneous
    drainage 77
intra-abdominal disease, CAT diagnosis
    41–79
intravenous hyperalimentation (IVH) 181–
    212
    amino acids 196, 211
    anergy 187
    cancer patients 212
    catheter insertion 200–2
    complications 207–11
    electrolytes 192, 197
    fat-free 194
    history 181, 182
    home 201, 205
    indications 189–91
    infants 201, 204
    infection 181
    infusion pump 203
    lifeline 182, 183
    lipid sources 193–5
    metabolic complications 209–11
    millipore filters in line 205
    new horizons 211, 212
    nutrient formula 191–4
    percutaneous subclavian puncture 200,
        202, 203, 208
    postoperative 190, 191
    preparation of solutions 199
    protein 195–7
    protocols 206, 207

septicaemia incidence 208, 209
sterilization 199, 200
trace elements 192, 198
trauma 185
vitamins 192, 197

jaundice
  obstructive, differential diagnosis 15
  surgical, causes 332

kidneys
  angiomyolipoma 62, 63
  in ascites 263, 264
  aspiration biopsy results 76
  cyst 61
  embolization and side-effects 105–7
  haemorrhage 19, 21
  mass lesion, calcified 62
  needle biopsy and diagnosis 75
  neoplasms 60, 61
  normal CAT scan 59, 60
  peritovenous shunt effects 292, 293
  renal cell carcinoma 62
  surgery and nephrectomy rate 105
kwashiorkor 186

laparoscopy
  diagnostic uses 29
  first description 28
laparotomy, small bowel malformation 94
leukopenia and 5-FU 151, 156
lipid
  daily requirements 193, 194
  intravenous hyperalimentation sources
    194
liquorice
  deglycyrrhizinized 244
  and dyspepsia 243
liver
  abscess 68
  adenoma 45
  aspiration biopsy results 76
  CAT scan, normal 42, 43
  cirrhosis 48, 49
  cystic disease 44
  diffuse disease 48–50
  fatty changes 48–9
  focal lesions 44–8
  haematoma 50
  haemorrhage and angiography 100–2
  hepatocellular carcinoma 46
  intravenous urographic contrast 43, 44
  metastatic tumours 46, 47

needle biopsy and diagnosis 75
peritoneovenous shunt effects 290–2
trauma 50, 100
lymphangiography 65

Mallory–Weiss tears 90
malnutrition 265, 266
mastectomy, relapse rates 175
MeCCNU 132, 133
  and B16 melanoma in mice 165
  colorectal cancer 157
  combination 157
Menghini needle biopsy 75, 76
menopause
  and chemotherapy dose modification 170
  and effective breast cancer therapy 167,
    168
methotrexate 147, 167
methylene blue in angiography 90, 94
metiamide 237
metrizamide 88
mid-arm circumference 187
Milan trial, National Cancer Institute
  breast cancer combination chemotherapy
    167–71
  chemotherapy regimen 167
  dose and age 170
  patients benefiting 167–9
  relapse rates 172
  therapy toxicity 177
mitomycin-C 144
mono-octanoin, stone dissolution 352
multimodal primary treatment 157
myelotoxicity 170
myolipoma, CAT scan 68

nephrectomy 103
nitrogen mustard 145
nutritional assessment 185–7
nutritional metabolism
  energy sources 183–5
  starvation 183, 184
  trace elements required 192
  trauma 184, 185
  vitamin requirements 192
nutritional therapy 188; see also intravenous
  hyperalimentation

obturator artery, bleeding control 111
oesophageal reflux 4, 7
oesophagoscopy 3–5
  biopsy and brushings 5
  corrosive injury 10

oesophagoscopy *(continued)*
  washings 4
oestrogen receptors and breast cancer che-
    motherapy 170
omentopexy 268
oophorectomy 175
Osler–Weber–Rendu syndrome 21

pancreas
  adenocarcinoma 53, 54
  cancer, antigenic markers 124–8
  common duct dilation 59
  diseases 16
  embolization, complications 101
  haemorrhage 101, 102
  neoplasm, CAT evaluation 54, 55
  normal, CAT scan 52, 53
  post surgery bleeding and cyanoacrylate
    101, 104
  pseudoaneurysms 89, 101
pancreatic juice, analysis and cancer 127
pancreatic oncofetal antigen and pancreatic
    cancer 125
pancreatitis
  chronic, calcium deposit 57
  complications 101
  diagnosis 55–9
  duct calculi 57
  emphysematous 58
  Gerota's fascia 60
  haemorrhagic 56
  multiple calcifications 58
  pseudocyst 56, 57
paracrine cell
  agonist–antagonist interplay at 222, 223
  secretion regulation 221
pepsin, inactivation of ulcerogen 220
peptic ulcer
  acid and pepsin role 220
  cause 219
  drug treatment 227–46
  healing, cell kinetics 226, 227
peptic ulcer, drug treatment
  antacids 240–2
  anticholinergic 229
  antipeptics 242, 243
  metabolic blockade 238–40
  mucosa protection 243–6
  prostaglandin effects 239
  receptor blockade 229–38
  secretion inhibition 228, 229, 238
  see also cimetidine
percutaneous drainage of abscesses 77

percutaneous transhepatic drainage 360,
    361
peritonitis
  cirrhotic ascites 268
  and liver failure 277
  and peritovenous shunt 276, 277
peritovenous shunt 257, 266, 269–304
  blood clots in vena cava 301–3
  breathing as motive force 270, 271
  cardiac disease and failure 295, 297–9
  cardiac output 293
  cavogram 273
  clotting in venous tubing 303
  complications 304–7
  contraindications 276, 277
  design requirements 269–74
  and disseminated intravascular coagula-
    tion 304–7
  failure 293–304
  fluid examination 279
  furosemide, post-surgery 287, 295
  haematocrit monitoring 288
  haemodilution effects 290, 291
  inadequate instruction 295
  indications for insertion 274–6
  insertion 277–88
    abdominal incision 279–81
    anaesthesia 278
    antibiotic use 280, 285
    cervical incision 281, 282
    infraclavicular incision in infants 285
    patency testing 282, 285, 286, 299, 300
    schematic 284
    tube passing 283, 284
  late failure 303
  late infection 303, 304
  liver effects 290–2
  long term results 293
  malplacement 294, 296
  occlusion 299, 300
  postoperative management 287–9
  pump, futility 273, 274
  renal function 292, 293
  results, immediate 289–93
  salt and diet 288, 289
  shuntogram 297, 299
  surgical procedure 278–87
  tube kinking, dye use 295, 297
  valve design 270, 271
  valve materials and properties 271–4
  valve requirements and fluids 270
  venous   pressure   and   angiographic
    patency test 300, 301

1-phenylalanine mustard
  breast cancer 167–9, 172
  and menses alteration 169
  relapse rates 169, 172
pitressin
  in diverticular haemorrhage 97, 98
  intravenous in gastrointestinal bleeding 86, 87, 90
pneumothorax 207
polyps, colorectal 22–5
postcholecystectomy syndrome 15
postpartum haemorrhage, embolotherapy 108
proctocolectomy 313
proctosigmoidoscopy 26
prostaglandins and gastric secretion inhibition 238, 245, 246
  clinical trials 240
  indomethacin-induced mucosa damage 245
  mode of action 239, 240
prostaglandin synthetase inhibitors and gastric mucosal damage 246
prostatic haemorrhage and surgery 107–9
protein
  in intravenous hyperalimentation diet 195–7
  uses in body 195
protein status, assessment 186, 187

radiation therapy
  as adjuvant in colorectal cancer 158
  in cervical carcinoma bleeding control 110
radiography in gastrointestinal disease 1
razoxane 145
renal see kidney
reproductive system, haemorrhage and sex 107–9
retroperitoneum
  abscess 71
  aspiration biopsy results 76
  fibrosarcoma 64
  lymph node disease 63
  lymphoma 64
  needle biopsy diagnosis 75
Roux-en-Y hepaticojejunostomy 363–7
  mortality 368
  Smith's modification 367, 368
  success rate 368, 369

sclerosing cholangitis 373–5

serum basic fetoprotein (BPF) 129
sigmoidoscopy 27, 28
smoking and false positive for pancreatic cancer 126
snare electrocautery 9
  colonic polyps 22–5
sodium cholate stone dissolution 351
sodium tetradecyl sulphate in gelatin, haemorrhage control 96
somatostatin 230
sphincter of Oddi fibrosis 375, 376
spleen
  aspiration biopsy results 76
  contusion recognition 113
  haemorrhage control 113, 114
starvation, metabolism in 183, 184
stomatitis and 5-FU 151
subclavian venepuncture 200, 202, 203
  complications 208
sucralfate 242, 243
sulpiride, ulcer healing 228, 229
sump syndrome 352
surgery
  biliary strictures 359–69
  and cancer staging, success 145
  common bile duct stones 352–4
  realization in ascites 257–307

tamoxifen 176
technetium 99m, red cell bleeding scan 96
tennagen 126
thiotepa
  colonic cancer adjuvant to resection 154
  and mastectomy 166
thrombocytopenia 156
thromboelastograms 306
tissue polypeptide antigen (TPA) in gastrointestinal malignancy 129, 130
trace elements
  daily requirements 192, 198
  effects of 198, 199
triangle of Calot 357, 358
triceps skinfold thickness 187
trimipramine and gastric ulcer healing 228
tri-potassium di-citrato-bismuthate, mucosal protection 245
tumour cell kinetics
  animal studies and chemotherapy 165, 166
  detectable size 164
  doubling time 165
  Gompertzian growth 165, 176
tumour size and sensitivity to therapy 177

ulcerative colitis 318
ultrasonography 65
  bile duct gallstones 333, 343
  biliary obstruction sites 332, 339–42
  biliary problems 51
  biliary tract obstruction 332–44
  biliary tree, normel 332, 336–8
  Budd–Chiari syndrome 260
  emphysematous pancreatitis 59
  gallbladder cholecystitis 332, 335
  renal masses 103
ureteric haemorrhage 105, 106
urinogenital tract haemorrhage 103–8; see
    also kidney, reproductive system
uterine haemorrhage, embolotherapy 108
uterine tumours 108

vaginal bleeding, control in cervical carcin-
    oma 110
vasopressin
  angiographic infusion 85, 90

hazard 14
  colonic diverticular bleeding 97
  infusion rates 86
  intra-arterial infusion 86
  stomach stress bleeding 91
vesicular haemorrhage 105, 106
vincristine 171
vitamin
  daily oral requirements 192, 197
  functions and intravenous hyperalimen
    tation 198
vitamin K 360

water, daily requirements 193

X-ray and colonoscopy indications 20

zinc deficiency 198, 199
Zollinger–Ellison syndrome 219
  cimetidine in 236, 237

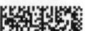